EAI/Springer Innovations in Communication and Computing

Series editor
Imrich Chlamtac, European Alliance for Innovation, Gent, Belgium

Editor's Note

The impact of information technologies is creating a new world yet not fully understood. The extent and speed of economic, life style and social changes already perceived in everyday life is hard to estimate without understanding the technological driving forces behind it. This series presents contributed volumes featuring the latest research and development in the various information engineering technologies that play a key role in this process.

The range of topics, focusing primarily on communications and computing engineering include, but are not limited to, wireless networks; mobile communication; design and learning; gaming; interaction; e-health and pervasive healthcare; energy management; smart grids; internet of things; cognitive radio networks; computation; cloud computing; ubiquitous connectivity, and in mode general smart living, smart cities, Internet of Things and more. The series publishes a combination of expanded papers selected from hosted and sponsored European Alliance for Innovation (EAI) conferences that present cutting edge, global research as well as provide new perspectives on traditional related engineering fields. This content, complemented with open calls for contribution of book titles and individual chapters, together maintain Springer's and EAI's high standards of academic excellence. The audience for the books consists of researchers, industry professionals, advanced level students as well as practitioners in related fields of activity include information and communication specialists, security experts, economists, urban planners, doctors, and in general representatives in all those walks of life affected ad contributing to the information revolution.

About EAI

EAI is a grassroots member organization initiated through cooperation between businesses, public, private and government organizations to address the global challenges of Europe's future competitiveness and link the European Research community with its counterparts around the globe. EAI reaches out to hundreds of thousands of individual subscribers on all continents and collaborates with an institutional member base including Fortune 500 companies, government organizations, and educational institutions, provide a free research and innovation platform.

Through its open free membership model EAI promotes a new research and innovation culture based on collaboration, connectivity and recognition of excellence by community.

More information about this series at http://www.springer.com/series/15427

Sara Paiva
Editor

Technological Trends in Improved Mobility of the Visually Impaired

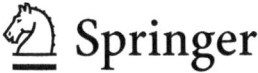 Springer

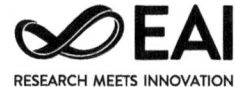

Editor
Sara Paiva
ARC4DigiT – Applied Research Center for
Digital Transformation, Instituto
Politécnico de Viana do Castelo
Viana do Castelo, Portugal

ISSN 2522-8595   ISSN 2522-8609   (electronic)
EAI/Springer Innovations in Communication and Computing
ISBN 978-3-030-16449-2   ISBN 978-3-030-16450-8   (eBook)
https://doi.org/10.1007/978-3-030-16450-8

This Springer imprint is published by the registered company Springer Nature Switzerland AG.
The registered company address is: Gewerbestrasse 11, 6330 Cham, Switzerland

Preface

The mobility of blind people assumes itself as an emerging area, where several scientific contributions have been made, much by the underlying social inclusion associated with it. Technology has the power to contribute to and assist the daily lives of visually impaired people, facilitating and promoting the more autonomous execution of tasks.

This book presents three main parts: a first one presenting states of the art and surveys that assess several aspects related to the mobility of blind people, namely related to smart cities, accessible context-aware systems, smart systems, ground plane checking, and recent trends in technologies and systems.

A second part focuses on more conceptual proposals for precise navigation systems, including a cloud video guidance system, a virtual vision architecture, a system that makes use of visible light communication, ambient intelligent environments, and the enhancement of cultural experiences.

Finally, a third part shows practical application cases in several parts of the world where mobility solutions are being tested and put into practice, such as IoT solutions in Africa, an autonomous mobility system in Italy, systems for blind children, audio-based mobile navigation systems, context-aware voice operated mobile guidance systems, or verbal indoor route descriptions for VIP travelers.

This book attracted contributors from all over the world, and I would like to thank all authors for submitting their works and also appreciate the reviewers for their review work. Also, a special thanks goes to EAI/Springer editorial team, fundamental for this book to see the light of day.

Viana do Castelo, Portugal   Sara Paiva

Contents

Part I
Literature Reviews and Surveys

Chapter 1
Smart Cities to Improve Mobility and Quality of Life of the Visually Impaired

Drishty Sobnath, Ikram Ur Rehman, and Moustafa M. Nasralla

1.1 Introduction

Visual function is classified according to four levels by the World Health Organization (WHO): normal vision, moderate vision, severe vision impairment and blindness (Texeira, Toledo, Amorim, Kofuji, & Rogério dos Santos, 2017). With approximately 38 million people suffering from blindness worldwide, and another 110 million suffering from visual impairment, research has focused on providing solutions that would allow those affected to improve their mobility and independently achieve daily activities, such as walking around cities safely, and performing other everyday tasks (Ramadhan, 2018). Visually impaired people (VIP) face various difficulties concerning urban mobility. The rapid pace of innovation and advances in technological research has given hope to the visually impaired in terms of finding ways to move around smart cities and enjoy a better Quality of Life (QoL). The term "smart city" was coined in the early 1990s to emphasise how city growth was pivoting towards technology, modernisation and globalisation (Gibson, Kozmetsky, & Smilor, 1992). Recent technological advancements have provided new opportunities to build smart cities that cater for the elderly population and

D. Sobnath
Research Innovation and Enterprise, Solent University, Southampton, UK
e-mail: drishty.sobnath@solent.ac.uk

I. U. Rehman (✉)
School of Computing and Engineering, University of West London, London, UK
e-mail: ikram_rehman@hotmail.com

M. M. Nasralla
Department of Communications and Networks Engineering, Prince Sultan University, Riyadh, Saudi Arabia
e-mail: mnasralla@psu.edu.sa

© Springer Nature Switzerland AG 2020
S. Paiva (ed.), *Technological Trends in Improved Mobility of the Visually Impaired*,
EAI/Springer Innovations in Communication and Computing,
https://doi.org/10.1007/978-3-030-16450-8_1

citizens with disabilities. The average age of the UK population is increasing; therefore, it is likely that the number of people with low vision or other visual impairment will increase concomitantly. In today's busy world, having access to information, performing everyday tasks independently, or engaging in education or employment is crucial. It is important to allow those people whose sight is deteriorating to have a normal life. With the help of ubiquitous computing, the engagement and interaction of VIP with other humans, as well as their surroundings, are achievable anytime and anywhere. The concept of "ubiquitous computing" can be defined as a model of human-to-computer interaction, in which the technology suits the natural environment of humans (Billah, Ashok, Porter, & Ramakrishnan, 2017; Hakobyan, Lumsden, O'Sullivan, & Bartlett, 2013). The invention of smartphones, along with continuous innovations in areas such as the Internet of Things (IoT), artificial intelligence (AI), augmented and virtual reality (AR/VR), cloud computing, embedded systems, remote sensors, wireless networks and robotics, has provided a remarkable cluster of functionalities and opportunities, which can support the mobility of VIP in a smart city setting (Skouby, Kivimäki, Haukipuro, Lynggaard, & Windekilde, 2014).

Furthermore, the amalgamation of the aforementioned technologies in a smart city setting would transform the lives of people with functional dependencies. Examples of healthcare applications that would benefit from the stated technologies include: remote health monitoring using wearable devices, remote diagnosis, remote surgery, and instant access to the emergency services. The ultimate goal of smart healthcare in a smart city setting is to bring healthcare to the user's home and bridge the gap between terrestrial boundaries (Hakobyan et al., 2013; Skouby et al., 2014). For VIP, smart cities have the potential to improve their QoL, reducing the challenges associated with their routine activities. As we are only now witnessing the beginning of the development of smart cities, such as Dubai, Singapore, New York and Beijing, current and future cities will continue to be adapted and tested, thereby potentially providing an experience closer to total accessibility for VIP if there is continual investment in this sector. In such complex ecosystems, specific sectors such as healthcare, education, environmental infrastructure and other public services are required to fulfil the specific needs of the population (Domingue et al., 2011). Smart cities also support the concept of sustainable economic growth, as well as the well-being of their citizens (Siano, Shahrour, & Vergura, 2018). They include, for example, more efficient ways of lighting buildings, contributing to a greener environment, safer public spaces and more interaction for the physically disabled (Siano et al., 2018). Their development relies on strong network infrastructure, the Internet or Web 2.0, and their success depends upon the collective intelligent workforce designing initiative, and cost-effective solutions. The European Commission is investing up to €1 billion in supporting the European Innovation Partnership on Smart Cities and Communities (EIP-SCC), which helps to bring together industries and citizens in at least 300 cities (European Commission, 2018a), and VIP will be one of the beneficiary groups of this project.

In recent times, advancements in Information and Communication Technology (ICT) and its associated services have facilitated the creation of a more cost-effective and sustainable environment. The implementation of ICT in a smart city context can provide personalised healthcare, social services and intelligent community services, to name just a few (Skouby et al., 2014). There are currently a number of EU projects working under the theme of Ambient Assisted Living (AAL) to improve the QoL of VIP, utilising ICT applications. The aim of such projects is to increase the level of autonomy indoors as well as outdoors, allowing them to carry out their daily activities without constraints. With the evolution of emerging IoT-enabled wireless technologies, the surge in the adoption of AI and big data analytics, the ability to recognise people or carry out routine activities can be envisaged as being feasible (Philip & Rehman, 2016).

Common problems for those with impaired sight are a lack of independence or mobility, social isolation and feelings of insecurity (Hakobyan et al., 2013). Social interaction plays a significant role in maintaining good physical, mental and emotional health for VIP, as demonstrated through research (Skouby et al., 2014). Thus, one of the key aspects of healthy living is to remain socially active and maintain relationships. Thanks to the development of new technologies, VIP are increasingly able to make social contact, communicate with family and friends in new ways, participate in their communities, and share learning, skills and experiences with others (Skouby et al., 2014). In order to decrease the fear of isolation for VIP, while simultaneously improving their mobility, smart cities would provide modern assistive technologies both indoors and outdoors, so that the visually impaired could benefit from full inclusion and integration in society (Hashem et al., 2016; Suryotrisongko, Kusuma, & Ginardi, 2017).

There are a number of opportunities and challenges in shaping these technologies, and this chapter provides a comprehensive review and recommendations on how a smart city can provide better QoL for VIP in the near future. This article delineates the areas into the following main categories: (1) public areas, (2) transport systems and (3) smart homes. The rest of the chapter is organised as follows. Section 1.2 provides related work. Section 1.3 discusses the application of crowdsourcing to help VIP in smart cities. In Sect. 1.4, we present IoT-based scenarios to assist VIP. Section 1.5 elaborates on potential AI- and VR/AR-enabled solutions. Finally, Sect. 1.6 concludes the chapter.

1.2 Related Work

There is huge potential to improve the mobility of visually impaired people (VIP) to allow them to detect obstacles by making use of the IoT and sensors, among other modern technologies, in a smart city setting. A number of studies have already tested the use of these technologies, showing possible ways to improve the independence of VIP. This section describes some existing solutions to help those people, and also shows how a smart city could improve upon these solutions and design its infrastructure to cater for an elderly population with disabilities, focusing on VIP.

1.2.1 Public Areas in Smart Cities for Visually Impaired People

Some of the challenges faced by elderly and VIP in cities and society today are mainly associated with mobility and navigating through known and unknown obstacles. In the public areas of smart cities, ICT solutions can help in mitigating the aforementioned challenges by providing solutions such as (Skouby et al., 2014):

(a) Audible and vibrotactile signal-based augmented systems for pedestrians, which would provide precise information about their location.
(b) A mobile assisted product recognition system for accessible shopping.
(c) Mobile assisted city apps adapted for visually impaired users.

The use of white canes or tactile devices is among existing solutions, but VIP very often still require other forms of support. Ramadhan (2018), in his study, developed a wearable smart system that consisted of a microcontroller board, different sensors, cellular network and a solar panel. This system was used to track the path of the VIP and alert them with a sound emitted through a buzzer, as well as wrist vibration, in the case of VIP being in noisy surroundings. The device also triggers an alarm if it detects that the person has tripped over, which alerts people nearby and can send the location information to their registered caregiver, if requested by the VIP. The sensors, operating only between the range of 2 and 4 m, include solar chargeable batteries. However, the solution still needs to be improved to detect obstacles up to head-level, as, currently, the user wears the device on his wrist. The system is also not capable of detecting fire, water, holes and stairs. With the application of AI and object recognition, as explained later in this chapter, the system can be improved to recognise the routes of users around smart cities, thus facilitating the mobility of VIP. For example, in a smart city setting where the network infrastructure is strong, assistive technologies can be exploited to assist people to move around. They can rely on devices and transport systems having voice command functions, through which they can enter their destination. Smart cities could also have touristic areas, having a voice describing the scene to help VIP to visualise places and feel included in their environment. These could be smart devices embedded with AI technologies, such as image recognition, which offer auditory clues to citizens. Google is currently developing an Android platform called Lookout (Musil, 2018), which will work with a camera device that can be fitted in a visually impaired person's shirt, and helps them to identify money, receive spoken navigational instructions and recognise the colour of objects. Similarly, smart cities can make use of related technologies both indoors and outdoors to more effectively guide the visually impaired.

Applications such as Seeing Eye GPS or BlindSquare are both mobile applications that make use of the Global Positioning System (GPS) to inform users of their location in moving from point A to B. However, they lack accuracy when navigating inside train stations and shopping malls, where the signals' strength is low. Here, Small Cells can be utilised to boost signal strength. Small Cells are low power base stations that can be installed in public spaces in a plug-and-play manner. Smart cities also present the possibility of equipping buildings with beacon-powered devices. Beacons are small, low-cost transmitters that can be fitted inside buildings, and they can send real-time information to mobile devices via Bluetooth Low Energy. Beacons work both indoors and outdoors, and can be placed, for example, at bus stops, entrances to buildings, and train platforms to inform VIP about specific areas (Fig. 1.1). VIP can therefore be notified via vibration or sound through their mobile devices. One existing example of the use of beacons is in the city of Warsaw in Poland: the city has developed a network of hundreds and thousands of beacon sensors to assist VIP to move around independently (Organisation for Economic Cooperation and Development, 2017). Nearly 85% of Warsaw's visually impaired population reported having strong dependence on family members or friends in order to carry out daily routine tasks, while over 80% are unemployed. The "Virtual Warsaw" project is expected to be completed in the city and extended to another 24 municipalities by 2021 (Organisation for Economic Cooperation and Development, 2017). Another application of beacons to help VIP has been deployed in the WAYFINDR application, which sends the user information about his proximity via audio instructions (Wayfindr, 2018).

Smart cities can also provide urban smart furniture or tactile floors to facilitate the movement of those with visual impairment. Tactile paving compensates for the absence of kerbs, and the visually impaired can make use of the information underfoot. However, it is important to note that this might not be beneficial to elderly citizens or those who suffer from diabetes, for example, as they may have reduced sensitivity in their feet (Sahin, Aslan, Talebi, & Zeray, 2015). Blister paving can provide warnings of potential hazards, or can be used for amenity purposes to give guidance. Smart cities could use a combination of radio frequency identification (RFID) device tags and GPS to allow white cane users to receive guidance when approaching places such as markets, cafes, theatres or subway stations. Mobile and talking tactile maps should be provided to VIP to improve their independence when moving around towns and cities. Physical maps could be designed to provide

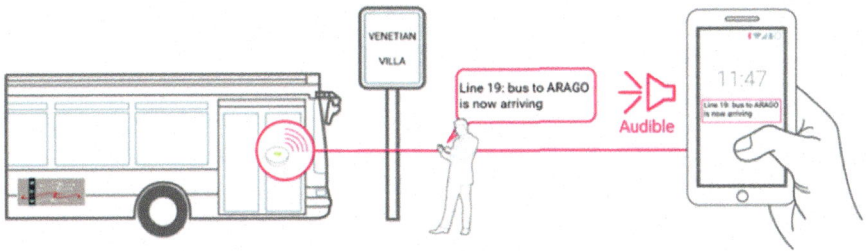

Fig. 1.1 Use of beacons as a potential solution (Jukna, 2017)

information about the positions of beacons, as previously described. The maps could further be linked to a mobile application, allowing citizens to feel confident when travelling alone in the city.

Additionally, smart cities can provide the latest technologies, such as the VoiceOver screen reader, to allow VIP to do their food shopping or visit the bank to deal with financial matters. Supermarkets can be equipped with devices to count money or recognise notes, and differentiate between various products, and all of this can be improved by using AI-based image recognition technologies. The OS X developed by Apple is already equipped with VoiceOver technologies, which allow users to have their text and application controls spoken aloud. At present, VIP are provided with various mobile applications, which they can use on their personal mobile devices to allow them to carry out daily tasks. A smart city, on the other hand, should provide services and applications that are user-friendly, as operating different applications from the mobile phone can be overwhelming for VIP.

1.2.2   Transport Systems in Smart Cities for Visually Impaired People

The public transport sector is another area where smart cities can be developed for VIP. Transportation presents various challenges at local, regional, national and international levels (Patricio, Haidee, Ciro, Telma, & Felipe, 2015). In recent years, mobile applications have already helped disabled people to use public transport in a more effective way, by receiving notifications from their mobile devices near bus stops to be alerted when a specific bus is approaching. However, many VIP still require human guidance to help them to identify the correct bus, or otherwise they may need to stop buses in order to enquire about the destination. Another challenge faced by VIP is the presence of more than one bus line at a busy bus station, therefore making it difficult for them to identify the relevant line. Applications such as CittaMobi have been used by visually impaired Brazilians to receive real-time vehicle scheduling, the best routes for their journeys, and other convenient tools, as described by some of its users (CittaMobi, 2018; Patricio et al., 2015). However, this application could be improved by enabling drivers to receive more information about passengers, filling the gap of the lack of interaction amongst services, users and applications (Patricio et al., 2015), which can be achieved in a smart city thanks to the sharing of data. Another application called GeorgiePhone, developed in the UK mainly for people suffering from low vision, consists of a bus tracking system, among other functionalities, to locate the nearest bus stop, read aloud the bus stop name every time the bus stops, and indicate bus arrival schedules. Another system, the Mobi+ project, implemented in the city of Clermont-Ferrand in France, provides an effective bus access service to people with disabilities and wheelchair users. The project consists of a wireless communication module with data exchange functionalities between buses and stations, and multi-alarm notification and multisensor surveillance to inform disabled passengers about the arrival of buses (Zhou, Hou, Zuo, & Li, 2012). RFID readers can be placed at smart bus stops, so that when passengers with a disability scan their tickets on these machines, the bus drivers are automatically updated about their passengers, improving data exchange and making provisions for those in need (Zhou et al., 2012). Since the elderly population is increasing at a fast pace, it is likely that the population of functionally dependent individuals will also increase in the next decade, hence more effective transport solutions must be developed as part of any smart city development project. Being able to move independently will also improve the QoL of VIP, as some studies have shown (García et al., 2015; Zhou et al., 2012).

Ubiquitous computing is also being adopted by car manufacturers in their design of future automobiles, with the aim of enabling those affected by low vision, such as the elderly population, to drive safely on the streets. Driverless car technologies take the needs of VIP into account. Self-driving cars make use of radars and lasers to check and make sure that the roads are clear (the Google self-driving car, for instance). A survey conducted by researchers at the University of Florida, with 38 visually impaired participants, showed optimistic results. The survey concluded that VIP endorsed the idea of self-driving cars, which they believe would overcome the challenges associated with their mobility (Brinkley, Posadas, Woodward, & Gilbert, 2017). However, the survey highlighted some concerns about the development of such technologies in terms of situational awareness, verification of desired location, parking options, safety and roadside assistance. The participants mentioned that there was a lack of consideration of the needs of individuals with visual impairment. In a smart city environment, legal and regulatory issues related to self-driving cars need to be addressed, and citizens need to be trained to respect the laws. The automated cars will need to effectively operate beside other, non-autonomous cars, which often are driven by unpredictable drivers who might not always be following the laws. These smart cars will also need to be supported by high-bandwidth mobile networks, since these vehicles work by collecting data from an array of sensors. Currently, these vehicles are also limited in terms of the data they can collect, and they are not equipped to know if there is a road blocked 10 m ahead. Subsequently, they still rely on human judgement when things have not been planned in advance. However, in a smart city environment, these smart cars can access data from other vehicles, also known as vehicle-to-vehicle communication (V2V), and from roadside units that can provide information about traffic, weather and blocked roads, among other information (Rathore, Ahmad, Paul, & Rho, 2016; Sichitiu & Kihl, 2008).

Some privacy and cybersecurity risks have already been identified concerning the development of such transport systems (Lim & Taeihagh, 2018). If proper protocols are implemented, then, in the long term, the use of smart vehicles can reduce environmental degradation, with low emissions of toxic gases and lower energy consumption. Studies have also shown that the use of automated vehicles by elderly people with low vision has the potential to reduce the amount of road accidents, since they rely on AI to interpret data and make decisions while adapting to changing conditions and eliminating human errors (West, 2016).

1.2.3   Homes of Visually Impaired People in Smart Cities

Smart cities also include the way homes are designed, which are commonly referred to as "smart homes". A smart home is considered to be an advanced automated or controlled home, as it makes use of AI technologies to become dynamic, more intelligent and learn from users' daily activities, thus allowing VIP to live independently (Skouby et al., 2014). Moreover, in the context of healthcare, smart homes will transform the way healthcare services are provided to their residents. Citizens with functional dependencies, including those with visual impairment, will be able to remotely connect to their preferred clinic from the comfort of their home. Solutions such as wearable sensors and sensor-based surveillance systems in smart home settings will track residents' health and notify emergency services, should immediate medical intervention be required. Smart health integrated in a smart home setting is a key player in reducing routine outpatient appointments, which in turn reduces needless travelling to the hospital, addressing the mobility issue associated with VIP (Skouby et al., 2014). Existing projects, for example, the GIRAF++ project, aim to offer an independent living experience to elderly citizens with low vision. This consists of sensors being implanted in smart homes to detect whether a person has issues with moving around, to detect falls, and also monitor some basic health vital signs. Web-enabled devices provide clear benefits, and motion sensors such as Microsoft Kinect can recognise the gestures of VIP in performing some remote tasks. It also has the ability to detect objects and faces, as stated in another study (Rahman, Poo, Amin, & Yan, 2015). Using such technologies can reduce indoor accidents and assist in finding objects around the house, if they are not in their usual place. Providing home Ambient Assisted Living (AAL) to help VIP is a challenge, and homecare systems need to be adapted to the growing elderly population by making use of recent developments in ICT (Mitchell, Liew, Gopinath, & Wong, 2018). Due to the rise in the number of VIP, there are greater demands for informal carers such as family and friends to look after them, and the coping capacity of these carers is decreasing (Pickard, Wittenberg, Comas-Herrera, Davies, & Darton, 2000; Simpson, Young, Donahue, & Rocker, 2010).

Smart cities should comprise smart homes and buildings equipped with audio and vibrotactile systems to improve the QoL and independence of their citizens. Besides, smart homes for VIP can be built to support their mobility inside their homes by making use of automated and smart devices. There are various tasks that could be automated in a smart home environment, whereby the visually impaired citizen would not need to be displaced to complete a task. Regarding the regulation of temperature in an indoor heating system, with a simple voice command, a visually impaired person can increase, decrease, switch on or turn off the heater in a smart home. Another popular tool that is useful for the visually impaired is a voice command assistant, such as "Amazon Echo Dot" or "Google Home", enabling access to music, audiobooks, news or weather updates. There are ways for VIP to be notified about events in the house, meaning that they do not need to move around to inspect things. For example, a water leak can be detected by sensors, switching off the oven can be done remotely via a smart switch, and even closing the gates can be achieved with automation. These are existing technologies that need to be considered to make a home smarter. People with low vision in a smart home would not need to switch lights on/off, as the presence of someone can be detected by passive infrared technologies. Window motors and sensors can be installed, being remotely controlled by wall switches, and monitoring the status of windows. Home appliances can be linked to smart switches that can also send notifications to remind the user to remotely turn them off. For the security and safety of VIP, smart smoke and CO_2 detectors can be connected to different devices, and warn the user or caregiver that smoke has been detected in the room.

Furthermore, regarding daily tasks such as gardening and cleaning, which involve the physical displacement of VIP, these can be enhanced with the use of robot floor cleaning or robot lawnmowers. A number of assistive technology tools have been implemented by companies such as Smartn Ltd, which allow disabled people to reshape their routine and lead a more independent life (Smartn, 2018). Some of these tasks were impossible prior to the advent of the smart home concept, which relies hugely on the strong network infrastructure.

The goal of designing smart homes is to safeguard VIP well-being in their own homes. Smart homes are embedded with assistive technologies, which enable them to provide such users with opportunities of independent living and reduce social isolation. Despite the fact that smart homes are stationary in nature, users inside these homes are mobile, thus they benefit from the embedded technologies around them (Hakobyan et al., 2013).

1.2.4 Mobile Assistive Vision Support Systems for Obstacle Detection and Space Perception

Over the years, assistive technologies have gone through several stages and forms, starting from a simple typewriter that helps VIP to write, to state-of-the-art mobile phone applications specifically developed for VIP to "see" and understand their surroundings.

Obstacle detection when navigating through urban spaces and space perception when navigating through open spaces are the two main solutions provided by mobile assistive technologies. The subsequent sections expand upon the aforementioned solutions, providing examples and use cases (Hakobyan et al., 2013):

Obstacle Detection

This solution comes under independent and safe navigation for VIP. The concept of safe navigation ensures that timely warning messages are sent to the respective users in order to make them aware of possible hazards in their path (Hakobyan et al., 2013). The traditional white cane obstacle detection method is relatively inexpensive, but it requires intensive training and significant effort by the user, who struggles to explore the area ahead of him. In Sect. 1.5, we have determined the challenges associated with the white cane approach. In the literature, several mobile assistive approaches of obstacle detection and avoidance have been proposed as augmented versions of the white cane method.

One such innovative approach is called SmartVision. It is a smartphone-based navigational support system, which operates by tracking the travelling path, along with detecting obstacles, utilising a navigational map. Such a navigational system surpasses the limited observational capabilities of the white cane by providing real-time and precise information about the obstacles on the route (Hakobyan et al., 2013). SmartVision is an outdoor use case that requires GPS support, which is prone to attenuation, particularly in adverse weather conditions. In such a case, the system would be regarded as unsafe for VIP. The risk of signal loss can be mitigated by using RFID tags instead of GPS. The RFID reader embedded within the white cane would detect RFID tags from its surroundings (e.g. pavements). In addition, there is a 3D camera (called a stereo camera, which consists of two lenses to stimulate the human binocular vision and capture 3D images) connected at chest level, a portable small computer worn in the shoulder, an earphone, and a small four-button device to explore the navigational menu. The addition of an audio interface provides verbal information about the route, obstacles en route, as well as points of interest (e.g. restaurants) en route. The vibrating device attached to the handle of the white cane works alongside an audio interface to alert VIP about the approaching obstacle. A similar prototype can be used in an indoor scenario, where Wi-Fi and the Global Information System (GIS) can be utilised to enable VIP to actively interact socially and obtain information inside their homes (Hakobyan et al., 2013).

The EU-funded EVA project, which stands for "Extended Visual Assistant", has addressed a twenty-first-century challenge in helping VIP to enjoy better QoL. The project has developed a high-tech glass with online connectivity, which was a low-cost solution as compared to training guide dogs, and also involves low energy consumption. With a stylish design, the glasses have a discreet camera, microphone, speaker and control buttons (European Commission, 2018b). It has been mentioned that the glasses will even be able to detect the proximity of cars in the future, allowing VIP to detect electric cars, which are usually more quiet (European Commission, 2018b). This could reduce the number of road accidents, while detecting a number of obstacles automatically and warning VIP.

Space Perception

In the previous system, we discussed navigation solutions that offer obstacle detection and avoidance. It is important to highlight that the navigation systems should not only focus on finding routes, but also should be able to perceive, interpret and comprehend information about VIP surroundings. Therefore, solutions incorporated under space perception systems such as MobileEye and LocalEyes would help VIP with their perception (Hakobyan et al., 2013).

The goal of MobileEye is to allow VIP to perceive, understand and interact with their surroundings, especially in situations where they are travelling alone. This can be achieved using embedded cameras in mobile phones, as well as text-to-speech conversion technology. Four subsystems are incorporated under MobileEye, which target different needs of VIP: (1) a mapper designed to distinguish different colours; (2) a software-based magnifier, used to facilitate reading; (3) a pattern recognition device to recognise objects such as money; and (4) a document retriever device used to extract a document from a database by simply scanning the keywords. The operations of the described software above are triggered through a voice message. The camera is activated by using double-clicks. In addition, the software automatically switches off after being idle for 2 min. However, the software can be further improved by increasing the response time, and by including the vibrational feature.

The other system, used to address space perception, called LocalEyes, operates through GPS, and provides a multimodal user-friendly interface. The services provided through LocalEyes include information about points of interest such as restaurants, coffee shops, pharmacies, shopping markets, etc.

1.3 Crowdsourcing to Help Visually Impaired People in Smart Cities

Crowdsourcing, which is another key factor in the developmental strategies of smart cities for the visually impaired, has gained some interest since the term was coined in the past decade. Crowdsourcing is a distributed problem-solving model achieved through the collaboration of various individuals via web-based platforms (Brabham, 2008). It is regarded as an alternative to enable public engagement and decision making. The EU has shown particular interests in using crowdsourcing methods to identify innovative solutions. One example of the use of crowds to help people with impaired vision is the "Be My Eyes" software program, which allows people with sight issues to request the help of someone who has no visual impairment and previously signed up as a volunteer via the platform. The software matches the person with a volunteer who can respond and help. Requests can range from checking expiry dates, distinguishing colours, reading instructions or navigating new surroundings. The visually impaired person simply has to point the phone to the object, or anything with which he requires assistance. The application currently has over one million volunteers, helping over 100,000 visually impaired people in 150 countries (Be My Eyes, 2018). Similarly, in a smart city environment, the government needs to encourage its citizens to collaborate via crowdsourcing to help people in need. The governmental infrastructure of smart cities should be accountable, responsive and transparent. Smart city crowdsourcing plays a vital role and can help in participatory planning, including the concept of open government, citizen reporting and can facilitate citizen-to-government support (Tooran, 2018). It does not only relate to technology, but focuses on collaborative approaches that create new ideas and increase efficiency, while saving resources. Crowdsourcing could be exploited to develop solutions for visually impaired people to navigate a smart city. This could assist them to locate landmarks, for example, by combining Google Street View (GSV) and online crowdsourcing, as stated in a study conducted in the US (Hara et al., 2015). The study involved 18 people with visual impairments informing the design of the proposed tool. The work used the collection of landmark descriptions, such as bus stop signs, benches, mail boxes, traffic poles, shelters or other physical objects, inserted by crowd workers in GSV. A smart device can then use GPS and text-to-speech to describe the necessary information to VIP. A smart city should be able to provide similar information to VIP in the future. Another example is the "Mobile Crowd Assisted Navigation" mobile application, developed and tested by a group of researchers to assist people with low vision to navigate. Reliable directions are given by an online volunteer community in real time via four arrow keys indicating right, left, forward or stop, which are then converted to audio instructions for the user (Olmschenk, Yang, Zhu, Tong, & Seiple, 2015).

Smart cities could assist VIP in different ways. We discussed earlier how the infrastructure and transportation system of a smart city are among the most important factors which can help VIP to enjoy a better lifestyle with improved mobility. The other identified capabilities involve sectors such as energy and utilities, public safety, health, housing and education (Korngold, Lemos, & Rohwer, 2017). Healthcare professionals have been estimated to be the fastest growing workforce in the United States, and they are important assets in a smart city, since in the next decade the elderly and disabled populations will increase (Korngold et al., 2017). To facilitate the jobs of these healthcare professionals, hospitals and other health infrastructure should exploit the use of IoT and smart mobile health technologies to support real-time data and provide personalised educational materials to citizens, including the VIP. There are already an estimated 36 million units of monitoring devices today, as compared to only three million units in 2011 (Korngold et al., 2017).

Future smart cities need to support the use of medical devices on the move for more effective monitoring and lower costs on hospital admissions for those suffering from chronic diseases.

Medical devices are gradually evolving to suit the needs of the VIP. However, these devices are still scarce (Heinemann, Drossel, Freckmann, & Kulzer, 2016). There are now state-of-the-art medical devices that allow patients to identify their medications. These medical devices include AccessaMed and Talking RX, which can be attached to box prescriptions to read aloud the recorded instructions by the pharmacist about the dosage of a medication, description of the pills as well as precautions or warnings (VisionAware, 2019). Digit-Eyes is yet another mobile application that can read QR codes containing prescription medication labels. These are not only useful for the visually impaired but also for the elderly patients who tend to have poor memory and poor vision.

The collection of patients' data via IoT technologies can further help innovators to improve existing systems using large sets of available data, and also allow VIP to comprehensively understand their personal health. This will encourage independent living. The visually impaired population suffering from chronic conditions would receive significant health benefits, and would not be required to make regular visits to the hospital for check-ups, since they could be assessed from their homes via the use of approved Bluetooth-enabled medical devices such as blood pressure monitors, digital thermometers, ECG via a smart vest, or weight scales that can send data automatically to a secure cloud.

Smart cities have the potential to decrease social isolation and empower VIP in various ways. Although many of these solutions have already been developed, many of them did not feature security aspects, and have not yet been tested or evaluated on a large scale. It is a key role of the government to encourage social innovation, and invest in technologies to improve the lives of VIP. By utilising the collection of data and connectivity, smart cities will provide new means of interaction, lifestyle management, and enable independent living. Through machine–machine communication, real-time monitoring, strong network infrastructure and crowdsourcing, smart cities can address some of the current problems faced by those with vision issues.

1.4 Internet of Things Applications for Visually Impaired People

1.4.1 IoT Architecture

IoT architecture consists of several layers used to facilitate cross-layer communication due to the different representation required at each layer. As mentioned in Domingo (2012), the IoT architecture consists of three layers, as shown in Fig. 1.2. These layers include the perception layer, network layer and application layer. Each layer's function is briefly described as follows:

(a) Perception layer: the main function of this layer is to identify the types of objects and collect perceptive information. This layer is constructed of sensors, actuators, controlling and monitoring devices (e.g. smartphones, tablets, PCs, PDAs, etc.), RFID tags and readers/writers.
(b) Network layer: the main function of this layer is to transmit information obtained from the perception layer. In addition, this layer is responsible for establishing the connectivity of the devices in the perception layer. Moreover, the network layer addresses the functionalities associated with wired and wireless networks, as well as the Internet.
(c) Application layer: this layer consists of innovative and smart solutions that employ IoT technology to support user applications.

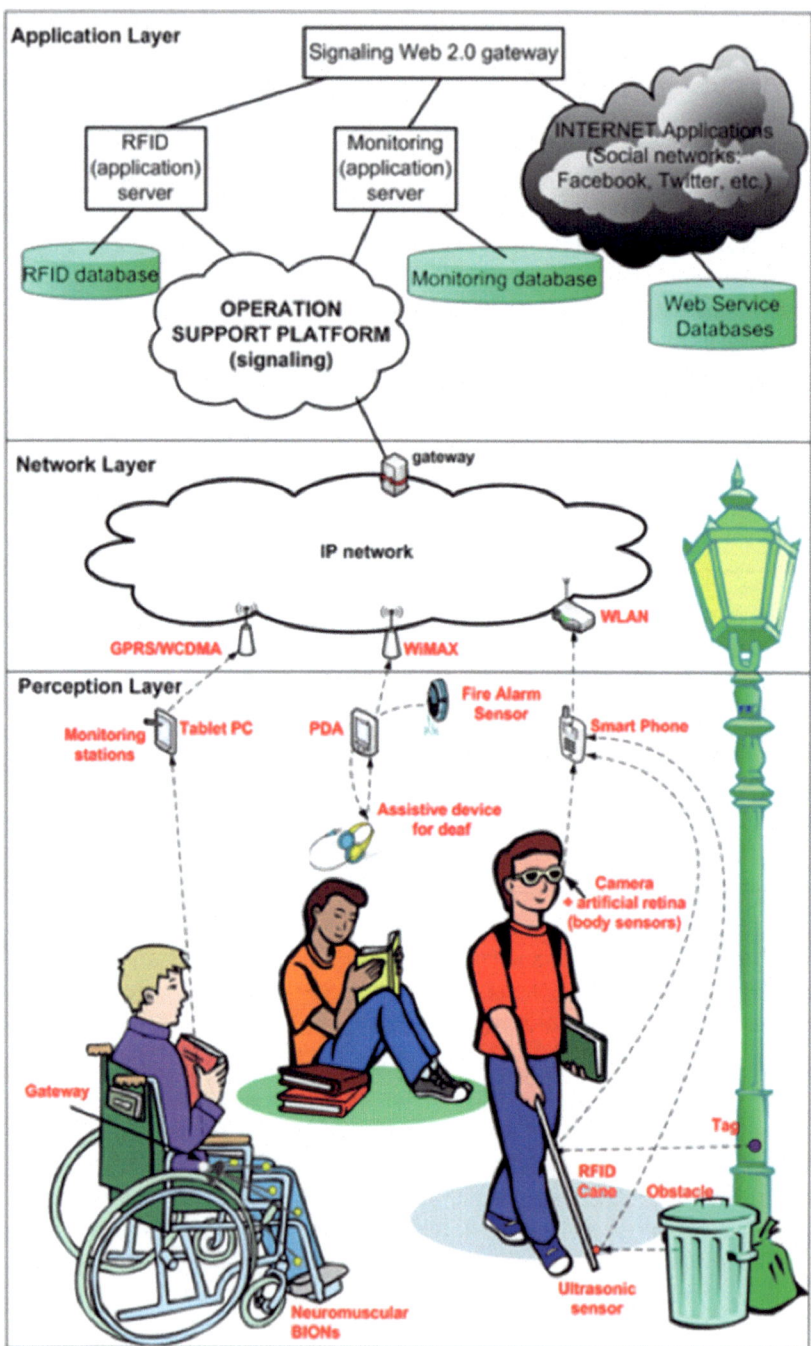

Fig. 1.2 IoT Layer Architecture (Domingo, 2012)

The authors in Domingo (2012) introduced several IoT applications for people with disabilities. These applications tend to show how IoT devices interact with each other to facilitate real-life scenarios, such as smart shopping, smart learning and smart home living.

Independent Shopping Scenario

Independent and safe mobility while shopping are the two main requirements for VIP in this particular scenario. According to a survey, VIP stated that a shopping centre is the most challenging environment in terms of space perception and in-store navigation, leading to a difficult shopping experience (Hakobyan et al., 2013).

IoT-based smart shopping, as shown in Fig. 1.3 (Domingo, 2012), meets the requirements of independent shopping and safe mobility by providing an in-store navigational system specifically designed for VIP. In addition, RFID tags distributed within the shopping centre connect to the RFID reader embedded in the smart white cane, which further connects to the VIP's smartphone via Bluetooth. This entire

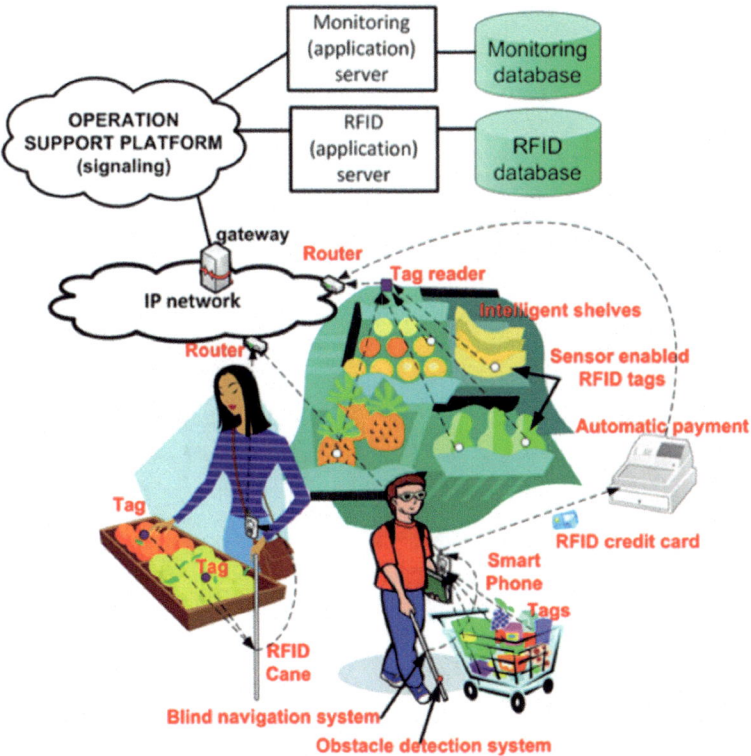

Fig. 1.3 Shopping scenario (Domingo, 2012)

setup helps VIP to keep track of their position and assists them with efficient in-store navigation (Domingo, 2012).

Smart Learning Scenario

The smart learning scenario, as shown in Fig. 1.4, has been proposed by the authors in Domingo (2012), who highlighted the importance of designing a smart interactive play environment and environmental learning systems for children with concomitant

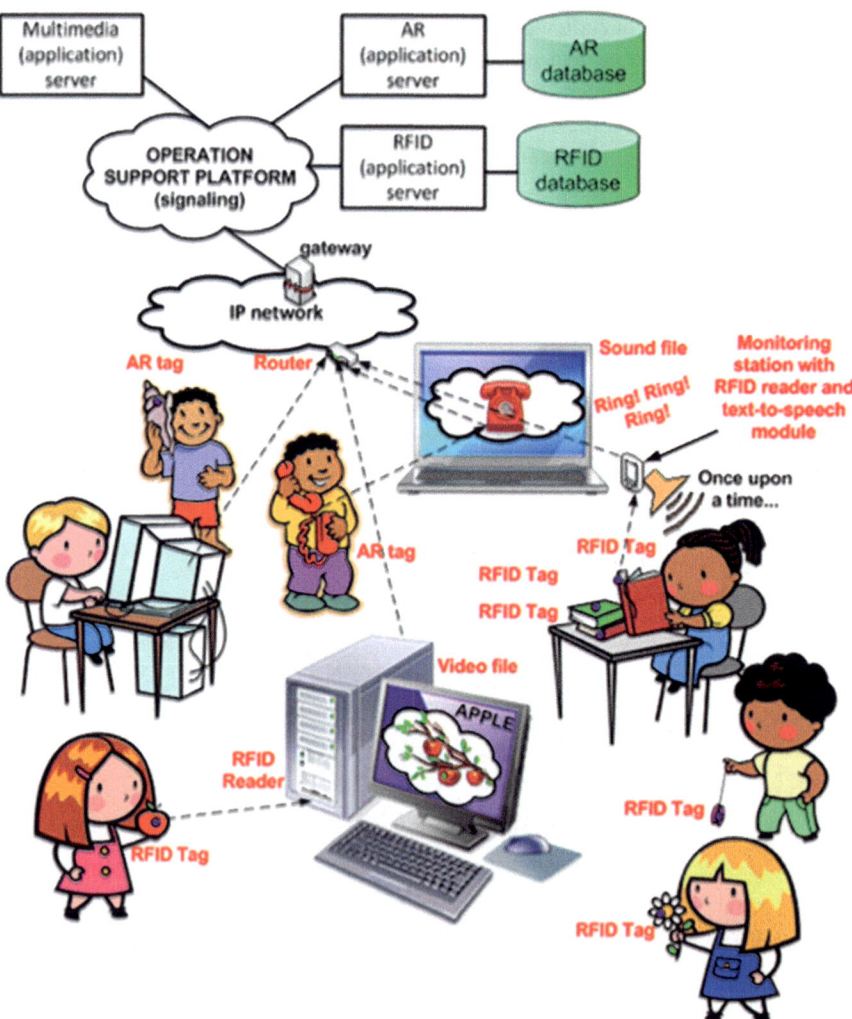

Fig. 1.4 Smart learning scenario (Domingo, 2012)

impairments. Their proposed design stimulates language and communication skills. The play and learning system consists of RFID technology, which is employed to distinguish between different objects such as toys. Moreover, the RFID tags attached to the toys are used to support children with concomitant impairments including visual impairment (Domingo, 2012). The proposed system is user-friendly, where an RFID reader is used to scan the tag and send the tag ID to the linked software, which in turn provides audible information about the scanned object.

Domestic Environment Scenario

Figure 1.5 shows the integration of technology and services in a smart home setting. Usually, a smart home involves the interaction of the objects using the home networking systems in order to enhance QoL. Home automation and control features are enabled by using devices such as automated appliances in kitchens, light and door controllers, indoor temperature controllers, water temperature controllers and home security devices (Domingo, 2012). Automated devices in smart homes are operated by sensors and actuators, which are embedded within home appliances. These embedded sensors monitor environmental conditions, process information collected via IoT devices, and communicate with other devices through wireless networks. After gathering information, local or cloud-based servers process the gathered information to provide a suitable service to users. For instance, in the case of fire being detected, actuators are triggered to address such an emergency situation (Domingo, 2012).

1.5   Artificial Intelligence (AI), Virtual Reality (VR) and Augmented Reality (AU) Solutions for Visually Impaired People

Recently, there has been increasing interest in applying AI and machine learning methods to the development of algorithms that will complement our lives. The aforementioned claim is supported by research, which states that AI, along with machine learning, is more reliable, consistent and efficient than the human brain, and naturally does not involve mood swings (Charlier & Kloppenburg, 2017). But what do we mean by AI? AI is an umbrella term, which is a sub-category of computer science. It encompasses machine learning algorithms, robotics, expert systems and language processing (Nayak & Dutta, 2017). The terms AI and machine learning are interchangeably used, and are often targeted towards the same goal (e.g. facilitating human interactions in an intelligent and efficient way without human intervention). Augmented reality (AR) and virtual reality (VR) also represent the next step in providing effective support to VIP either inside their homes, whilst they are navigating the streets, or within a smart environment (Katz et al., 2012; Wilson,

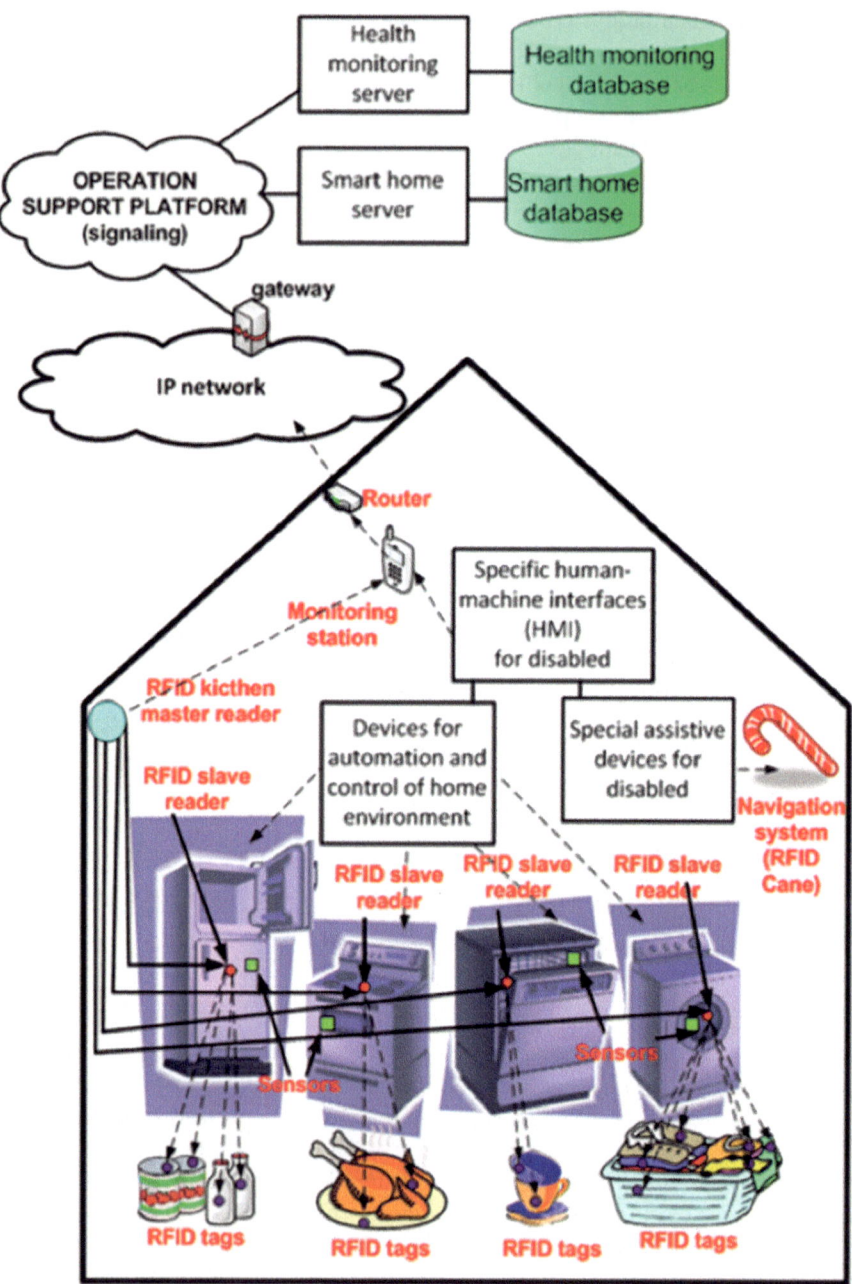

Fig. 1.5 Domestic environment scenario (Domingo, 2012)

Foreman, & Stanton, 1997). VR is a completely simulated environment, which does not link with the real world. It provides an interactive computer-generated environment that allows users to perform a number of tasks. VR is successfully used for flight and driving simulators, training in medicine, and overcoming a number of psychological issues. However, despite its excellent features, it is very limited for VIP. On the other hand, AR combines simulation and overlays with the real world environment. A new concept has emerged called mixed reality (MR), where not only is digital simulation merged with the real world, but also the digital objects can interact with each other. Microsoft introduced the HoloLens mixed reality glasses in 2016, which were expensive, with high resource requirements (Moemeka & Moemeka, 2015). Many other companies have also invested in this sector, and a number of AR glasses models are available, such as Google Glass and Epson Moverio, which provide mobility solutions for VIP. The HoloLens and Google Glass technologies may be integrated with Google Maps, allowing VIP to navigate the streets, while AR glasses can read signs and provide feedback to the user about their surroundings.

AI, AR and VR are no longer concepts associated with the future. They are very much in our present, and have been widely adopted in recent years. Classic examples of AI-based applications—of which most of us are unaware—are right in front of us. These include Apple's Siri, Tesla's self-driving and collision detection, Facebook's face recognition software, Netflix's movie recommendations, banks' fraud detection mechanisms, to name just a few (Charlier & Kloppenburg, 2017). Healthcare is one of many domains in which AI is prevailing, revolutionising healthcare delivery. In terms of diagnostic precision, these intelligent systems imitate a medical expert's diagnostic experience, and provide diagnoses with a high degree of accuracy. An eye-opening demonstration between human doctors and AI-assisted machines was conducted by the Royal College of Physicians. Based on 100 sample medical scenarios, the AI-enabled machines scored better than human doctors in terms of diagnostic accuracy, with a high score of 98% (Olson, 2018).

Similarly, people with functional disabilities such as visual impairment will benefit from AI. However, such AI methods need to be embedded into state-of-the-art IoT devices in order to fully exploit AI capabilities. Furthermore, it is essential for AI-enabled devices to aid in real time, as non-real-time support may not serve the purpose of anytime and anywhere access, defined earlier in this chapter. Although emerging technologies such as IoT may provide backend information and data, the front end or consumer-centred device would be AR-based smart glasses, providing valuable information to users during their daily routine both inside and outside their homes.

After researching the literature, as described earlier in this chapter, we found studies which investigated means to improve the QoL of VIP. Such studies utilised ultrasonic sensors, microcontrollers, webcams and audio feedback mechanisms to assist navigation through obstacles (Cardin, Thalmann, & Vexo, 2007; Dunai, Lengua, Tortajada, & Simon, 2014; Gharani & Karimi, 2017; Jonnalagedda et al., 2014; Lee, Chen, Sung, & Lu, 2014; Poggi & Mattoccia, 2016). However, they proposed bulky prototypes, which may be questionable with regard to the aspects of usability and user experience. In addition, these studies lacked the integration of AI in their tactile vision systems. Besides, concerns of mobility and affordability were also associated with the proposed systems.

In recent times, AI-enabled intelligent vision systems have gained in popularity in academic, research and industrial communities, which jointly work together to improve QoL for those with visual impairment. Innovative AI-based solutions that mostly emphasise navigation and obstacle detection have been proposed. These include road crossing assistance, guide drones, locating and identifying bus stops, navigational tools to travel between indoor and urban outdoor spaces, computer vision and VR/AR tools to complement human vision, to name just a few. The success of the aforementioned projects was made possible due to the advent of emerging IoT devices (e.g. image and object capturing devices), and AI and machine learning techniques (e.g. neural networks, Fuzzy Inference Systems and deep learning, etc.). Besides navigation and obstacle detection, social interaction is another paradigm that has found hope in AI-enabled solutions for VIP. Solutions such as the "Social Assistant", which incorporates cameras and vibrating belts as input devices, have been found useful in providing visual cues that correspond to facial expressions, hand gestures and head nodding of the social partner. The responses provide verbal feedback to the person with visual impairment.

Furthermore, in the years to come, the concept of an AI-enabled "Social Assistant" will evolve into an AI-enabled "Personal Assistant" that already knows the voice, and facial and physical attributes of people one interacts with regularly. Embedded expression recognition features would recognise facial expressions (e.g. angry and humorous expressions). Moreover, finding people would be possible. Such intelligent solutions are revolutionary in their use to benefit VIP, leading to improved QoL. However, these solutions require further testing and validation in terms of user acceptance and satisfaction, which is a gap that needs to be filled.

The concept of smart cities is a new paradigm that aims to overcome the aforementioned gap by endorsing the idea of smart living, utilising the best available features of AI, such as pattern recognition, expert prediction and robotics. Furthermore, smart homes, smart streets and smart transportation, being the sub-categories of smart cities, will revolutionise ambient assisted living, especially for VIP. In a smart city setting, the connectivity between IoT-enabled smart devices and next generation wireless networks, along with the concept of context-awareness, will play an indispensable role in augmenting the QoL of VIP. According to Gharani and Karimi (2017), the term context refers to "any information that can be used to characterise the situation of an entity, where an entity can be a person, place, or object that is considered relevant to the interaction between a user and an application, including the user and application themselves". The distinctive features of context-aware systems are their ability to operate without user interaction, and their ability to gather contextual information from a user's environment and adapt to it accordingly. Such systems can be easily integrated into a smart city setting, which makes them suitable candidates for healthcare applications, and, in particular, for assisted ambient living for the visually impaired.

Considering a user's environment, where the user is a person with visual impairment, the following characteristics have been identified as influencing context-awareness:

(a) Physical and temporal characteristics (e.g. location)
(b) Social interactions
(c) Economic characteristics (e.g. affordability)
(d) Competency (e.g. ability to carry out a task)
(e) Technical characteristics

The government, businesses and policy makers need to incorporate the identified characteristics in a smart city context to provide strong interaction between visually impaired citizens and their environment.

Traditional white cane sticks and guide dogs form a basis from which AI-enabled systems can learn. Primarily, white cane sticks and guide dogs are widely used by VIP for navigation and the detection of obstacles in their surroundings. White cane sticks only detect obstacles below the waistline, and do not provide precise information about a user's surroundings, such as irregular objects, objects above waist-level, and the distance between the user and the object. To address these limitations, smart sticks and guide drones have been proposed. Such innovative solutions represent a step forward in reducing injuries associated with traditional vision support systems. However, these proposals are not completely AI-enabled, which is a major research gap, especially in a smart city context, which is all about AI-enabled smart living. To attain user acceptance with respect to AI-enabled smart sticks and guide drones, the following requirements need to be met:

(a) Provide real-time feedback, which should be haptic or tactile to ensure timely steering.
(b) Provide contextual information about the user's environment.
(c) Provide a pattern recognition feature to identify obstacles and/or objects.
(d) Provide precise distance information between the user and the obstacle.
(e) Provide information to other commuters about their presence in the vicinity.
(f) Provide reliability.
(g) Aid in terms of verbal as well as sensory instructions/commands.
(h) Provide a distinction between different objects as well as people.

Microsoft has recently launched "Canetroller", a virtual haptic cane, which provides visually impaired users with different types of feedback, namely vibrotactile, spatial 3D auditory and resistance feedback, in a virtual environment setup (Zhao et al., 2018). Participants can use the virtual cane to identify virtual objects, such as a crossing, a bin or a table, in a virtual environment set up in an empty room. The study showed that Canetroller was a promising tool that enabled visually impaired participants to navigate through virtual spaces, and this could help them in orientation and mobility training (Zhao et al., 2018).

Furthermore, in designing AI-enabled vision support systems, it is crucial to involve VIP themselves in the design process. Such a methodology will enable developers to customise a design to suit their requirements. In addition, it may be necessary to include their carers in the design process, as they will provide input for the AI system to understand and prioritise the activities that VIP can/cannot do on their own. Once the user requirements have been gathered, customising an AI-based solution should be straightforward, in any domain, whether indoors or outdoors. To elaborate further on the AI aspect of smart cities, it is important for AI-enabled devices and/or software to be trained in order to replicate traditional approaches used by VIP intelligently and without much human intervention.

1.6   Conclusion

The features that should be considered in building smart cities for VIP include smart homes, smart transportation, social interactions and smart healthcare, which need to be supported by proper legislation. In a smart city setting, VIP located indoors should be able to identify obstacles and the distance between them, switch appliances on and off, and capture anomalies. Outdoors, they should be guided through pedestrian crossings, and ultimately be provided an optimal route to their desired destination without any hindrance. When using public transportation, they should be able to identify bus stops, be notified about bus arrivals, and be directed towards vacant seats.

Smart city adoption is inspired by the fact that people's QoL will be enhanced, along with the environment becoming more disabled-friendlier. Technological advancements can enhance the ability of individuals to fully participate in social activities and live independently. Moving in this direction will provide ease of accessibility and support for all levels of citizens. Moreover, ICT-based technologies are more manageable when implemented in smart cities, with sensing and monitoring capabilities, along with the utilisation of data-driven approaches. In a generation of connected technologies, our developed smart cities will show their readiness and potential to align with this evolution, and facilitate the path towards a technological future.

With the advent of AI, artificial and tactile intelligent vision systems must incorporate image recognition features, obstacle detection, collision detection and fall detection in a single prototype. In addition, such prototypes should be user-friendly, accessible, and adhere to safety, security and privacy requirements. While there are a number of technologies available in the market that offer a promising future for the application of AR in a smart city for the visually impaired, they are far from the reach of normal consumers, due to a number of constraints, including high prices, limited programmes and a lack of research in the industry. The size of the proposed AR glasses is also a consideration, as they need to accommodate a camera, projection display, battery and the processor.

The creation of smart cities is still in its infancy with regard to assisted living for visually impaired people. For an intelligent vision support system, it is important to recognise and prioritise the essentials that VIP associate with improved QoL. User acceptance in terms of accessibility, privacy and security are prerequisites for such intelligent and guided vision support systems to find sustainable success in the field of healthcare.

Acknowledgements Dr. Drishty Sobnath would like to acknowledge the Research, Innovation and Enterprise department of Solent University for supporting this work.

Dr. Ikram Ur Rehman would like to acknowledge the CU Coventry for its support. Also, he appreciates the support from Ajaz Ali for his valuable insights for this chapter.

Dr. Moustafa Nasralla would like to acknowledge the management of Prince Sultan University (PSU) for the valued support and research environmental provision which have led to completing this work.

References

Be My Eyes. (2018). *Be my eyes - Bringing sight to blind and low-vision people*. Retrieved November 27, 2018, from https://www.bemyeyes.com/

Billah, S. M., Ashok, V., Porter, D. E., & Ramakrishnan, I. V. (2017). Ubiquitous accessibility for people with visual impairments: Are we there yet? In *SIGCHI Conference Human Factors in Computer Systems* (pp. 5862–5868). New York, NY: ACM. https://doi.org/10.1145/3025453.3025731

Brabham, D. C. (2008). Crowdsourcing as a model for problem solving an introduction and cases. *Convergence: The International Journal of Research into New Media Technologies and Singapore, 14*(1), 75–90. https://doi.org/10.1177/1354856507084420

Brinkley, J., Posadas, B., Woodward, J., & Gilbert, J. E. (2017). Opinions and preferences of blind and low vision consumers regarding self-driving vehicles: Results of focus group discussions. In *19th International ACM SIGACCESS Conference*. New York, NY: ACM. https://doi.org/10.1145/3132525.3132532

Cardin, S., Thalmann, D., & Vexo, F. (2007). A wearable system for mobility improvement of visually impaired people. *Visual Computer., 23*, 109. https://doi.org/10.1007/s00371-006-0032-4

Charlier, R., & Kloppenburg, S. (2017). *Artificial intelligence in HR: A no brainer*. London: PwC.

CittaMobi. (2018). *CittaMobi*. Retrieved November 26, 2018, from https://www.cittamobi.com.br/home/

Domingo, M. C. (2012). An overview of the internet of things for people with disabilities. *Journal of Network and Computer Applications, 35*, 584–596. https://doi.org/10.1016/j.jnca.2011.10.015

Domingue, J., Galis, A., Gavras, A., Zahariadis, T., Lambert, D., Cleary, F., ... Nilsson, M. (2011). The future internet. In D. Hutchison, T. Kanade, J. Kleinberg, A. Kobsa, & F. Mattern (Eds.), *Lecture notes in computer science*. Berlin: Springer. https://doi.org/10.1007/3-540-68339-9_34

Dunai, L. D., Lengua, I. L., Tortajada, I., & Simon, F. B. (2014). Obstacle detectors for visually impaired people. In *2014 International Conference on Optimization of Electrical and Electronic Equipment, OPTIM 2014*. Washington, DC: IEEE. https://doi.org/10.1109/OPTIM.2014.6850903

European Commission. (2018a). *General Assembly of the European Innovation Partnership on Smart Cities and Communities (EIP-SCC)*. Brussels: European Commission. Retrieved November 22, 2018, from https://ec.europa.eu/info/events/energy-events/general-assembly-european-innovation-partnership-smart-cities-and-communities-eip-scc-2018-jun-27_en

European Commission. (2018b). *New smart glasses can talk to the blind*. Brussels: European Commission. Retrieved November 23, 2018, from https://cordis.europa.eu/result/rcn/230142_en.html

García, C. R., Quesada-Arencibia, A., Cristóbal, T., Padrón, G., Pérez, R., & Alayón, F. (2015). An intelligent system proposal for improving the safety and accessibility of public transit by highway. *Sensors, 15*, 20279–20304. https://doi.org/10.3390/s150820279

Gharani, P., & Karimi, H. A. (2017). Context-aware obstacle detection for navigation by visually impaired. *Image and Vision Computing., 64*, 103. https://doi.org/10.1016/j.imavis.2017.06.002

Gibson, D. V., Kozmetsky, G., & Smilor, R. W. (1992). *The Technopolis phenomenon: Smart cities, fast systems, global networks.* Lanham, MD: Rowman & Littlefield Publishers. Retrieved from https://books.google.co.uk/books?id=_NxMwZfAafYC&printsec=frontcover&dq=The+Technopolis+Phenomenon:+Smart+Cities,+Fast+Systems,+Global+Networks.+Rowman+%26+Littlefield,+New+York+(1992)&hl=en&sa=X&ved=0ahUKEwjP5eL11-XeAhWGxYsKHQTlB3sQ6AEIKjAA#v=onepage&q=T

Hakobyan, L., Lumsden, J., O'Sullivan, D., & Bartlett, H. (2013). Mobile assistive technologies for the visually impaired. *Survey of Ophthalmology., 58*, 513. https://doi.org/10.1016/j.survophthal.2012.10.004

Hara, K., Azenkot, S., Campbell, M., Bennett, C. L., Le, V., Pannella, S., ... Froehlich, J. E. (2015). Improving public transit accessibility for blind riders by crowdsourcing bus stop landmark locations with google street view. *ACM Transactions on Accessible Computing (TACCESS), 6*(2), 5. https://doi.org/10.1145/2717513

Hashem, I. A. T., Chang, V., Anuar, N. B., Adewole, K., Yaqoob, I., Gani, A., ... Chiroma, H. (2016). The role of big data in smart city. *International Journal of Information Management., 36*, 748. https://doi.org/10.1016/j.ijinfomgt.2016.05.002

Heinemann, L., Drossel, D., Freckmann, G., & Kulzer, B. (2016). Usability of medical devices for patients with diabetes who are visually impaired or blind. *Journal of Diabetes Science and Technology, 10*(6), 1382–1387. https://doi.org/10.1177/1932296816666536

Jonnalagedda, A., Pei, L., Saxena, S., Wu, M., Min, B.-C., Teves, E., ... Dias, M. B. (2014). *Enhancing the safety of visually impaired travelers in and around transit stations.* Pittsburgh, PA: Carnegie Mellon University.

Katz, B. F. G., Kammoun, S., Parseihian, G., Gutierrez, O., Brilhault, A., Auvray, M., ... Jouffrais, C. (2012). NAVIG: Augmented reality guidance system for the visually impaired. *Virtual Reality., 16*, 253. https://doi.org/10.1007/s10055-012-0213-6

Korngold, D., Lemos, M., & Rohwer, M. (2017). *Smart cities for all: A vision for an inclusive, accessible urban future.* San Francisco, CA: BSR. Retrieved from http://smartcities4all.org/wp-content/uploads/2017/06/Smart-Cities-for-All-A-Vision-for-an-Inclusive-Accessible-Urban-Futur...-min.pdf

Jukna, L. (2017). *Smart cities for the blind.* London: Living Map. Retrieved December 4, 2018, from https://www.livingmap.com/smart-city/smart-cities-for-the-blind/

Lee, C. L., Chen, C. Y., Sung, P. C., & Lu, S. Y. (2014). Assessment of a simple obstacle detection device for the visually impaired. *Applied Ergonomics., 45*, 817. https://doi.org/10.1016/j.apergo.2013.10.012

Lim, H. S., & Taeihagh, A. (2018). Autonomous vehicles for smart and sustainable cities: An in-depth exploration of privacy and cybersecurity implications. *Energies, 11*(5), 1062. https://doi.org/10.3390/en11051062

Mitchell, P., Liew, G., Gopinath, B., & Wong, T. Y. (2018). Age-related macular degeneration. *The Lancet., 392*, P1147. https://doi.org/10.1016/S0140-6736(18)31550-2

Moemeka, E., & Moemeka, E. (2015). Leveraging cortana and speech. In *Real world windows 10 development.* New York, NY: Apress. https://doi.org/10.1007/978-1-4842-1449-7_12

Musil, S. (2018). *Google developing Lookout app to aid the visually impaired - CNET.* Retrieved November 23, 2018, from https://www.cnet.com/news/google-developing-lookout-app-to-aid-the-visually-impaired/

Nayak, A., & Dutta, K. (2017). Impacts of machine learning and artificial intelligence on mankind. In *Proceedings of 2017 International Conference on Intelligent Computing and Control, I2C2.* Washinton, DC: IEEE. https://doi.org/10.1109/I2C2.2017.8321908

Olmschenk, G., Yang, C., Zhu, Z., Tong, H., & Seiple, W. H. (2015). Mobile crowd assisted navigation for the visually impaired. In *2015 IEEE 12th Intl Conf on Ubiquitous Intelligence and Computing and 2015 IEEE 12th Intl Conf on Autonomic and Trusted Computing and 2015 IEEE 15th Intl Conf on Scalable Computing and Communications and Its Associated Workshops (UIC-ATC-ScalCom)* (pp. 324–327). Washinton, DC: IEEE. https://doi.org/10.1109/UIC-ATC-ScalCom-CBDCom-IoP.2015.69

Olson, P. (2018). *This AI just beat human doctors on a clinical exam.* Jersey City, NJ: Forbes.

Organisation for Economic Cooperation and Development. (2017). *Embracing innovation in government global trends.* Paris: OECD. Retrieved from https://www.oecd.org/gov/innovative-government/embracing-innovation-in-government.pdf

Patricio, M., Haidee, L., Ciro, L., Telma, R., & Felipe, F. (2015). Analysis and proposed improvements in the support for the visually impaired in the use of public transportation. In *SMART 2015: The Fourth International Conference on Smart Systems, Devices and Technologies* (pp. 414–415). Copenhagen: IARIA XPS Press. Retrieved from https://webcache.googleusercontent.com/search?q=cache:ufklXUFk6uAJ:https://www.thinkmind.org/download.php%3Farticleid%3Dsmart_2015_3_20_40084+&cd=1&hl=en&ct=clnk&gl=uk

Philip, N. Y., & Rehman, I. U. (2016). Towards 5G health for medical video streaming over small cells. In *IFMBE Proceedings.* Cham: Springer. https://doi.org/10.1007/978-3-319-32703-7_214

Pickard, L., Wittenberg, R., Comas-Herrera, A., Davies, B., & Darton, R. (2000). Relying on informal care in the new century? Informal care for elderly people in England to 2031. *Ageing and Society., 20*, 745. https://doi.org/10.1017/S0144686X01007978

Poggi, M., & Mattoccia, S. (2016). A wearable mobility aid for the visually impaired based on embedded 3D vision and deep learning. In *Proceedings - IEEE Symposium on Computers and Communications.* Washington, DC: IEEE. https://doi.org/10.1109/ISCC.2016.7543741

Rahman, M., Poo, B., Amin, A., & Yan, H. (2015). Support system using microsoft kinect and mobile phone for daily activity of visually impaired. In *Transactions on engineering technologies* (pp. 425–440). Dordrecht: Springer. https://doi.org/10.1007/978-94-017-9588-3_32

Ramadhan, A. J. (2018). Wearable smart system for visually impaired people. *Sensors, 13*(3), 834. https://doi.org/10.3390/s18030843

Rathore, M. M., Ahmad, A., Paul, A., & Rho, S. (2016). Urban planning and building smart cities based on the internet of things using big data analytics. *Computer Networks., 101*, 63. https://doi.org/10.1016/j.comnet.2015.12.023

Sahin, Y. G., Aslan, B., Talebi, S., & Zeray, A. (2015). A smart tactile for visually impaired people. *Journal of Trends in the Development of Machinery and Associated Technology, 19*, 101.

Siano, P., Shahrour, I., & Vergura, S. (2018). Introducing smart cities: A transdisciplinary journal on the science and technology of smart cities. *Smart Cities., 1*, x. https://doi.org/10.3390/smartcities1010001

Sichitiu, M. L., & Kihl, M. (2008). Inter-vehicle communication systems: A survey. *IEEE Communications Surveys and Tutorials., 10*, 88. https://doi.org/10.1109/COMST.2008.4564481

Simpson, C., Young, J., Donahue, M., & Rocker, G. (2010). A day at a time: Caregiving on the edge in advanced COPD. *International Journal of Chronic Obstructive Pulmonary Disease, 5*, 141–151. Retrieved from https://www.ncbi.nlm.nih.gov/pmc/articles/PMC2898087/?tool=pmcentrez&report=abstract

Skouby, K. E., Kivimäki, A., Haukipuro, L., Lynggaard, P., & Windekilde, I. (2014). Smart cities and the ageing population. In *32nd Meeting of WWRF, Marrakech, Morocco.* Retrieved from https://pdfs.semanticscholar.org/d7a5/84f867996dbdf78a34697523c537dae218bc.pdf

Smartn. (2018). *Smart Home quality of life package for the visually impaired.* Salisbury: Smartn. Retrieved December 4, 2018, from https://smartn.co.uk/product/smart-home-quality-of-life-package-for-the-visually-impaired/

Suryotrisongko, H., Kusuma, R. C., & Ginardi, R. H. (2017). Four-hospitality: Friendly smart city design for disability. *Procedia Computer Science, 124*, 615. https://doi.org/10.1016/j.procs.2017.12.197

Texeira, C., Toledo, A. S., Amorim, A. d. S., Kofuji, S. T., & Rogério dos Santos, V. (2017). Visual impairment and smart cities: Perspectives on mobility. *JOJ Ophthalmology, 3*, 555613. https://doi.org/10.19080/JOJO.2017.03.555613

Tooran, A. (2018). Crowdsourced smart cities versus corporate smart cities. In *The 4th PlanoCosmo International Conference* (Vol. 158, p. 12046). Bristol: IOP Publishing. https://doi.org/10.1088/1755-1315/158/1/012046

VisionAware. (2019). *Products and devices to help you identify your medications*. Arlington, VA: VisionAware. Retrieved January 4, 2019, from http://www.visionaware.org/info/essential-skills-2/managing-your-medication/products-and-devices-to-help-you-identify-your-medications/235

Wayfindr. (2018). *About Wayfindr*. London: Wayfindr. Retrieved from https://www.wayfindr.net/about-wayfindr

West, D. M. (2016). *Moving forward: Self-driving vehicles in China, Europe, Japan, Korea, and the United States*. Washington, DC: Brookings Institution. https://doi.org/10.1049/cce:20070305

Wilson, P. N., Foreman, N., & Stanton, D. (1997). Virtual reality, disability and rehabilitation. *Disability and Rehabilitation., 19*, 213. https://doi.org/10.3109/09638289709166530

Zhao, Y., Bennett, C. L., Benko, H., Cutrell, E., Holz, C., Morris, M. R., & Sinclair, M. (2018). Enabling people with visual impairments to navigate virtual reality with a haptic and auditory cane simulation. In *Proceedings of the 2018 CHI Conference on Human Factors in Computing Systems - CHI '18*. New York, NY: ACM. https://doi.org/10.1007/BF00652898

Zhou, H., Hou, K.-M., Zuo, D., & Li, J. (2012). Intelligent urban public transportation for accessibility dedicated to people with disabilities. *Sensors, 12*, 10678–10692. https://doi.org/10.3390/s120810678

Chapter 2
A Survey on Accessible Context-Aware Systems

Iyad Abu Doush, Issam Damaj, Mohammed Azmi Al-Betar,
Mohammed A. Awadallah, Ra'ed M. Al-khatib, Alaa Eddin Alchalabi,
and Asaju L. Bolaji

2.1 Introduction

The widespread of small devices with computing and sensing capabilities enables
collecting different information about our daily activities and about ourselves.

I. A. Doush (✉)
Department of Computer Science and Information Systems, American University of Kuwait,
Salmiya, Kuwait

Computer Sciences Department, Yarmouk University Irbid, Jordan
e-mail: idoush@auk.edu.kw

I. Damaj
Electrical and Computer Engineering Department, Rafik Hariri University, Mechref, Lebanon
e-mail: damajiw@rhu.edu.lb

M. A. Al-Betar
Department of Information Technology, Al-Huson University College, Al-Balqa Applied
University, Al-Huson, Irbid, Jordan
e-mail: mohbetar@bau.edu.jo

M. A. Awadallah
Department of Computer Science, Al-Aqsa University, Gaza, Palestine
e-mail: ma.awadallah@alaqsa.edu.ps

R. M. Al-khatib
Department of Computer Science, Yarmouk University, Irbid, Jordan
e-mail: raed.m.alkhatib@yu.edu.jo

A. E. Alchalabi
School of Electrical Engineering and Computer Science, University of Ottawa, Ottawa, ON,
Canada

A. L. Bolaji
Department of Computer Science, University of Ilorin, Ilorin, Nigeria
e-mail: lbasaju@fuwukari.edu.ng

© Springer Nature Switzerland AG 2020
S. Paiva (ed.), *Technological Trends in Improved Mobility of the Visually Impaired*,
EAI/Springer Innovations in Communication and Computing,
https://doi.org/10.1007/978-3-030-16450-8_2

Mark Weiser, the godfather of ubiquitous computing, identified three key aspects of his famous vision: context-aware computing, ambient intelligence, and ambient monitoring of people and things (Weiser 1999). Indeed, context-aware systems (CAS) can recognize the surrounding environment in which they are executed (Alegre, Augusto, & Clark 2016). Abowd and Mynatt (2000) identified the minimum information for understanding context as the five W's: who, what, where, when, and why. Information can be collected using different kinds of devices. The collected information (raw data) has to be classified to recognize the context information (Sanchez, Lanza, Olsen, Bauer, & Girod-Genet 2006; Rana, Hume, Reilly, Jurdak, & Soar 2016). The raw (sensor) data is retrieved directly from the data source, while the context information means processing the raw data by adding metadata.

The way that CAS are developed can be affected by the amount of data to be processed, and the reasoning level that the application is expected to perform. The approaches that can be used to develop CAS are, first, the *no-application* style, in which a system performs all the necessary actions to make the application itself aware without any application boundaries among acquisition, preprocessing, storing, and reasoning. Second, the *implicit* style, which uses libraries, frameworks, and tool-kits to perform context acquisition, preprocessing, storing, and reasoning. Lastly, the *explicit* style, which uses context management infrastructure or middleware solutions in order to have a separation between context management and its application (Ahn & Kim 2006). Context reasoning can be classified into Exact and Inexact as shown in Fig. 2.1 (Zhang, Huang, Lai, Liang, Zou, & Guo 2013).

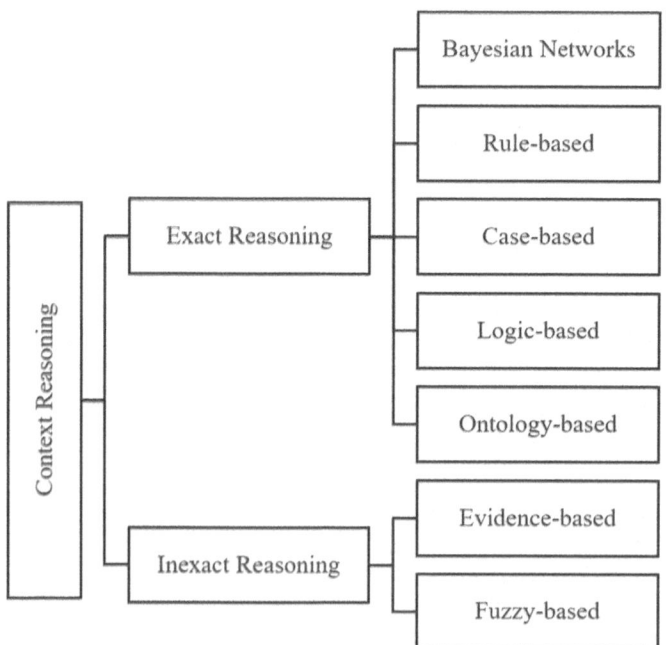

Fig. 2.1 The taxonomy of context reasoning (Zhang et al. 2013)

In CAS, context information is used to take an action according to a predefined event and at a specific timing of interactions. The way the actions are designed can take three forms (Abowd, Dey, Brown, Davies, Smith, & Steggles 1999). Actions can be *presentation*-based, where the context to select is based on what information and services are to be presented. For instance, an action to produce a shopping list through the smart refrigerator while the user is in the supermarket. Furthermore, actions can be designed according to the *execution* of services per the user context. For example, the action to turn on the air-condition at home when the user leaves office. Moreover, action designs can be based on *tagging* sensor data with context information to be processed at a later time. The timing of CAS interactions can be classified into *personalization*, *passive* (automatic), and *active* (Barkhuus & Dey 2003). In personalization, the users set manually the preferences or expectations, such as setting home temperature to a specific level. Passive timing relies on the continuous monitoring of the environment; here, the system provides users with suitable options (e.g., list of discounted products on the mobile when entering a shop). Furthermore, CAS interaction timing is considered *active* when the system monitors the environment continuously and acts autonomously (e.g., smoke detection in a room). The user interaction in CAS has evolved from one-to-one, in which one user interacts with one device, to reach many-to-many in which many users interact with many devices in different environments (See Fig. 2.2) (Grguric, Gil, Huljenic, Car, & Podobnik 2016).

According to the latest report issued by the World Health Organization (WHO) in 2011 (World Health Organization WHO), over a billion people (i.e., 15% of the

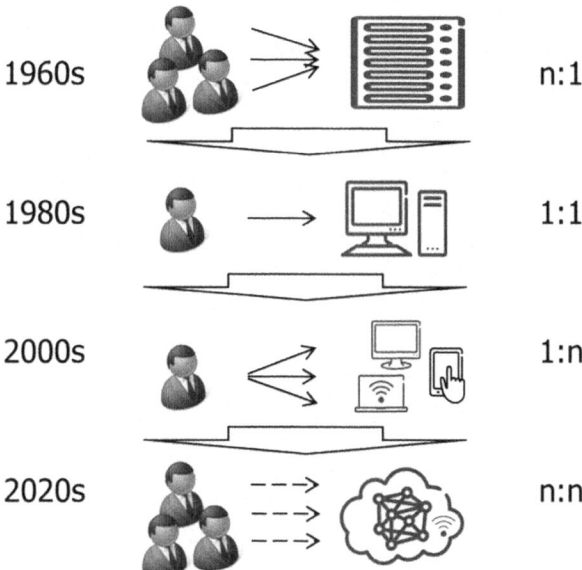

Fig. 2.2 Evolution of the interaction over the years (Grguric et al. 2016)

world population) have a kind of disability. With no doubt, people with disabilities can utilize CAS to accomplish tasks and be supported to overcome different difficulties when dealing with a variety of environments. For example, indoor and outdoor context-aware navigation systems can help blind people to reach different locations to perform daily activities. In the work environments, a CAS can help deaf people by enabling their communication with colleagues. CAS can help people with cognitive disabilities (e.g., people with memory impairment) in completing scheduled tasks, such as taking medicine or attending a doctor appointment (Jarrah & Doush 2014). An *accessible context-aware system* can be defined as a system that collects information about the user or the surrounding environment in order to understand the user situation and predict his/her interest, then personalize the information presentation based on the user needs. Despite the significantly large number of research investigations in the area of CAS, only a small number is available in the market. In this paper, a comprehensive literature survey for the state-of-the-art CAS for people with disabilities is provided. An extensive survey of the literature is conducted by examining relevant articles from the main academic databases, such as *IEEE Xplore, Science-Direct, Springer*, and *ACM* digital library, and using the scholarly literature search engine *Google Scholar*. The keywords used in the search include "context-aware system disability," "context-awareness accessible/accessibility system," "accessible/accessibility context-aware system," "accessible/accessibility mobile context-aware," "personalized ubiquitous system," "accessible location-based system," and "context-aware systems" associated with the keywords "blind," "deaf," "cognitive impairment/disability," and "motor impairment/disability." In addition, the keyword "context-aware survey" is used to look for other aspects studied in other surveys. The retrieved papers are within the period from 2007 to 2017. We find 144 papers and selected from them 46 papers. Relevant papers were shortlisted based on their titles and abstract. The shortlisted papers are then reviewed, for inclusion in the survey, based on the presented methodology, system architecture, and completeness of the evaluation framework.

We classify the investigation according to the type of disability. In addition, the strategies for making CAS accessible and the interaction models are identified. We analyze and evaluate the systems proposed, and suggest patterns for CAS contexts, interactions, and strategies for accessibility. Moreover, we highlight the lessons learned from existing systems and identify possible future directions. To the best of our knowledge, this is the first research effort that provides a thorough survey of CAS for people with disabilities. The presented survey differs from existing ones in specifically classifying CAS according to the type of disability they support. The survey analyzes the systems in terms of system context, context type, system purpose, learning algorithm, context detection technology, type of disability, evaluation methods, task complexity, deployment complexity, and accuracy. In order to present the strategies for making context-aware systems accessible, we link the type of disability to different types of application type, input and output methods, target-users evaluation, and limitations.

The paper is organized as follows. Section 2.2 presents the research objectives and methodology of the survey. Section 2.3 summarizes a large collection of CAS per type of disability. In Sect. 2.4, a thorough discussion is presented to analyze state-of-the-art solutions, strategies for making CAS accessible, interaction models per type of disability, and existing similar surveys of CAS. Section 2.5 identifies opportunities for improvement, concludes the paper, and sets the ground for future works.

2.2 Research Objectives and Methodology

In CAS, the computing system dynamically adapts itself to the user circumstances (Nijdam, Han, Kevelham, & Magnenat-Thalmann 2010). The context information must be accurately and timely gathered, then it needs to be inserted into the system to enable awareness (Lee, Choi, & Elmasri 2009). To that end, CAS can automatically respond to dynamic changes and make adequate interventions. CAS is usually contextualized based on use. Indeed, the use of CAS is highly common in applications that involve people with disabilities. Important characteristics of CAS include their classification according to context, context data acquisition, interaction models, and strategies for making CAS accessible. Different classification schemes, according to context, are available for CAS, which include the following:

- **Active context**: which influences the behavior of the application as it autonomously changes the application behavior according to the sensed information (Morse, Armstrong, & Dey 2000).
- **Passive context**: which prevents updated context or sensor information to be available to the user, but allows the user to decide how to change the application behavior according to the observed context (Morse et al. 2000).
- **Primary context**: which are the contexts that characterize the situation of a particular entity (e.g., location, time, and activity) (Schilit, Adams, & Want 1994).
- **Secondary context**: this type of context can be derived from a primary context by identifying high-level information (e.g., environment and relationships) (Schilit et al. 1994).

CAS design depends on the conditions and the special requirements of a system. CAS requirements include knowing the number of potential users, the type of used sensors and actuators, and the resources in the used computing devices, such as personal computers (PCs), tablets, and smartphones. In CAS design, context data acquisition plays the important role in specifying the architectural model of the system. There are three different approaches on how to acquire context data (Chen 2004), namely the following:

- **Direct sensor access**: this approach is used when devices consist of locally built-in sensors, such as smartphones sensors, GPS, and accelerometer.
- **Middleware infrastructure**: the middleware approach conducts a layered architecture into context-aware systems with the notion of hiding low level sensing details.

– **Context server**: this distributed approach allows remote data resources. It facilitates concurrent access of multiple sensor data which are collected and moved into a context server. Such operation enables the reuse of sensors data.

To enable CAS adoption for a wide-range of users, it is important to provide resources according to the user preferred type of interaction. The classification of people with disabilities can be as follows (Cavender, Trewin, & Hanson 2008):

– **Visual impairment**: represents a kind of losing vision (e.g., low vision, blind, and color blindness).
– **Hearing impairment**: represents losing the ability to hear partially or totally in one or both ears.
– **Motor impairment**: represents the restriction or inability of muscle control or person movement.
– **Cognitive impairment**: represents psychological and mental impairment either from childhood or as a result of aging.

An interaction model can be defined as how the interaction techniques are combined to define the user's perspective of the interaction "look and feel" (Beaudouin-Lafon 2000). Interaction models of CAS are user- and disability-context-specific. Common interaction models comprise signs, sounds, text, images, videos, vibrations, sips and puffs, etc. To make a CAS accessible, disability-specific interaction models should be augmented to the system to provide a user-friendly interface for people with special needs.

A CAS can be used by a person with disability in different situations. For example, help a blind person during indoor navigation or automatically turn on speech-to-sign-language translator in a government office. In order to make CAS accessible for people with disabilities, we must think about providing the information using an accessible interface. In some cases, the CAS can help users by adding extra information about the surrounding environment (e.g., a blind person is stopping near an item in a museum and hear details about that item). In other cases, the CAS needs to remove extra information (e.g., a person with cognitive disability can get help by eliminating non-essential images from a navigated website). CAS can help deaf people in different domains, such as learning environments and working environments. In such environments, the communication between deaf people and non-deaf people using CAS can enable the communication between the two persons in real time.

In this investigation, we survey a large set of systems, approaches, and frameworks, and we aim at achieving the following research objectives: identify context-specific models, identify the interaction models for different kinds of disability, identify strategies for making CAS accessible, and present a thorough discussion on CAS contexts, interactions, and strategies for accessibility. In addition, propose patterns for CAS contexts, interactions, and strategies for accessibility, critique and evaluate best practices in the field, and identify areas for future research.

The adopted survey methodology organizes the literature review per target users. We classify investigations according to disability type. In addition, we analyze the surveyed systems in terms of the context type, technology used, learning algorithm, user interface, and the provided system analysis evaluation. The survey is concluded by a rich discussion, and a set of recommendations and conclusions that well describe the current system patterns and plots future directions.

2.3   Disabilities and Context-Awareness

Disabilities and context-awareness have been the target of many modern applications. Main interests comprise areas, such as blind and visual impairment, deaf, motor disabilities, cognitive disabilities, and more. In the following subsections, important system developments and applications are identified with a focus on context-specific models, interaction models for different kinds of disability, and the strategies for making CAS accessible. The following subsections focus on presenting the proposed systems. More specifically, critical appraisals are thoroughly presented in Sect. 2.4.

2.3.1   Blind and Visually Impaired

Doush, Alshattnawi, Al-Tamimi, Alhasan, and Hamasha (2017) propose an approach to help blind people to complete indoor navigation using a smartphone. The proposed system uses different communication technologies, such as Wi-Fi, Bluetooth, and radio-frequency identification. The system allows for detecting an object located in a shelf with a minimum distance of 10 cm between objects. The mobile phone provides users with voice instructions of the path with the least number of hazards.

Mirri, Prandi, Salomoni, Callegati, and Campi (2014) propose a novel geospatial mapping service in order to help the blind people by providing personal paths. The proposed system provides the personal paths based on collecting the related data from users and bus companies. On the user side, the system collects data by sensing and using crowdsourcing data provided by the system users in order to map barriers and facilities they face in the real environment. On the bus companies side, the system considers the open data provided by buses to know the actual facilities, arrival times, and stop times. For the evaluation purposes, the authors tested the proposed system on real data extracted from Bologna and Italy with different user profiles. The investigated user profiles include motor impairment, elderly, blind, and visually impaired users. The proposed system provides a path that is tailored according to the user's needs and preferences using real-time data. The proposed system achieves satisfactory results as compared with mainstream geospatial mapping services. The authors identify future directions to enhance the system including collecting user behavior, applying machine learning techniques, and using the dynamic method to update the results automatically according to the user profile.

Santoro, Paterno, Ricci, and Leporini (2007) propose a preliminary-interaction mobile system for a museum guide with diverse accessibility options. The system supports the needs and preferences of different users with visual impairment. The aim of the proposed system is providing effective and natural interactions with the environment through the combination of multiple inputs, such as gesture, location, images, and voice. Moreover, the proposed system provides different levels of accessibility. The developed system has different versions that include basic navigation, navigation with audio feedback, navigation using tilt, and navigation with audio and tilt.

Ivanov (2012) presents an indoor navigation system for blind people. The system has several advantages including the use of 4-dimensional modeling of buildings. The supported multi-dimensional modeling comprises a 3-dimensional building model, objects geometry, and the status of all sensors. Sensors are distributed building-wide to monitor doors status, windows status, fire, etc. in real time. The purpose of the system is to improve the navigation process based on the position, shape, and the characteristics of all objects. Moreover, the system uses a planning algorithm to get the optimal route for the blind user. Furthermore, the system supports automatic re-routing in the case of emergency, such as fire. In addition, the proposed system uses an algorithm to detour obstacles. Moreover, the system can be used to search for people or objects within the building.

Ghorbel, Kadouche, and Mokhtari (2007) present a new strategy for enhancing the accessibility of the blind people in their living environments. The presented strategy includes two defined actors. Firstly, a user actor that can access the user profile which includes the user needs and preferences. The second actor can diversify existing services and their contents, personalize the system according to the user profile, and discover the context in the visited environment. The system is initially deployed in Europe (Fig. 2.3).

Chaudary and Pulli (2014) propose a smart outdoor navigation system for the blind and visually impaired people. A visually impaired person can independently walk around in urban sidewalks using an augmented guidance cane. The prototype of the proposed system is designed using four components. The system components are an augmented guidance cane, a magnet points trail, a metallic trail, and a pulsing magnet apparatus. A user of the system uses a white cane with a small reader. In the sidewalks, the magnet points and metallic trails are installed. Accordingly, the user can walk around independently by sensing the magnet points using the smart cane. To enable detecting specific locations, the pulsing magnet apparatus is installed on the verge at all points of interests, such as post office, shopping mall, bar, and coffee shops. When a user reaches any point of interest, a serialized vibration is emitted from the pulsing magnet apparatus that, in turn, vibrates the cane and displays the name as serialized Braille code.

Pereira, Nunes, Vieira, Costa, Fernandes, and Barroso (2015) introduce blind guide, an intelligent system based on ultrasound sensors, which can be used to help blind users for obstacles detection. This system is used to guide people who are blind in indoor or outdoor navigation. Blind people face a variety of obstacles, which are considered as active threats. The head level obstacles like upper balconies are

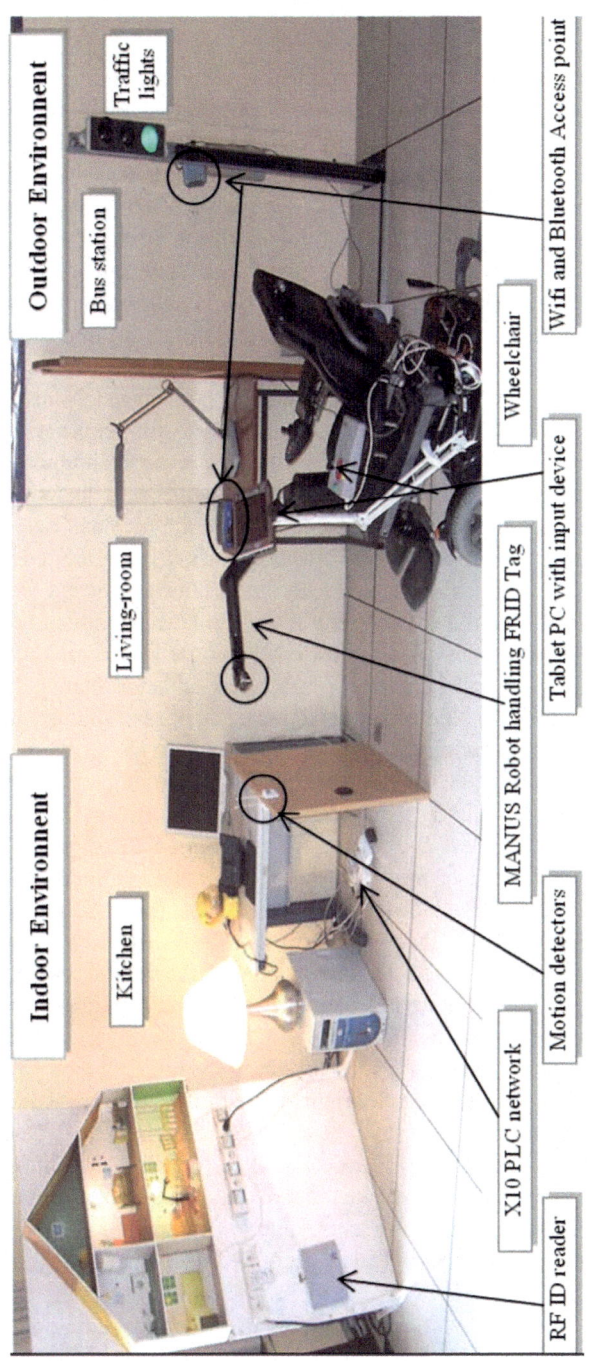

Fig. 2.3 Laboratory condition and experimentation demonstrator (Ghorbel et al. 2007)

among the most dangerous kinds of obstacles; such obstacles cannot be detected using white canes or by a guide dog. The blind-guide system is proposed to detect all kinds of obstacles. The system consists of a jacket with sensors and two knee strips with sensors.

Zhan, Faux, and Ramos (2015) propose a novel pervasive system called "smart glasses," which recognizes daily human activities from a wearable device. The system uses contextual information to classify subjects' daily livings using vision and head motion data. The system can be used in both indoor and outdoor environments. The system is built using a framework consisting of an accelerometer, head camera, and safety goggles. The purpose of the system is to provide caregivers with the ability to track daily activities of a specific person, such as a disabled or an elderly person. In addition, the system can be programmed for assistance purposes, such as scheduling medicine reminders. The system was evaluated on two different types of users, elderly and disabled. The accuracies achieved by the system are acceptable with values of 90.04% for elders and 77.07% for people with disability.

Doush, Alshattnawi, and Barhoush (2015) propose a mobile application to assist blind users in performing location-based tasks that need to be completed in a predefined order. The proposed application localizes the user and detects the start point and the end point of each location-based task using GPS coordinates. It helps the user by providing information according to his/her current location using vibration and speech. The paper presents a set of guidelines that can be used when building an accessible mobile user interface for people who are blind to perform ordered tasks. The system is evaluated on three blind-folded sighted users and on 11 blind persons. The results point out on the importance of minimizing the number of instructions given during the navigation. The version with the minimum number of instructions results in a better navigation accuracy when compared to the standard version.

Aly (2014) introduces MND_{WSN}, a monitoring and navigation system to help people who are blind, deaf, or motor disabled. They can use their smartphones to navigate around and move from the start point to the end point without any external help. This system is based on installing many wireless sensor networks (WSN) as sensed nodes that are fixed in each destination point at the floor. The communication between the nodes is performed via Bluetooth and Zigbee modules. The system is located on the main server on the ground floor of a building. Here, the server follows up the movement of a disabled person and observes any deviation in navigation. The system is evaluated on a three-floor university building which is equipped with WSN-nodes and cameras. The system can alert the disabled participant by verbal alert only for blind, picture aid only for deaf, and picture with verbal for wheelchair users. Ten people with disabilities evaluated the proposed system for planning seven different trips with a total number of trips equal to 70 trips. The success rate using the proposed system equals 90% and it becomes only 55.7% without using the proposed system.

2.3.2 Motor Disabled

Rantanen, Vanhala, Tuisku, Niemenlehto, Verho, Surakka, Juhola, and Lekkala (2011) introduce a lightweight, wearable, and wireless gaze tracker with integrated selection command source for human–computer interaction. The main purpose of the system is to control a computer with mobility, for example, using a mouse or a keyboard, and without the use of hands. The prototype mainly targets disabled people with limited body control. The presented prototype allows the user to use head motions and facial gestures to communicate and control their computers without the need for conventional interaction devices. The wireless gaze tracking is accomplished by using a video-based method.

Tavares, Barbosa, Cardoso, Costa, Yamin, and Real (2016) present Hefestos as an intelligent system that enables pervasive accessibility. The system employs user profiles (Wagner, Barbosa, & Barbosa 2014), context-awareness (Mehra 2012), and trails management (Silva, Rosa, Barbosa, Barbosa, & Palazzo 2009) to help people with disabilities and the elderly in completing their daily activities. The system can be integrated with different technologies by using a personal assistant agent which can support different kinds of disabilities. The Hefestos context is part of the physical environment in which the user is located, such as a building, a room, or a region within the city. In addition, the system can be used to manage static resources which are in fixed locations, such as parking areas. The system can also be used for dynamic resources that can be in different locations, such as a public accessible bus moving in the city. Furthermore, the system can be used in both indoor and outdoor environments. The main building blocks of the system include web services (user profiles, special needs, contexts, and trails), a multi-agent system (accessibility assistant, communication assistant, and personal assistant) (Padgham & Winikoff 2004), an administrative site, and an ontology. The ontology is used to standardize the terms used in the proposed system and to make it easier to communicate between multiple agents. The collected information is used to provide users with the resources needed to improve their accessibility. The proposed ontology is then applied on a wheelchair and controlled through a mobile phone. Ten users evaluated the system in terms of technology acceptance; 96% agreed that it is easy to use and 98% agreed on its usefulness.

Mortazavi, Pourhomayoun, Ghasemzadeh, Jafari, Roberts, and Sarrafzadeh (2015) introduce a pilot application, which uses a wearable accelerometer to calculate the metabolic equivalent of task (MET) of exergaming movements using active video games. The target end-users for the system are identified as people suffering from chronic conditions. The accelerometer helps to obtain data that is used in calculating the energy expenditure and MET in order to record the user activity levels. The system focuses mainly on two types of contextual information, namely the activity type and the sensor location. The contextual information is vital for improving the quality of data and reasoning about each activity level. The system requires an indoor physical environment in which the user places a series of accelerometers on their hip, ankle, and feet. The combined information from the aforementioned sensors is processed to calculate the energy expenditure and the corresponding MET for each activity. Indeed, the proposed system presents an approach for improving the quality of information in a wireless health monitoring system by integrating contextual information within the data processing flow.

Zhu and Sheng (2011) present a smart assisted living (SAIL) system. SAIL is an intelligent system that provides human–robot interactions for elderly and disabled people. The system gathers meaningful context information of daily activity recognition and provides it to remote healthcare professional. In addition, this investigation focuses on solving the two most common problems with human–robot interactions including hand gesture and daily activity recognition. The SAIL context is a part of the physical environment in which the user is located, such as a building or a room. The framework of the system consists of a body sensor network, a companion robot, a PDA, and a remote health provider. The body sensor network collects user's contextual information, such as motion detection and vital signs. The collected data then gets transmitted to the companion robot via a wireless connection using the Zigbee protocol. At this point, the data is processed on the robot to detect human intentions and health conditions. A smartphone is used as an access point for consulting the healthcare professional. The hand gesture recognition uses lightweight and resource-aware algorithms for distinguishing between different gestures. Finally, the motion data from different peripherals are combined to detect 13 different activities including sitting, standing, and lying down.

Margetis, Antona, Ntoa, and Stephanidis (2012) elaborate the need that emerges from enabling accessible user interaction in modern ambient intelligence (AmI) environments. The investigation includes the identification of the main obstacles which limits the provision of alternate and personalized accessibility solutions in AmI environments. The presented work focuses on people with disabilities and elders. The investigation includes the presentation of ontology-based user and interaction modeling, ready-to-use accessibility solutions, accessible applications— all in the context of AmI environments.

Kleinberger, Becker, Ras, Holzinger, and Muller (2007) develop an assisted living laboratory which is used to train people with motor disability to handle modern interfaces. The authors identify the main challenges of future interfaces in assisted living and the adequate technological environment for testing. Several challenges are identified including system adaptivity and heterogeneity, and the ethical, social, medical, and technological constraints due to the special needs of people with motor disability.

Abbate, Avvenuti, Bonatesta, Cola, Corsini, and Vecchio (2012) introduce a fall detection system which uses smartphones or external sensors for monitoring the movements of the patients. The system uses classification techniques in order to avoid false alarms and to provide stable and accurate readings. The target user of the system is identified as people with motor disability or elderly who frequently turn out to be alone for an extended period of time. The collected information from the system can be used to provide an efficient and remote caregiving service for the people with motor disability or elderly. Ten users evaluated the system in terms of importance, usability, and technology acceptance. The general evaluation of the volunteers is positive.

Lustrek, Gjoreski, Vega, Kozina, Cvetkovic, Mirchevska, and Gams (2015) present a fall detection system for people with motor disability or elders using location sensors and accelerometers. The system introduces 1–4 wearable tags that can be detected using location sensors. The location sensors monitor user activities and location in a premise. The readings from location sensors are augmented with the information from an accelerometer to accurately detect falls. The confidence system requires either a single location-based tag, which is mandatory on the chest, or three additional tags on the chest, waist, and ankles. It is of high importance that the system differentiates between safe falls such as lying on the bed from possible life-threatening falls by adding the context data into the equation. The difference between the accuracy when using a single tag and three additional tags is 2.2% in favor of the 4-tag system. Since the difference in accuracy is almost minimal between the two system arrangements, the use of a single location-based tag is recommended as it is more comfortable to the user.

Aloulou, Mokhtari, Tiberghien, Biswas, and Yap (2014) propose a system that focuses mainly on people with motor disability with chronic decline. The provided solution aims at minimizing the level of stress and burden suffered by the caregivers as the disease evolves. The framework of the system is developed on the bases of sensory information and first-order logic rules. The system performs an environment discovery to detect and connect with new sensors and interaction devices deployed in the environment. The discovery and connection of the model are performed using Zigbee as the wireless peripheral. The information from these entities is used for monitoring the behavior of the patient with respect to the context. Contextual information allows the framework to select the best possible assisting system for the patient and the most suitable device for a given situation. Users are given notification and alerts and are encouraged to solve their problems on their own. However, if the user does not respond after a specific given time, the caregivers are notified about the situation.

Bozgeyikli, Bozgeyikli, Clevenger, Raij, Alqasemi, Sundarrao, and Dubey (2015) introduce a system that uses virtual reality (VR) for vocational rehabilitation (VR4VR) aimed at enabling job coaches to use virtual reality environments to safely train individuals with disabilities on job skills. VR enables safe immersion of potential employees in a different range of scenarios they may encounter before they face them in real life. The system is designed to support three types of disabilities: autism spectrum disorder (ASD), traumatic brain injury (TBI), and severe mobility impairment (SMI), such as stroke or spinal cord injury patients. While increasing the complexity of the tasks, reinforcement is also used to make the user repeat the already gained knowledge. A reward system to encourage the engagement with the system is also designed. For each environment, there are various tasks that are designed specifically considering the needs of the three disability groups. The training tasks include warehouse tasks, hotel room tasks, and grocery store tasks. While the user is performing these tasks, interactive prompts and feedback are given via visual and auditory aids to assist and reinforce learning.

2.3.3   Cognitive Disabled

Maxhuni, Muñoz-Meléndez, Osmani, Perez, Mayora, and Morales (2016) present a smart system for detecting bipolar disorder episodes. The system uses voice and motor activity for classifying the type of episode suffered by the patient. The proposed system assists healthcare professionals and patients in real-time detection of episodes. The paper also discusses the inefficiencies found in the current literature, which requires the user to fill a questionnaire on their current suffering state.

Lin, Zhang, Connelly, Ni, Yu, and Zhou (2015) present an intelligent system that detects trajectory disorientation. The system uses real-world GPS datasets to assist people suffering from dementia in navigational tasks. The collected GPS dataset helps in graphically visualizing the trajectory model, which allows the computational methods to successfully classify the disorientations. The system can be useful in providing alerts and reminders to cognitively impaired patients with memory loss when they suffer from being lost in an unfamiliar environment. The system is evaluated using ten individuals and achieved an accuracy of 95% with 3% false rate.

Okoshi, Nozaki, Nakazawa, Tokuda, Ramos, and Dey (2016) propose Attelia, a middleware that detects breakpoints of users mobile interactions to deliver notifications accordingly. The system detects active user times based on phone data, no external sensors are required. The proposed system allows users to have an effective and adaptive notification cycle. The Attelias context is part of the usual computing environment of users, such as social media, email, or any notification enabled application. The system monitors user's smartphone activities and classifies breakpoints. Notifications to the user are given at the identified breakpoints. The system consists of a physical device that receives the notifications, a middleware application for monitoring user activities, and a classifier that monitors breakpoints of applications. The system is optimized to reduce the number of notifications received by the user at an unwanted time.

Saunier and Balbo (2009) propose an environment operational model that can be used to enable the regulated interactions in the issue of multi-party communications and context-awareness known as environment as active support of interaction (EASI). It enables each agent to actively modify the environment based on its interaction needs. The proposed EASI solution focuses to avoid the massive over-loading that has been shown in the existing state-of-the-art mobile alerting system (MAS) models, like the overhearing which is any possible heard communications from unpredicted agents. The proposed EASI model adapts three filters (direct, hierarchy, and indirect) with matching algorithm to regulate a complex interaction in multi-party communications. The authors show that their model provides a suitable framework for the regulation of MAS interactions, as well as proposing an algorithm and assess with an example stemming from the ambient intelligence domain. The model performance is evaluated on a bus network system and compared with the classic broadcast.

Ramos, Oliveira, Satoh, Neves, and Novais (2018) propose an orientation system with augmented reality interface using a mobile phone to help people with cognitive disabilities. The system can notify the user to change direction before making a mistake. It also helps caregivers to remotely track the user location.

2.3.4   Hearing Disabled

Hasan, Chipara, Wu, and Aksan (2014) evaluate hearing aids with different auditory contexts. The auditory contexts are based on the listening activity, room size, and the speakers' location. The AudioSense (Hasan, Lai, Chipara, & Wu 2013) audio evaluation tool is used to investigate the performance of different hearing aids. The users are asked to evaluate different aspects of what they listened to.

Chaudary & Pulli (2014) introduce smart outdoor navigation system for the deaf–blind. The system uses guidance cane with a small reader for magnet points. The system requires the installation of metallic trails, then the user can sense the magnet points using the smart cane.

Aly (2014) introduces a monitoring and navigation system to help people who are blind, deaf, or motor disabled. The system can alert the disabled participant by verbal alert only for blind, picture aid only for deaf, and picture with verbal for wheelchair users.

Tavares et al. (2016) propose user profiles and trails management to help people with disabilities and the elderly in completing their daily activities. The system can be used in both indoor and outdoor environments. The system uses an ontology to make it easier to communicate between multiple agents. The collected information is used to provide users with the resources needed to improve their accessibility. The proposed ontology can be used to identify the interfaces needed for the deaf.

Kbar, Abidi, Hammad Mian, Al-Daraiseh, and Mansoor (2016) developed an interface for searching and communicating for a person with disability in a university. They used event-behavior algorithm to predict the user action pattern. The used technologies are RFID and Wi-Fi to track users and identify their movement patterns. The user can utilize the system to search the university campus, communicate using SMS, email, chatting, notification, and event booking. The user profile is used to present the user with correct modalities and suitable user interface. The system is proposed to be used by all kinds of disabilities.

2.4   Discussion

2.4.1   Analysis of the State-of-the-Art Solutions

Many solutions are proposed in the literature to provide accessible CAS. The main challenges to CAS include providing the right information to the right person, at the right time, and in the right place and way (Fischer 2012). In other words, the challenges comprise providing accurate information, according to a specific disability type, in a timely fashion, per a specific location, and in a safe way. Effective CAS aim at avoiding overloading users with information during the system interactions.

In the analysis of the state-of-the-art solutions, the indicators and discussion are based on the context, context type, system purpose, learning algorithm, context detection technology, type of disability, evaluation methods, task complexity, deployment complexity, and accuracy. We are comparing to look for similarities and differences, common patterns, topic span, and topic concentrations. In Table 2.1, the analysis of 16 different CAS is presented, and in Table 2.2 we investigate seven CAS. Although the survey presented in this paper includes a variety of references, a small subset provides concrete information on all the identified analysis indicators as presented in the tables.

The analysis reflects that previous research works provide solutions mainly for blind (Margetis et al. 2012; Pereira et al. 2015; Doush et al. 2017; Zhan et al. 2015) and motor disabled (Tavares et al. 2016; Abbate et al. 2012; Lustrek et al. 2015). However, only a few solutions are proposed for other types of disabilities including deaf people (Chaudary & Pulli 2014; Kbar et al. 2016; Tavares et al. 2016; Aly 2014), autism spectrum disorder and severe mobility impairment (Bozgeyikli et al. 2015), cognitive-disabled (Lin et al. 2015), chronic neuro-cognitive disorders (Aloulou et al. 2014), disabled people with limited body control (Rantanen et al. 2011), bipolar disorder (Maxhuni et al. 2016), and people with chronic conditions (e.g., obesity and asthma) (Mortazavi et al. 2015). Only three solutions are claimed to be universally accessible which covers the major three types of disabilities, namely blind, deaf, and motor disabled (Aly 2014; Zhu & Sheng 2011; Kbar et al. 2016).

In order to capture the context of the user, several learning algorithms and techniques are proposed in the literature. In Tavares et al. (2016), an ontology is used to standardize the terms used. Many solutions rely on classifying user's context data (Hinze & Buchanan 2005; Margetis et al. 2012; Zhan et al. 2015; Lin et al. 2015; Abbate et al. 2012; Aloulou et al. 2014; Mortazavi et al. 2015). Other investigations propose the use of navigation systems which utilizes routing algorithms to help users during navigation (Aly 2014; Doush et al. 2017). Moreover, other investigations use machine learning techniques to classify the user situation as in Lustrek et al. (2015), or to classify the user gesture (Zhu & Sheng 2011).

Although users do not prefer to hold or use extra equipment, as this may limit their movement, using special hardware devices is sometimes essential. Many state-of-the-art solutions need special hardware to be used by the user, such as magic wand (Margetis et al. 2012), smart cane (Chaudary & Pulli 2014), ultrasound sensors at the user body (Pereira et al. 2015), head mounted display (Bozgeyikli et al. 2015), head motion sensor and camera (Zhan et al. 2015), wearable motion sensor (Mortazavi et al. 2015), body sensor network (Zhu & Sheng 2011), camera for facial movement detection (Rantanen et al. 2011), and shelf reader device (Doush et al.

Table 2.1 CAS general features

System	Context	Type	Purpose	Learning algorithm	Detection tech.	Disability
Hefestos (Tavares et al. 2016)	I; O	Pervasive accessible resources (e.g., wheelchair ramps)	Assist in daily activities	User profiles; trails management; ontology; multi-agent	Mobile phone; 3G; Wi-Fi; Bluetooth	Motor disabled; other
AmI (Margetis et al. 2012)	I; O	Accessible resources	Use *magic wand*; control electric-devices	User monitoring to manage and analyze requirements	*Magic wand*; PC; mobile	Blind; visually-impaired
Smart sys. (Chaudary & Pulli 2014)	O; urban	POIs identification; urban	Independent movement for a blind person	Navigation based on sensing	Smart cane; magnet points; trails	Blind and deaf; blind
MND$_{WSN}$ (Aly 2014)	I	Accessible resources	Guidance; navigation; movement and deviation monitoring	Optimal routing; Dijkstras shortest path; safe routing	Mobile phone; 3G/Wi-Fi, Zigbee; Bluetooth	Blind; deaf; motor disabled
Blind guide (Pereira et al. 2015)	I; O	Obstacles detection	Autonomous navigation	Simple data acquisition	Ultrasound sensors on shoulders and knees	Blind
VR4VR (Bozgeyikli et al. 2015)	I	Assisted training	Assist trainer; job training	Simple data acquisition	Virtual reality; gamification; head-mounted display; gesture control	Autism; brain injury; mobility impairment
Smart glasses (Zhan et al. 2015)	I; O	Use contextual information to classify daily activities	Track daily activities	Context information; image recognition, analysis, and classification	Mobile phone; camera; 3G; Wi-Fi; accelerometer; Bluetooth; safety goggles	Blind
Disorientation (Lin et al. 2015)	I; O	GPS navigation	Trajectory and disorientation detection	Contextual information; graphical model generation; irregularities detection in trajectories	Mobile phone; 3G; Wi-Fi; Bluetooth	Cognitively-impaired

(continued)

Table 2.1 (continued)

System	Context	Type	Purpose	Learning algorithm	Detection tech.	Disability
Fall (Abbate et al. 2012)	I; O	Motion tracking; location identification	Fall detection	Identify irregular motion to detect falls	Mobile phone; accelerometer; 3G; Wi-Fi; Bluetooth	Motor disabled
Confidence (Lustrek et al. 2015)	I	Fall detection	Identify irregular motion to detect falls	Signal pattern recognition; users activity recognition; support vector machine (SVM); random forest algorithm	Location sensors; accelerometer; mobile phone	Motor disabled
Assistive living (Aloulou et al. 2014)	I	User activity tracker	Caregiver assistive services	Simple data acquisition	Mobile phone; 3G; Wi-Fi; Zigbee	Chronic neuro-cognitive disorders
Exergaming (Mortazavi et al. 2015)	I	Energy consumption measurement in physical activities	Activity monitoring	Simple data acquisition	Exergaming (wearable motion sensor); accelerometer; 3G; Wi-Fi	Obesity; hypertension; diabetes; hyperlipidemia; heart failure; asthma; depression
SAIL (Zhu & Sheng 2011)	I	Daily activity recognition	Monitoring user activities	Neural network and hidden Markov model to classify gesture.	Mobile phone; 3G; Wi-Fi; Bluetooth; body sensor network	Motor disabled; others
Eye gaze (Rantanen et al. 2011)	I	Facial movements and gestures	Computer control	Simple data acquisition	Video transmitter; camera; data communication	Motor disabled
Bipolar (Maxhuni et al. 2016)	I; O	Speech and movement monitoring during conversation	Classify the mood of the user	Simple data acquisition	Mobile phone; accelerometer; microphone; GPS; magnetometer	Bipolar disorder
ISAB (Doush et al. 2017)	I	Navigate to locate an item on a shelf	Navigate the user to reach an item in a shelf	Modified Dijkstra algorithm	Wi-Fi; mobile phone; RFID reader and tags; Bluetooth	Blind

Note that I and O means I(ndoor) and O(utdoor)

Table 2.2 Context detection evaluation

System	Evaluation method	Task complexity	Deployment complexity	Accuracy
Hefestos (Tavares et al. 2016)	Usefulness; ease-of-use	Suggestion of accessible resources based on a wheelchair location	A mobile application that communicate with a server to provide accessible resources	NA
MND$_{WSN}$ (Aly 2014)	Usefulness; ease-of-use	Correct navigation deviation	A mobile application that communicate with a server for autonomous navigation	90%
Smart glasses (Zhan et al. 2015)	Usefulness; ease-of-use	Provides contextual information using body worn sensors and cameras	A mobile application that classifies sensor information to recognize activities	77.4%
Disorientation (Lin et al. 2015)	Usefulness; ease-of-use	Alerts in case irregularities are detected in users trajectory	A mobile application that retrieves location, produce a graphical model, and compute irregularities	95%
Fall (Abbate et al. 2012)	Usefulness; ease-of-use	Fall alert using an accelerometer	A mobile application that detect falls	90%
Confidence (Lustrek et al. 2015)	All fall scenarios have been covered in lab tests, while the real life tests resulted in few false fall detection alarms	Trip; fall; slow fall; sitting fall; no-fall; lay; quick sit	Radio tag and 3 accelerometer are worn by the user to identify if s/he falls	80–100%
ISAB (Doush et al. 2017)	Simple testing of the indoor features	Locating user; help the user to find an item in a shelf	A mobile phone that utilizes installed localization technologies (i.e., RFID tags, RFID reader, Bluetooth module, and Wi-Fi routers) to help the user find an item in a shelf	Reach an object in a shelf within 10 cm

2017). Other solutions do not require the user to have a special hardware as it relies on setting up the environment and using only the mobile phone to assist the user (Aly 2014; Tavares et al. 2016; Lin et al. 2015; Abbate et al. 2012; Lustrek et al. 2015; Maxhuni et al. 2016).

Various solutions are proposed in the literature to support CAS applications. User profiling is used to provide the user with suitable interaction, resources, and identified special interests. For example, user profiles can help during navigation to reach accessible resources (Tavares et al. 2016; Margetis et al. 2012; Aly 2014), tourism sights (Hinze & Buchanan 2005), or points of interest (POI) in a city (Chaudary & Pulli 2014). Furthermore, other systems are proposed to guide blind users through, and warning them about, obstacles (Pereira et al. 2015). The use of virtual reality gamification can help in training different users with disabilities to acquire the skills needed for different jobs or it can help the rehabilitation of the patient. Such systems rely on using the gestures and the user movement to complete the training task (as in Bozgeyikli et al. 2015) or it can be used to restore the health of the user. Moreover, object recognition is used by different systems to notify users about the surrounding environment. The graphical information from the environment is used to classify and recognize objects to help blind users (as in Zhan et al. 2015). In addition, many systems are proposed to help blind or visually impaired users during navigation. Several systems are used to detect user disorientation (as in Lin et al. 2015), while others provide users with step-by-step directions to reach into a specific object located in a shelf (Doush et al. 2017). Several CAS are proposed to help the motor disabled. Other systems are proposed to help in providing alarms for motor disabled caregivers (e.g., if the person fall down Abbate et al. 2012; Lustrek et al. 2015). Other systems can track user activities and report them to the caregiver (Aloulou et al. 2014; Mortazavi et al. 2015; Zhu & Sheng 2011). The eye gazing control systems can be used by people with limited body control. Such systems can help in identifying user intention using a predefined pattern of eye movements (Rantanen et al. 2011).

In most cases, the evaluations of CAS are scenario based, where users test the different functionalities of a system. The users are asked to perform a sequence of tasks to understand usability and/or accessibility of the CAS (Manzoor, Truong, & Dustdar 2008). This method is more effective than inspecting each system component separately as the context of the usage is taken into consideration (Doush, Bany-Mohammed, Ali, & Al-Betar 2013b).

2.4.2 Strategies for Making Context-Aware Systems Accessible

In order to present the strategies for making CAS accessible, we link the type of disability to different types of Application, input and output methods, target-users evaluation, and limitations. We are comparing to look for similarities and differences, common patterns, system evaluation depth and reliability, and challenges. In Table 2.3, the strategies for making CAS accessible of fourteen different systems

Table 2.3 CAS accessibility features

System	Disability	App. type	Output	Input	Evaluation	Limitations
Hefestos (Tavares et al. 2016)	Motor disabled, other	Mobile app.	Mobile phone screen	Mobile phone screen	10 users	Limited to tests on wheelchair, specific in disability type, reduced context-awareness
AmI (Margetis et al. 2012)	Blind, visually impaired, elderly	Magic wand	Voice	Magic wand	One blind teacher	Requires holding special hardware, tests limited to one user
Smart system (Chaudary & Pulli 2014)	Blind and deaf, blind	N/A	Cane vibration	Smart cane	N/A	Requires holding special hardware
MND$_{WSN}$ (Aly 2014)	Blind, deaf, motor disabled	Mobile app.	Mobile phone screen	Mobile phone with touch screen	10 users, 7 trips for each user, 70 trips in total	Complex setup, complex data collection, limited to indoor use6
Blind guide (Pereira et al. 2015)	Blind	N/A	Buzzer sound	Ultrasound sensor	Two blind users	Unable to detect head-level obstacles due to sensor positioning, requires holding special hardware, still in design stages
Smart glasses (Zhan et al. 2015)	Blind and deaf, blind	Mobile app.	Mobile phone screen	Accelerometer and camera	5 elderly, 30 disabled patients	Phone is placed over eyeglasses which limits use duration due to heavy weight
Disorientation (Lin et al. 2015)	Cognitively impaired	Mobile app.	Mobile phone screen	GPS coordinates using a mobile phone	10 users	No testing in application, tests are limited to GPS traces and healthy adults
Fall (Abbate et al. 2012)	Motor disabled	Mobile app.	Mobile phone screen	Mobile phone screen; accelerometer	10 users aged above 65	Limited testing

Table 2.3 (continued)

System	Disability	App. type	Output	Input	Evaluation	Limitations
Confidence (Lustrek et al. 2015)	Motor disabled	Mobile app.	Fall reports	Location sensor, accelerometer	Two tests: 12 user and 10 users	Ergonomics and appearance
Exergaming (Mortazavi et al. 2015)	Obesity, hypertension, diabetes, hyperlipidemia, heart failure, asthma, depression	Video game	Monitor or TV	Accelerometer	6 healthy male subjects	Testing is limited to the same age group, different activity levels require additional user inputs.
SAIL (Zhu & Sheng 2011)	Motor disabled, others	Personal digital assistant	Mobile phone screen, web-interface	Mobile phone screen	Evaluated by the authors	No testing in application
Eye gaze (Rantanen et al. 2011)	Motor disabled	N/A	Monitor	Camera head mount	10 healthy users	Limited testing to healthy users, significant errors
Bipolar (Maxhuni et al. 2016)	Bipolar disorder	Mobile app.	Mobile phone screen	Accelerometer, microphone	5 users	Testing is limited to a controlled environment
ISAB (Doush et al. 2017)	Blind	Mobile app.	Mobile phone screen, voice	Mobile phone screen	20 blind users	Connection losses among system components, requires holding special hardware, inaccuracies in obstacle avoidance

are summarized. In all systems, outputs depend on the type of disability of the user. For visually impaired or blind; the output can be voice (Margetis et al. 2012; Aly 2014), cane vibrations (Chaudary & Pulli 2014), and buzzer-sound alerts for obstacles (Pereira et al. 2015). Furthermore, for elderly or cognitive-impaired users, voice alerts are used for disorientation from the saved traces (Lin et al. 2015), and voice directions and vibrations on a mobile phone (Doush et al. 2017). Moreover, pictures are used for deaf users (Aly 2014). Indeed, several state-of-the-art solutions provide CAS based on using mobile applications (Tavares et al. 2016; Aly 2014; Zhan et al. 2015; Lin et al. 2015; Abbate et al. 2012; Lustrek et al. 2015; Maxhuni et al. 2016; Doush et al. 2017).

Evaluating the proposed system through their targeted users is essential to prove its effectiveness and efficiency in the application. In the surveyed literature, a small number of systems are found to evaluate effectiveness or efficiency through ten or more target users (Tavares et al. 2016; Aly 2014; Lustrek et al. 2015; Doush et al. 2017). In additions, several investigations are evaluated on a very small number of target users (e.g., one or two users (Margetis et al. 2012; Pereira et al. 2015; Zhu & Sheng 2011), five users (Maxhuni et al. 2016), or six users (Mortazavi et al. 2015)). Moreover, other investigations do not present any target-user evaluations (Chaudary & Pulli 2014). In evaluations, the small numbers of target users limit the reliability of the presented measures of system effectiveness including usability, reliability, accuracy, accessibility, to name but a few. Hefestos (Tavares et al. 2016) is the only system that is evaluated in terms of ease-of-use and usefulness. The evaluation is based on the technology acceptance model (TAM) (Marangunić & Granić 2015). The results show that the ease-of-use is 96% and the usefulness is 98%.

Several CAS relies on using sensors as inputs. For example, sensors can be embedded on smart canes as in Chaudary and Pulli (2014), ultrasound sensors can be used to detect obstacles as in Pereira et al. (2015), and location sensors and accelerometers are adopted for fall detection in Lustrek et al. (2015). In addition, smart phone cameras and accelerometers are used as inputs in Zhan et al. (2015), accelerometers only in Mortazavi et al. (2015), and data from accelerometer and microphones in Maxhuni et al. (2016). Other systems use GPS coordinates of user traces (Lin et al. 2015), a head mount with camera (Rantanen et al. 2011), and Wi-Fi signal strength to locate a user (Doush et al. 2017).

2.4.3 *Interaction Models of Different Types of Disability*

Interaction models of CAS are strongly related to the user needs including the type of disability. The modality provided to the user, through the CAS, identifies the needed interaction channels. Each type of disability requires different kind of user modalities. For example, people with visual impairment can benefit from using speech directions, alert sounds, sonification sounds, and vibration to communicate with the user (Doush & Pontelli 2013). Moreover, communication with people with hearing impairment can be done through converting spoken words into sign

Table 2.4 Interaction modalities for different types of disabilities

Communication direction	Interaction modality	Hearing	Visual	Motor	Cognitive
Input to the system	Voice recognition	X	X	X	X
	Voice to text	X	X	X	X
	Keyboard and mouse	X			X
	Gesture	X	X	X	X
	Brain–computer interface	X	X	X	X
	Body motion detection	X	X	X	X
	Sign language	X			
	Braille keyboard		X		
Output from system	Text to voice		X	X	X
	Display screen	X		X	X
	Vibration	X	X	X	X
	Flashing light or LED	X		X	X
	Sonification		X	X	X
	Alert sound		X	X	X
	Sign language	X			
	Magnification		X		

language, provides closed captioning to videos, converting gestures of the sign language into text, and shows alert messages in specific situations. Furthermore, people with motor impairment, in most cases, can interact with the CAS using normal input methods. However, users who have limb amputation can utilize specialized equipment, such as sip and puff. People with cognitive impairment can rely on using alerts on specific situations, reminders for events, images, and sounds, and repeating notifications in the case of emergency.

The collected data about users, such as the type of disability and the surrounding environment, aids in identifying the user context, appropriate actions, and the interaction model (Fischer 2012). Several state-of-the-art investigations exploit user profiling to provide the user with a suitable interaction (Tavares et al. 2016; Margetis et al. 2012; Aly 2014; Chaudary & Pulli 2014). Indeed, profiling enables the development of accessible CAS for people with disabilities with an interaction model that is tailored to the needs of the user. Table 2.4 shows the interaction channels for different people with disabilities. Such categorization can help in identifying the suitable interface to be provided based on the user profile and it can assist the user in providing the modality that is relevant to the user situation.

2.4.4 Existing Reviews on Context-Aware Systems

Closely related work on reviewing CAS include (Zhang et al. 2013; Fischer 2012; Verbert, Manouselis, Ochoa, Wolpers, Drachsler, Bosnic, and Duval 2012; Truong

& Dustdar 2009; Baldauf, Dustdar, & Rosenberg 2007; Li, Eckert, Martinez, & Rubio 2015; Bettini, Brdiczka, Henricksen, Indulska, Nicklas, Ranganathan, and Riboni 2010; Bellavista, Corradi, Fanelli, & Foschini 2012). The identified work differs from our survey in the method adopted and aim. Verbert et al. (2012) presents a survey of context-aware recommender systems (CARS) that are deployed in technology enhanced learning (TEL) environments. The investigation is divided into, firstly, the presentation of a context framework that identifies context dimensions for the analysis and development of CARS for TEL. Secondly, the investigation includes an in-depth analysis of CARS as deployed in educational settings. Systems analysis provides insight on the utilization of current prototypes to evaluate the potential impact of the approaches on the learning process. The work includes the identification of weaknesses in the use of contextual data and validations in real experiments.

Truong and Dustdar (2009) present a survey that aims at studying and analyzing the current techniques and methods employed in context-aware web service systems (CAWSS). A discussion of the future trends and proposition of further steps on making web services systems context-aware is presented. The paper analyzes existing CAWSSs based on the techniques they support, such as context information modeling, context sensing, distribution, security and privacy, and adaptation techniques. The analysis includes examining existing systems based on application domains, system type, mobility support, multi-organization support, and level of web services implementation. The findings include confirming increased support of CAWSSs; however, limitations are identified as related to system interoperability, security, and operations in multi-organizational environments. Comparing between different methods of distributing context data is presented by Bellavista et al. (2012).

Additional survey work is presented in the literature. The systematic investigation of context-awareness in ubiquitous media is presented by Zhang et al. (2013). The proposition of a reference framework from a systematic viewpoint is identified by studying the functionalities and services of context-awareness. Sub-viewpoint groups are created by extracting functionalities from services such as context modeling, preprocessing, reasoning, inconsistency and detection, and resolution. Furthermore, the author presents an overview of the state of the art of existing context-awareness efforts by following the proposed reference model. An investigation on common architecture and conceptual design principles of CAS is done by Baldauf et al. (2007). The authors present an abstract layered architecture for CAS. In addition, several existing middleware and server-based techniques are used to reduce the complexity of developing applications. Fischer (2012) proposes the development of a multi-dimensional framework for CAS to address the challenge in transcending existing frameworks. The framework is based on insights derived from the development and assessment of a variety of different systems that have been proposed previously. Li et al. (2015) compare between different technical aspects of eleven context-aware middleware architectures. The results show that none of the examined context-aware middleware architectures succeeded in satisfying all the settings needed to develop CAS. The requirements for context modeling and reasoning along with a comparison between state-of-the-art methods used to model and reason contexts are examined by Bettini et al. (2010).

The main conclusions and recommendations (Zhang et al. 2013; Fischer 2012; Verbert et al. 2012; Truong & Dustdar 2009; Baldauf et al. 2007; Li et al. 2015; Bettini et al. 2010) include the following challenges:

– Creating an infrastructure for rapidly building context-aware media applications (Zhang et al. 2013).
– Designing programming abstractions and systematic development tools (Zhang et al. 2013).
– Developing large-scale context-aware applications that support wider user movements and heterogeneous devices (Zhang et al. 2013).
– Understanding the design trade-offs, the promises, and the pitfalls between adaptive and adaptable systems, information delivery and information access technologies, and contextualized information representations and serendipity (Fischer 2012).
– Using contextual data need to be tackled to increase uptake of CARS, and validate research efforts in realistic trial experiments in TEL recommender systems (Verbert et al. 2012).
– Enabling the development of context-aware web services through improved distributed context management, security and privacy techniques as well as interoperable representations for context information (Truong & Dustdar 2009).
– Supporting enhanced security and privacy in CAS (Baldauf et al. 2007).
– Using a general standard, automatically develop the system inference rules, and full deployment of the CAS in real-world environments (Li et al. 2015).
– The availability of a powerful modeling and reasoning framework which can satisfy the need of presenting high-level context and resolve the uncertainty of context information (Bettini et al. 2010).
– Handling of distributed, often uncertain context data from many sources (i.e., aggregation and filtering) (Bellavista et al. 2012).

2.4.5   The Proposed Multi-Layer CAS Framework

Limited work has been reported in the literature to provide a multi-layer framework for rapidly prototyping CAS for people with disability. Therefore, the research community needs to focus on creating frameworks for developing accessible CAS. Ideas and methods can be incorporated based on recent advancements in internet-of-things (IoT) architectures. Any proposed framework needs to tailor the user interaction based on a predefined set of user profiles with the requirements needed for each kind of disability. In addition, the provided framework needs to take into consideration the concept of assistive service continuity (Ghorbel et al. 2007) to keep track of the user activities in different environments and helping the user accordingly across different settings.

Figure 2.4 presents our multi-layer CAS framework that supports people with disabilities. The suggested framework comprises a physical, communication and network, and application layers. We sort the layers according to the level of abstraction. The physical layer includes the hardware infrastructure of the system, such as sensors, actuators, and data acquisition systems. Technologies such as wearable devices, BANs, rapid prototyping hardware boards, and seamless interfaces are found to be trending. Moreover, the communication and network layer includes modern and trending standards, such as Wi-Fi, Bluetooth, Zigbee, and Cloud. An interpretation sublayer supports the application layer and comprises

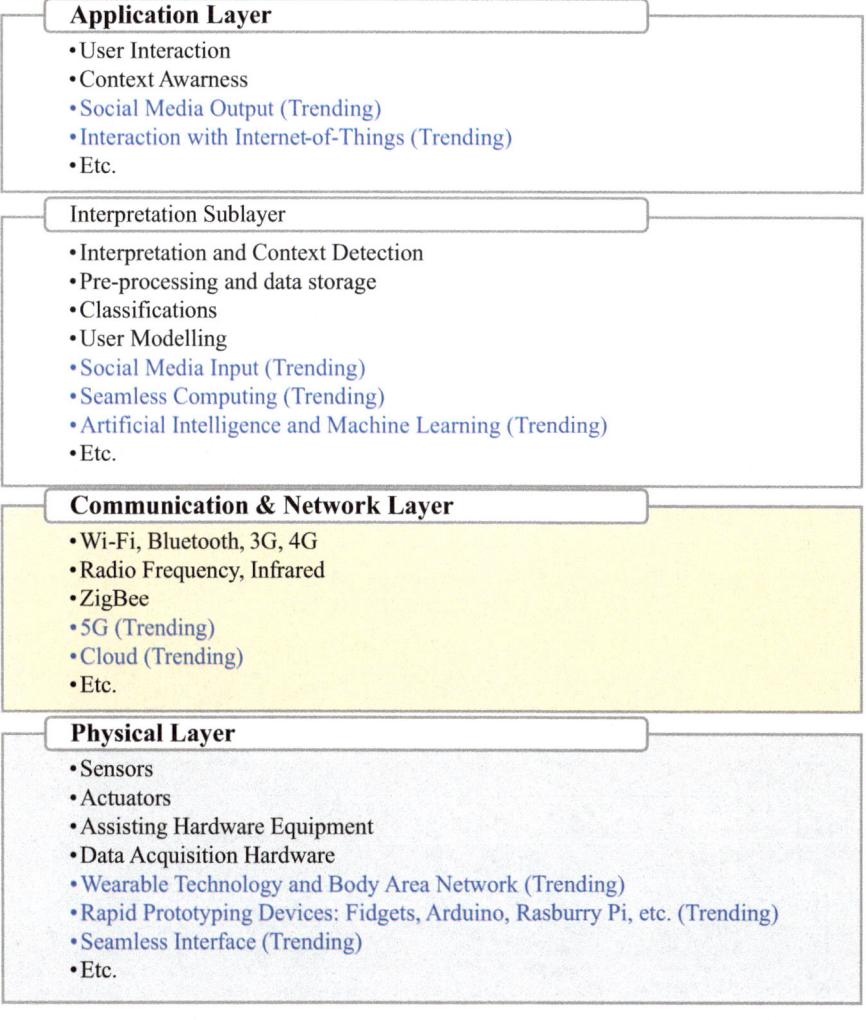

Application Layer
- User Interaction
- Context Awarness
- Social Media Output (Trending)
- Interaction with Internet-of-Things (Trending)
- Etc.

Interpretation Sublayer
- Interpretation and Context Detection
- Pre-processing and data storage
- Classifications
- User Modelling
- Social Media Input (Trending)
- Seamless Computing (Trending)
- Artificial Intelligence and Machine Learning (Trending)
- Etc.

Communication & Network Layer
- Wi-Fi, Bluetooth, 3G, 4G
- Radio Frequency, Infrared
- ZigBee
- 5G (Trending)
- Cloud (Trending)
- Etc.

Physical Layer
- Sensors
- Actuators
- Assisting Hardware Equipment
- Data Acquisition Hardware
- Wearable Technology and Body Area Network (Trending)
- Rapid Prototyping Devices: Fidgets, Arduino, Rasburry Pi, etc. (Trending)
- Seamless Interface (Trending)
- Etc.

Fig. 2.4 The proposed CAS multi-layer framework

the interpretations, context detections, classifications, user modeling, preprocessing, and data storage. We observe social media input, seamless computing, and the use of artificial intelligence as trending technologies. The application layer is responsible for user interaction, demonstrating context-awareness, etc. We consider exploiting existing smart IoT systems and access to social media within the deployment environment as trending features that drive future CAS for people with disability. The social network can be used to improve information classification and tagging in the environment. Furthermore, it can help in tracking user activity patterns to provide seamless interaction. Future CAS can rely on the social network user engagement to provide semantic data (Doush & Pontelli 2010; Doush et al. 2012; Doush & Al-Bdarneh 2013) for different contexts. Although such use of social network has been proposed in the past (von Ahn et al. 2006; Eagle & Pentland 2006), the number of investigations is still limited. An example deployment of the proposed CAS framework is presented in Fig. 2.5.

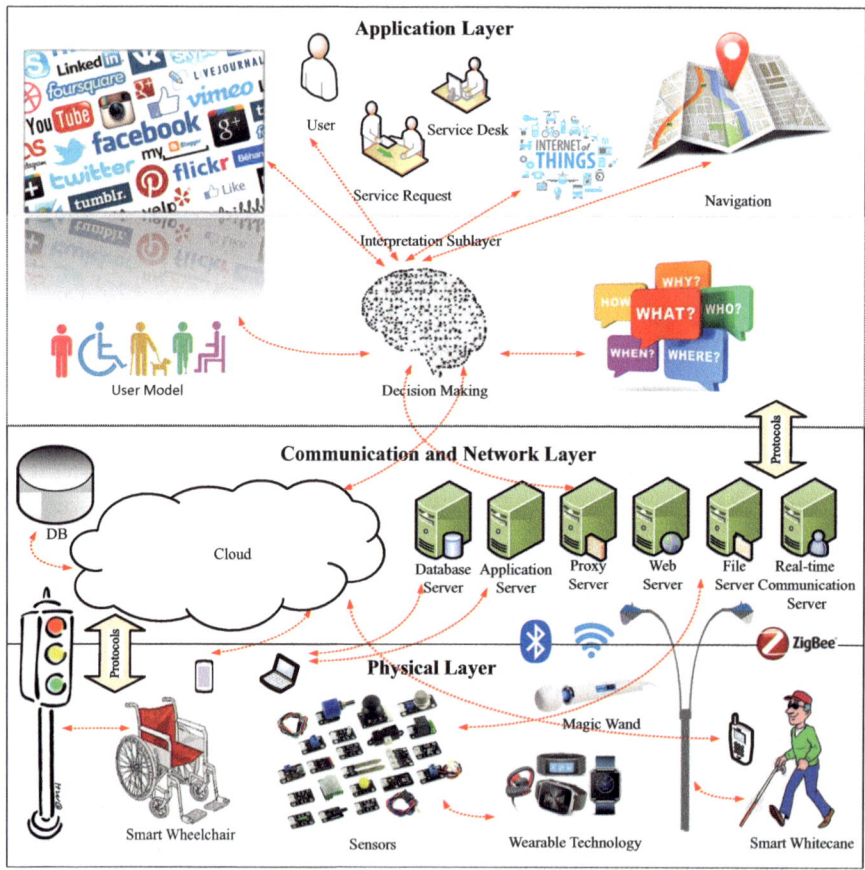

Fig. 2.5 Example deployment of a modern CAS framework that supports people with disabilities

2.5   Conclusions and Future Work

This survey paper presents the current research works and best practices in the area of accessible CAS. We study and analyze a large number of accessible CAS for different types of disabilities. The systems are viewed in terms of the context type they tackle, the disability type, and the interaction model used to present the context information. Out of the surveyed systems, a small subset presents CAS for people with disabilities and provides concrete information on all the proposed analysis indicators. Most of the proposed CAS are for blind and people with motor impairment, only one CAS targets deaf users, and two systems are presented as universally accessible for different kinds of disabilities. To that end, the need arises for developing CAS for the excluded groups of users, such as deaf. In addition, universally accessible CAS that target different kinds of disabilities need to be further investigated.

At present, mobile phones highly enable pervasiveness and ubiquitousness, and can be equipped with impressive sensors. State-of-the-art mobile phones support Wi-Fi, 4G, Bluetooth, and NFC technologies—to name but a few. Modern mobile phones can include accelerometers, ambient light sensors, GPS sensors, compasses, proximity sensors, pressure sensors, and combined cameras and microphones (Al-Qudah, Doush, Alkhateeb, Maghayreh, and Al-Khaleel 2014). The embedded sensors can be used for gathering relevant information, detect contexts, and recognize activities. Thus, each user pattern of activities can be predicted and assisted. The majority of the present-day CAS either use a mobile phone or need the user to hold special hardware to collect context information. In our opinion, seamless CAS are trending and will become prevalent in the near future; users will no longer need to hold extra devices or even mobile phones. However, the use of mobile phones is still one of the most appealing technologies at the present time for CAS for people with disabilities. Indeed, the use of mobile phones enables the deployment of CAS in different environments.

According to the surveyed CAS, the type of the disability determines the output. For users who are visually impaired and blind, the output can take the form of voice, vibrations, and buzzer-sound alerts. Users who are deaf rely on pictures as an output from CAS. Moreover, users who are cognitive impaired depend on voice commands and vibrations. We observe universal CAS that can rapidly adapt to different disabilities, and customize its interaction, as a promising research direction. In addition, the available variety of modern wearable technologies and body area networks (BANs) can enable advanced automatic detection of user actions and environments, and intervene accordingly. For example, CAS can save energy consumption of hardware by automatically putting the BAN in a sleep mode—if the blind person stops moving for a period of time. Wearable technologies can absolutely increase the accuracies of detection and interventions, and provide a safer and more reliable system to use.

Developing effective and truly accessible CAS require solid evaluations and validations. The surveyed systems include 16 accessible CAS; however, only 4 systems evaluate effectiveness. Most commonly, the verification tests include 10 or more target users. In many cases, the testing was done on healthy people. To that end, thorough analysis and testing, and solid evaluations of CAS for people with disability must be performed for any developed system.

The limitations of the proposed systems in the literature can be summarized in the following: the inability to detect the surrounding environment accurately, the system requires holding special hardware, and the limited testing of the proposed CAS with the target users. These limitations need a focus of the research community on using the internet-of-things to collect information accurately about the surrounding environment and this can lead to better serving the user. The booming research in the area of body area network can help in allowing the CAS to sense the user information without the need to hold special hardware. One of the important aspects when developing CAS that can serve people with disabilities is to involve users in the system design by involving them in all stages of the system development in order to tackle the problems they encounter.

A few research work is done in the area of using user profiles to provide users with the suitable communication channel for interaction. More research work to be done in the area of adaptive interfaces for people with disabilities which can collect data about users and the surrounding environment to provide the user with the suitable interaction.

Several opportunities for future work can be identified from the presented survey. The focus of future work should be on improving the security aspects of CAS (Lukowicz et al. 2012; Damaj 2007; Al-Chalabi, Essa, Shahzad, & Damaj 2015), exploiting modern and hybrid high-performance computing systems (Damaj & Diab 2001; Damaj & Kasbah 2018; Kasbah, Damaj, & Haraty 2008), using advanced sensors, performing reliable verifications, enabling customizations and adaptation (El-Shafei, Shalati, Rehayel, & Damaj 2014; Doush, Alkhateeb, Maghayreh, & Al-Betar 2013a), providing points of interest based on accessibility levels (Santos, Almeida, Martins, Gonçalves, & Martins 2017), and more. According to Domingo (2012), the use of body and nanosensors can help people with visual impairment to recognize faces or expressions. The deaf person can be notified using visual (e.g., light) or vibrotactile signals when detecting sounds or smoke. Using body sensors, actuators, and neurochips can help in user movements by detecting intention when moving specific muscles, such technology can help people with paralyzed limbs. Furthermore, a question remains on how much information a system needs to save to accurately intervene. Information organization and semantic tagging are required to provide more beneficial information to the user through the CAS and to minimize the amount of data that has to be saved, such investigations can make future systems more efficient in terms of time and space. CAS can help people with disabilities to be more involved in the events in their surrounding environments. A different approach is suggested in Novais and Carneiro (2016) to develop CAS by considering behavioral cues. The contextual data are collected using geo-location, sensor, system and network logs, user interactions, and social connections.

The dynamic mobile environment makes the amount of generated context data huge which increase the level of uncertainty. Bobek and Nalepa (2017a,b) propose

HMR+ language which can model the context in an efficient manner and allow resolving any uncertainty in an intelligent way. The rules defined using this language are assigned a certainty factor that stands for the rule confidence level. Online knowledge discovery methods (e.g., Hoeffding trees) are suggested to minimize mobile power and storage consumption.

There are several additional future improvements for CAS. For instance, CAS that provide assistance for people with disabilities need to be accurate and with minimal mistakes. However, we can differentiate between "understandable mistake" and "incomprehensible mistake" (Lukowicz et al. 2012). For example, if walking is classified as running, then we would consider this as an understandable mistake. On the other hand, if the system classifies sleeping as running, then this is considered as an incomprehensible mistake. Moreover, smart cities can provide a future direction in considering more complex contexts (Leem & Kim 2013; Shin 2009). For example, the system can be used with dynamic resources (e.g., emergency medical assistance and public transportation). Modern CAS can benefit from the advancement in speech recognition and computational linguistics towards increased system seamlessness (Damaj, Imdoukh, & Zantout 2017).

References

Abbate, S., Avvenuti, M., Bonatesta, F., Cola, G., Corsini, P., & Vecchio, A. (2012). A smartphone-based fall detection system. *Pervasive and Mobile Computing, 8*(6), 883–899.

Abowd, G. D., Dey, A. K., Brown, P. J., Davies, N., Smith, M., & Steggles, P. (1999). Towards a better understanding of context and context-awareness. In *Proceedings of the 1st International Symposium on Handheld and Ubiquitous Computing, HUC '99* (pp. 304–307). London: Springer.

Abowd, G. D., & Mynatt, E. D. (2000). Charting past, present, and future research in ubiquitous computing. *ACM Transactions on Computer-Human Interaction, 7*(1), 29–58.

Ahn, S., & Kim, D. (2006). *Proactive context-aware sensor networks* (pp. 38–53). Berlin: Springer.

Al-Chalabi, A. E., Essa, S., Shahzad, H., & Damaj, I. (2015). A wearable and ubiquitous NFC wallet. In *2015 IEEE 28th Canadian Conference on Electrical and Computer Engineering (CCECE)* (pp. 152–157). Piscataway: IEEE.

Al-Qudah, Z., Doush, I. A., Alkhateeb, F., Maghayreh, E. A., & Al-Khaleel, O. (2014). Utilizing mobile devices' tactile feedback for presenting braille characters: An optimized approach for fast reading and long battery life. *Interacting with Computers, 26*(1), 63–74.

Alegre, U., Augusto, J. C., & Clark, T. (2016). Engineering context-aware systems and applications: A survey. *Journal of Systems and Software, 117*(suppl. C), 55–83.

Aloulou, H., Mokhtari, M., Tiberghien, T., Biswas, J., & Yap, P. (2014). An adaptable and flexible framework for assistive living of cognitively impaired people. *IEEE Journal of Biomedical and Health Informatics, 18*(1), 353–360.

Aly, W. H. F. (2014). MNDWSN for helping people with different disabilities. *International Journal of Distributed Sensor Networks, 10*(7), 489289.

Baldauf, M., Dustdar, S., & Rosenberg, F. (2007). A survey on context-aware systems. *International Journal of Ad Hoc and Ubiquitous Computing, 2*(4), 263–277.

Barkhuus, L., & Dey, A. (2003). *Is context-aware computing taking control away from the user? Three levels of interactivity examined* (pp. 149–156). Berlin: Springer.

Beaudouin-Lafon, M. (2000). Instrumental interaction: An interaction model for designing post-wimp user interfaces. In *Proceedings of the SIGCHI Conference on Human Factors in Computing Systems, CHI '00* (pp. 446–453).

Bellavista, P., Corradi, A., Fanelli, M., & Foschini, L. (2012). A survey of context data distribution for mobile ubiquitous systems. *ACM Computing Surveys, 44*(4), 24:1–24:45.

Bettini, C., Brdiczka, O., Henricksen, K., Indulska, J., Nicklas, D., Ranganathan, A., & Riboni, D. (2010). A survey of context modelling and reasoning techniques. *Pervasive and Mobile Computing, 6*(2), 161–180.

Bobek, S., & Nalepa, G. J. (2017a). Uncertain context data management in dynamic mobile environments. *Future Generation Computer Systems, 66*, 110–124.

Bobek, S., & Nalepa, G. J. (2017b). Uncertainty handling in rule-based mobile context-aware systems. *Pervasive and Mobile Computing, 39*, 159–179.

Bozgeyikli, L., Bozgeyikli, E., Clevenger, M., Raij, A., Alqasemi, R., Sundarrao, S., et al. (2015). Vr4vr: Vocational rehabilitation of individuals with disabilities in immersive virtual reality environments. In *Proceedings of the 8th ACM International Conference on Pervasive Technologies Related to Assistive Environments, PETRA '15* (pp. 54:1–54:4).

Cavender, A., Trewin, S., & Hanson, V. (2008). General writing guidelines for technology and people with disabilities. *ACM SIGACCESS Accessibility and Computing, 1*(92), 17–22.

Chaudary, B., & Pulli, P. (2014). Smart cane outdoor navigation system for visually impaired deaf-blind and blind persons. *Journal of Communication Disorders, Deaf Studies and Hearing Aids, 125*(2), 1–9.

Chen, H. (2004). *An Intelligent Broker Architecture for Pervasive Context-Aware Systems.* Ph.D. Thesis, University of Maryland, Baltimore County.

Damaj, I. (2007). Higher-level hardware synthesis of the Kasumi cryptographic algorithm. *Journal of Computer Science and Technology, 22*(1), 60–70.

Damaj, I., & Diab, H. (2001). Performance analysis of extended vector-scalar operations using reconfigurable computing. In *ACS/IEEE International Conference on Computer Systems and Applications, 2001* (pp. 227–232). Piscataway: IEEE.

Damaj, I., Imdoukh, M., & Zantout, R. (2017). Parallel hardware for faster morphological analysis. *Journal of King Saud University - Computer and Information Sciences.* https://doi.org/10.1016/j.jksuci.2017.07.003. http://www.sciencedirect.com/science/article/pii/S1319157817301611

Damaj, I., & Kasbah, S. (2018). An analysis framework for hardware and software implementations with applications from cryptography. *Computers & Electrical Engineering, 69*, 572–584.

Domingo, M. C. (2012). An overview of the internet of things for people with disabilities. *Journal of Network and Computer Applications, 35*(2), 584–596.

Doush, I. A., Alkhateeb, F., Maghayreh, E. A., & Al-Betar, M. A. (2013a). The design of RIA accessibility evaluation tool. *Advances in Engineering Software, 57*, 1–7.

Doush, I. A., Alkhateeb, F., Maghayreh, E. A., Alsmadi, I., & Samarah, S. (2012). Annotations, collaborative tagging, and searching mathematics in e-learning. CoRR abs/1211.1780.

Doush, I. A., Alshattnawi, S., Al-Tamimi, A., Alhasan, B., & Hamasha, S. (2017). ISAB: Integrated indoor navigation system for the blind. *Interacting with Computers, 29*(2), 181–202.

Doush, I. A., Alshattnawi, S., & Barhoush, M. (2015). Non-visual navigation interface for completing tasks with a predefined order using mobile phone: a case study of pilgrimage. *International Journal of Mobile Network Design and Innovation, 6*(1), 1–13.

Doush, I. A., & Al-Bdarneh, S. (2013). Automatic semantic generation and Arabic translation of mathematical expressions on the web. *International Journal of Web-Based Learning and Teaching Technologies, 8*(1), 1–16.

Doush, I. A., Bany-Mohammed, A., Ali, E., Al-Betar, M. A. (2013b). Towards a more accessible e-government in Jordan: An evaluation study of visually impaired users and web developers. *Behaviour & IT, 32*(3), 273–293.

Doush, I. A., & Pontelli, E. (2010). Integrating semantic web and folksonomies to improve e-learning accessibility. In *Proceedings of 12th International Conference on Computers Helping People with Special Needs, ICCHP 2010, Vienna, Austria, July 14–16, 2010, Part I* (pp. 376–383).

Doush, I. A., & Pontelli, E. (2013). Non-visual navigation of spreadsheets - enhancing accessibility of Microsoft Excel™. *Universal Access in the Information Society, 12*(2), 143–159.

Eagle, N., & (Sandy) Pentland, A. (2006). Reality mining: Sensing complex social systems. *Personal and Ubiquitous Computing, 10*(4), 255–268.

El-Shafei, M., Shalati, A. A., Rehayel, M., & Damaj, I. (2014). HOBOT: A customizable home management system with a surveillance robot. In *IEEE 27th Canadian Conference on Electrical and Computer Engineering, CCECE 2014, Toronto, ON, Canada, May 4–7, 2014* (pp. 1–7).

Fischer, G. (2012). Context-aware systems: The 'right' information, at the 'right' time, in the 'right' place, in the 'right' way, to the 'right' person. In *Proceedings of the International Working Conference on Advanced Visual Interfaces, AVI '12* (pp. 287–294)

Ghorbel, M., Kadouche, R., & Mokhtari, M. (2007). User & service modelling in assistive environment to enhance accessibility of dependent people. In *International Conference on Information and Communication Technologies and Accessibility, ICTA '07, April, Hammamet, Tunisia.*

Grguric, A., Gil, A. M. M., Huljenic, D., Car, Z., & Podobnik, V. (2016). *A survey on user interaction mechanisms for enhanced living environments* (pp. 131–141). Cham: Springer International Publishing.

Hasan, S. S., Chipara, O., Wu, Y. H., & Aksan, N. (2014). Evaluating auditory contexts and their impacts on hearing aid outcomes with mobile phones. In *Proceedings of the 8th International Conference on Pervasive Computing Technologies for Healthcare, ICST (Institute for Computer Sciences, Social-Informatics and Telecommunications Engineering)* (pp. 126–133)

Hasan, S. S., Lai, F., Chipara, O., & Wu, Y. H. (2013). Audiosense: Enabling real-time evaluation of hearing aid technology in-situ. In *2013 IEEE 26th International Symposium on Computer-Based Medical Systems (CBMS)* (pp. 167–172). Piscataway: IEEE.

Hinze, A., & Buchanan, G. (2005). Context-awareness in mobile tourist information systems: challenges for user interaction. In *International Workshop on Context in Mobile HCI at the Conference for 7th International Conference on Human Computer Interaction with Mobile Devices and Services.*

Ivanov, R. (2012). RSNAVI: An RFID-based context-aware indoor navigation system for the blind. In *Proceedings of the 13th International Conference on Computer Systems and Technologies, CompSysTech '12* (pp. 313–320)

Jarrah, S. I., & Doush, I. A. (2014). *Context Detection Using Machine Learning to Assist Smartphone Users with Memory Impairment.* Master's thesis, Yarmouk University, Jordan.

Kasbah, S.J., Damaj, I.W., & Haraty, R. A. (2008). Multigrid solvers in reconfigurable hardware. *Journal of Computational and Applied Mathematics, 213*(1), 79–94. https://doi.org/10.1016/j.cam.2006.12.031

Kbar, G., Abidi, M. H., Hammad Mian, S., Al-Daraiseh, A. A., & Mansoor, W. (2016). A university-based smart and context aware solution for people with disabilities (USCAS-PWD). *Computers, 5*(3), 18.

Kleinberger, T., Becker, M., Ras, E., Holzinger, A., & Muller, P. (2007). Ambient intelligence in assisted living: Enable elderly people to handle future interfaces. In C. Stephanidis (Ed.) *Universal access in human-computer interaction. Ambient interaction, lecture notes in computer science* (vol. 4555, pp. 103–112). Berlin: Springer.

Lee, H., Choi, J. S., & Elmasri, R. (2009). A classification and modeling of the quality of contextual information in smart spaces. In *2009 IEEE International Conference on Pervasive Computing and Communications* (pp. 1–5).

Leem, C. S., & Kim, B. G. (2013). Taxonomy of ubiquitous computing service for city development. *Personal and Ubiquitous Computing, 17*(7), 1475–1483.

Li, X., Eckert, M., Martinez, J. F., & Rubio, G. (2015). Context aware middleware architectures: Survey and challenges. *Sensors, 15*(8), 20570–20607.

Lin, Q., Zhang, D., Connelly, K., Ni, H., Yu, Z., & Zhou, X. (2015). Disorientation detection by mining GPS trajectories for cognitively-impaired elders. *Pervasive and Mobile Computing, 19*, 71–85.

Lukowicz, P., Nanda, S., Narayanan, V., Albelson, H., McGuinness, D. L., & Jordan, M. I. (2012). Qualcomm context-awareness symposium sets research agenda for context-aware smartphones. *IEEE Pervasive Computing, 11*(1), 76–79.

Lustrek, M., Gjoreski, H., Vega, N. G., Kozina, S., Cvetkovic, B., Mirchevska, V., Gams, M. (2015). Fall detection using location sensors and accelerometers. *IEEE Pervasive Computing, 14*(4), 72–79.

Manzoor, A., Truong, H. L., & Dustdar, S. (2008). *On the evaluation of quality of context* (pp. 140–153). Berlin: Springer.

Marangunić, N., Granić, A. (2015). Technology acceptance model: A literature review from 1986 to 2013. *Universal Access in the Information Society, 14*(1), 81–95.

Margetis, G., Antona, M., Ntoa, S., & Stephanidis, C. (2012). Towards accessibility in ambient intelligence environments. In *Ambient intelligence* (pp. 328–337). Berlin: Springer.

Maxhuni, A., Muñoz-Meléndez, A., Osmani, V., Perez, H., Mayora, O., & Morales, E. F. (2016). Classification of bipolar disorder episodes based on analysis of voice and motor activity of patients. *Pervasive and Mobile Computing, 31*, 50–66.

Mehra, P. (2012). Context-aware computing: Beyond search and location-based services. *IEEE Internet Computing, 16*(2), 12–16.

Mirri, S., Prandi, C., Salomoni, P., Callegati, F., & Campi, A. (2014). On combining crowd-sourcing, sensing and open data for an accessible smart city. In *2014 Eighth International Conference on, Next Generation Mobile Apps, Services and Technologies (NGMAST)* (pp. 294–299). Piscataway: IEEE.

Morse, D. R., Armstrong, S., & Dey, A. K. (2000). The what, who, where, when, why and how of context-awareness. In *CHI'00 Extended Abstracts on Human Factors in Computing Systems, CHI EA'00* (pp. 371–371)

Mortazavi, B., Pourhomayoun, M., Ghasemzadeh, H., Jafari, R., Roberts, C. K., & Sarrafzadeh, M. (2015). Context-aware data processing to enhance quality of measurements in wireless health systems: An application to MET calculation of exergaming actions. *IEEE Internet of Things Journal, 2*(1), 84–93.

Nijdam, N. A., Han, S., Kevelham, B., & Magnenat-Thalmann, N. (2010). A context-aware adaptive rendering system for user-centric pervasive computing environments. In *Melecon 2010, 15th IEEE Mediterranean Electrotechnical Conference* (pp. 790–795)

Novais, P., & Carneiro, D. (2016). The role of non-intrusive approaches in the development of people-aware systems. *Progress in Artificial Intelligence, 5*(3), 215–220.

Okoshi, T., Nozaki, H., Nakazawa, J., Tokuda, H., Ramos, J., & Dey, A. K. (2016). Towards attention-aware adaptive notification on smart phones. *Pervasive and Mobile Computing, 26*, 17–34. Thirteenth international conference on pervasive computing and communications (PerCom 2015).

Padgham, L., & Winikoff, M. (2004). *Developing intelligent agent systems: A practical guide*. New York: Wiley.

Pereira, A., Nunes, N., Vieira, D., Costa, N., Fernandes, H., & Barroso, J. (2015). Blind guide: An ultrasound sensor-based body area network for guiding blind people. *Procedia Computer Science, 67*, 403–408. Proceedings of the 6th international conference on software development and technologies for enhancing accessibility and fighting info-exclusion.

Ramos, J., Oliveira, T., Satoh, K., Neves, J., & Novais, P. (2018). Cognitive assistants—an analysis and future trends based on speculative default reasoning. *Applied Sciences, 8*(742), 1–23.

Rana, R., Hume, M., Reilly, J., Jurdak, R., & Soar, J. (2016). Opportunistic and context-aware affect sensing on smartphones. *IEEE Pervasive Computing, 15*(2), 60–69.

Rantanen, V., Vanhala, T., Tuisku, O., Niemenlehto, P. H., Verho, J., Surakka, V., Juhola, M., & Lekkala, J. (2011). A wearable, wireless gaze tracker with integrated selection command source for human-computer interaction. *IEEE Transactions on Information Technology in Biomedicine, 15*(5), 795–801.

Sanchez, L., Lanza, J., Olsen, R., Bauer, M., & Girod-Genet, M. (2006). A generic context management framework for personal networking environments. In *3rd Annual International Conference on Mobile and Ubiquitous Systems - Workshops, 2006* (pp. 1–8).

Santoro, C., Paterno, F., Ricci, G., & Leporini, B. (2007). A multimodal mobile museum guide for all. In *Mobile Interaction with the Real World (MIRW 2007)*. pp. 21–25.

Santos, F., Almeida, A., Martins, C., Gonçalves, R., & Martins, J. (2017). Using POI functionality and accessibility levels for delivering personalized tourism recommendations. *Computers, Environment and Urban Systems*. https://doi.org/10.1016/j.compenvurbsys.2017.08.007

Saunier, J., & Balbo, F. (2009). Regulated multi-party communications and context awareness through the environment. *Multiagent and Grid Systems, 5*(1), 75.

Schilit, B., Adams, N., & Want, R. (1994). Context-aware computing applications. In *Proceedings of the 1994 First Workshop on Mobile Computing Systems and Applications, WMCSA '94* (pp. 85–90).

Shin, D. H. (2009). Ubiquitous city: Urban technologies, urban infrastructure and urban informatics. *Journal of Information Science, 35*(5), 515–526.

Silva, J., Rosa, J., Barbosa, J., Barbosa, D. N. F., & Palazzo, L. A. M. (2009). Content distribution in trial-aware environments. In *Proceedings of the XV Brazilian Symposium on multimedia and the web, WebMedia '09* (pp. 15:1–15:8). New York: ACM.

Tavares, J., Barbosa, J., Cardoso, I., Costa, C., Yamin, A., & Real, R. (2016). Hefestos: An intelligent system applied to ubiquitous accessibility. *Universal Access in the Information Society, 15*(4), 589–607.

Truong, H. L., & Dustdar, S. (2009). A survey on context-aware web service systems. *International Journal of Web Information Systems, 5*(1), 5–31.

Verbert, K., Manouselis, N., Ochoa, X., Wolpers, M., Drachsler, H., Bosnic, I., & Duval, E. (2012). Context-aware recommender systems for learning: A survey and future challenges. *IEEE Transactions on Learning Technologies, 5*(4), 318–335.

von Ahn, L., Ginosar, S., Kedia, M., Liu, R., & Blum, M. (2006). Improving accessibility of the web with a computer game. In *Proceedings of the SIGCHI conference on human factors in computing systems, CHI '06* (pp. 79–82)

Wagner, A., Barbosa, J. L. V., & Barbosa, D. N. F. (2014). A model for profile management applied to ubiquitous learning environments. *Expert Systems with Applications, 41*(4, Part 2), 2023–2034.

Weiser, M. (1999). The computer for the 21st century. *SIGMOBILE Mobile Computing and Communications Review, 3*(3), 3–11. https://doi.org/10.1145/329124.329126

World Health Organization (WHO). (2011). Retrieved 30 October 2017, http://www.who.int/disabilities/world_report/2011/en/

Zhan, K., Faux, S., & Ramos, F. (2015). Multi-scale conditional random fields for first-person activity recognition on elders and disabled patients. *Pervasive and Mobile Computing, 16*, 251–267. Selected papers from the twelfth annual IEEE international conference on pervasive computing and communications (PerCom 2014).

Zhang, D., Huang, H., Lai, C. F., Liang, X., Zou, Q., & Guo, M. (2013). Survey on context-awareness in ubiquitous media. *Multimedia Tools and Applications, 67*(1), 179–211.

Zhu, C., & Sheng, W. (2011). Wearable sensor-based hand gesture and daily activity recognition for robot-assisted living. *IEEE Transactions on Systems, Man, and Cybernetics - Part A: Systems and Humans, 41*(3), 569–573.

Chapter 3
Smart Systems to Improve the Mobility of People with Visual Impairment Through IoM and IoMT

Raluca Maria Aileni, George Suciu, Victor Suciu, Sever Pasca, and Jean Ciurea

3.1 Introduction

Smart systems designed for people suffering from visual impairments can be integrated as personal equipment, implants or in common transport systems, and lead to mobility improvement. The architecture and integrated mode (invasive, non-invasive) of the smart wearable systems are dependent on the health status of the patient and age.

The WHO's report regarding blindness and vision impairment (Vision Impairment and Blindness, 2018) estimates that approximately 1.3 billion have a form of vision impairment and the people are over the age of 50 years. According to the International Classification of Diseases 11 (2018), vision impairments are:

- Distance vision (441.5 million people)

  - Mild vision impairment (188.5 million people);
  - Moderate–severe vision impairment (217 million people);
  - Severe impairment—blind (36 million people);

- Near vision (826 million people)

According to the WHO (World Health Organization), the principal causes of visual impairment are uncorrected refractive errors, glaucoma, age-related macular degeneration (AMD), cataract, diabetic retinopathy, corneal opacity, and trachoma. In Europe, around 9.6% of the population is affected by visual impairment.

R. M. Aileni (✉) · G. Suciu · V. Suciu · S. Pasca
Faculty of Electronics, Telecommunication and Information Technology, Politehnica University of Bucharest, Bucharest, Romania

J. Ciurea
Neurosurgery Department, Bagdasar-Arseni Hospital, Bucharest, Romania

© Springer Nature Switzerland AG 2020
S. Paiva (ed.), *Technological Trends in Improved Mobility of the Visually Impaired*,
EAI/Springer Innovations in Communication and Computing,
https://doi.org/10.1007/978-3-030-16450-8_3

The invasive integration and rehabilitation for people with visual impairment and blindness involve neuroscience and advanced prosthetics technologies such as neural implants MEA (multielectrode array) for cortical stimulation, implantable visual prosthesis microsystems (Bionic Eye, Argus II (Second Sight)) and retinal prosthetics (Retina Implant, Pixium Vision). These implants generate patterns of light that can be interpreted as visual patterns to improve the mobility, object localization and quality of life.

Nowadays, over a billion people are estimated to be living with disabilities. The lack of support services make them overly dependent on their families and prevent them from being socially included. A good solution is to use Mobile Assistive Technologies (MAT) to perform tasks in everyday lives, but one of the most important and challenging tasks is to create a solution which offers the assistance and support they need to achieve a good quality of life and allows them to participate in social life. This paper reviews researches within the field of MATs to help people with visual impairment in their daily activities like navigation and shopping (Elgendy & Lanyi, 2018).

Today, the blind and visually impaired are among the biggest groups of disabled people in the world. We can specify that a limited number of available smart technologies are dedicated to the care of persons with disabilities. The blind and the visually impaired still need to rely on other people in their daily navigation. There are a few applications, which are intended to ease the lives of the visually impaired and blind, but there are no very actively used devices and/or applications, which would benefit their mobility and independence, and which would be affordable at the same time. The author believes that by combining the existing technologies in a smart way and looking at the future of Internet of Things solutions, it is possible to come out with a smart, cost-efficient solution. There have been companies producing a variety of technologies for the blind and visually impaired segment. The most usual approach is that a regular device has been updated or modified for their use among visually impaired people. Screen reader or technologies, which transmit the message in a suitable form, are the most frequent examples. Many examples require multiple devices to work and there are successful examples of using a computer, but those are not focused on navigation (Ounapuu, 2016).

Five forces of today's solutions:

- Mobile—The product is mobile, as the devices can be used anywhere, anytime, by anyone.
- Social media—The social media perspective is created through the web application that also serves as a communication platform of the users. Live navigation data is fed for the community building purposes, in order to develop the navigation of the community of blind and visually impaired people, but also contribute to the navigation of everyone. Therefore, the public interest can be high also among the non-visually impaired, as the benefit of improved maps is evident.

- Data (Big Data)—The amounts of data sent from and to the device is enormous, as it happens on the go. Location data, error messages, messages exchanged via the voice command create a lot of useful data which can be used in the field of Connected Health, Connected Car, Connected Cities, Connected Living etc.
- Sensors—The device is equipped with sensors that detect the environment's dangerous objects to allow the person with visual impairment to know the distances etc.
- Location—Real-time location is used, as the GPS locating is a necessary tool for device usability. Location services enable improving locating the person in rural areas, where currently the navigation and location services are not so advanced yet.

A variety of tech-fuelled solutions are now enabling the visually impaired to experience their world in a more customized, intuitive, and independent way by creating solutions that are low cost and accessible to the roughly two million Britons living with some form of visual impairment.

Before developing his project Neatebox a few years ago, Gavin Neate formerly worked for Guide Dogs for the Blind helping, visually impaired individuals adjust to their guide dogs. After learning how blind people experienced the world, he recognized a problem with the conventional way that they interact with crosswalks. His idea uses something similar to iBeacon technology to enable a blind person to interact with a control box wirelessly, via an app on their phone.

A similar idea is London's Wayfindr app, in prototype phase, which was developed in partnership with the Royal London Society for the Blind's (RLSB) Youth Forum and ustwo, a product design studio. Also, using iBeacon technology, the app triangulates the user's position using their smartphone and then transmits instructions audibly, based on where the user wants to go. It is specifically targeted at London's roughly 9000 youth who are visually impaired and who report that they often suffer from a sense of lack of independence if they can't navigate public transport on their own.

Another tech solution to visual impairment, coming from MIT's Media Lab, refers to the fact that as technology advances, people are spending more and more time on tablets and digital devices. While trying to develop 3D screens that can be watched without special glasses, co-creator Gordon Wetzstein said he stumbled on the potential for another major solution.

Not designed specifically for blind people, but rather anyone with minor to major visual impairments, a prototype for vision correcting displays for e-readers, tablets or laptops has been developed to correct severe impairments, using a protective sleeve or cover glass (Huang, Wetzstein, Barsky, & Raskar, 2016).

However, for all people suffering from visual impairment (mild, moderate, severe, bling) the assistive technologies for mobility must offer the information about appropriate paths, dangers, distances, critical events, and interest points (hospitals, airports, train, railways, taxi and bus stations). Because in case of the visual impairment the reading acuity is lower, this inconvenient can be reduced by wearable voice-controlled virtual assistants.

3.2 Visual Impairments – Types and Causes

In this chapter, we will address the essential factors related to visual impairments, namely types of visual impairments, causes that lead to these types of affections, symptoms, most appropriate kind of treatment and diagnosis.

3.2.1 Types of Visual Impairments

Before analyzing the types of affections in the area of visual impairment, we must define what a visual impairment is.

Visual Impairment affections relate to a condition in which an individual's capacity to recognize things or objects are not healthy. The function of the eye for various reasons becomes limited.

Visual impairment affection can be anything covering from not being able to see near or far off things to partial or complete blindness. The capacity of an individual to recognize objects is termed as the visual acuity of the person and is a basis for diagnosing a person with Visual Impairment (Dandona & Dandona, 2006).

Therefore, the most common types of Visual Impairments are:

– Hypermetropia or farsightedness is a common affection where an individual is not able to see objects that are far away from him or her;
– Myopia or nearsightedness is another type of visual impairment in which an individual is not able to see accurately the objects that are near to him or her;
– Complete blindness is a severe condition that limits the individual sight capacity. Thus, the person is not able to see anything at all from both eyes.

Persons who have Partial Blindness are not able to see to some extent from one eye. Approximately one person in three has some form of vision-reducing eye disease by the age of 65. The most common causes of vision loss among the elderly are age-related macular degeneration, glaucoma, cataract, and diabetic retinopathy. Impairment due to medical conditions like diabetes causes diabetic retinopathy, which damages the retina to the extent that the ability of an individual to see gets significantly, affected (ePainAssist, 2018).

Accessibility and autonomy are fundamental needs for people with visual impairments wishing to enjoy their rights as citizens and to access buildings, premises, and other facilities. Dealing with the possibility of autonomously performing activities of daily living, two main aspects are mandatory: autonomous mobility and living independently. The literature is rich in attempts to provide technical solutions to improve the quality of life and autonomy for visually impaired people.

3.2.2 Cause of Visual Impairments

In order to perform a proper diagnosis of visual impairment affections, it is necessary to examine the leading causes. There are many causes for Visual Impairment, some are acquired, and some are congenital. The primary conditions which lead to Visual Impairment are:

- Eye Injury: A direct blow or injury to the eye, especially injuries to the cornea which are quite common, may result in Visual Impairment.
- Inherited Conditions: There are also cases in which Visual Impairment is an inherited condition. One such medical condition that is an inherited Visual Impairment is retinitis pigmentosa (Facts About Retinitis Pigmentosa, 2018). Stargardt disease (Tanna, Strauss, Fujinami, & Michaelides, 2017) is the most common form of inherited juvenile macular degeneration, occurring in one in every 8000–10,000 people worldwide. It causes a gradual loss of central vision. It is usually developed during childhood or adolescence, resulting in a loss of the central part of the visual field.
- Infectious eye diseases can involve the eyelids, conjunctiva, cornea, or other areas within the eye. Serious complications sometimes include cataract, glaucoma, retinal detachment, or vision loss. Uveitis (Uveitis/Infectious Diseases, 2018) refers to inflammation of the uvea, the middle layer of the eyeball, and this layer refers to the iris, ciliary body, and choroid.

The cornea is a frequent site of infection, especially from the herpes simplex virus, which is the most common reason in the U.S. for corneal blindness.

- Cataract is a medical condition originated by an accumulation of calcium in the lens of the eyes resulting in Visual Impairment. Cataract, more encountered in the elderly population, is mostly due to natural aging and wear and tear of the eyes. In the United States, cataract is one of the leading causes of blindness in the elderly population.
- Diabetic Retinopathy: Is a common affection in people with diabetes, while the blood sugar becomes significantly uncontrolled that the condition affects the retina of the eye causing Visual Impairment and ultimately leading to complete blindness in some cases.
- Glaucoma: is a medical condition and is caused by increased pressure on the optic nerves and thus damaging the optic nerve resulting in Visual Impairment. This condition is seen mostly in the elderly population but is also noticed in babies who are born with this condition.
- Macular Degeneration: This is an age-related medical condition determined by the progressive loss of vision in one eye or both and is caused due to natural degeneration of the macula.

3.2.3   Diagnosis of Visual Impairment Affections

The diagnosis of the cause of Visual Impairment starts with a history taking of the patient in which the physician inquires about when the symptoms started and how bad is the eyesight.

In order to do this, the ophthalmologist carries out a series of tests to determine the cause of the Visual Impairment and formulate the best treatment plan. Firstly, an eye examination is performed in which the ophthalmologist will inspect the eyelids, conjunctiva, cornea, and lens. Depending on what the ophthalmologist observed on the first examination the following tests are carried out:

– Snellen's Test: Also known as the Snellen's acuity test (Currie, Bhan, & Pepper, 2000), determines the patient's ability to recognize the letters shown on a Snellen chart; the patient' reads out random letters displayed in a progressively shortened manner.

  The test score resulted after this type of examination consists of two numbers. The first number implies the distance from where the patient was able to recognize the letters correctly and the second number is how far a healthy individual can be from the chart to read out the letters on the chart correctly. Typical testing distances for the Snellen chart are 20 ft and 6 m. If a subject can read a line at 20 ft and the "normal" observer can see the same line at 40 ft, then the subject has 20/40 Snellen acuity. Two drawbacks to the Snellen chart are that the chart has a different number of letters on each line and the size change of letters is not constant between lines. The Bailey-Lovie and ETDRS charts overcome these weaknesses by having a logarithmic reduction in letter size from line to line and a constant number of letters on each line. Visual acuity is sometimes specified in terms of LogMAR acuity to give a continuous number for it (Schwiegerling, 2004).

– Visual Field Test: A visual field test is an eye examination that can detect dysfunction in central and peripheral vision that is caused by various medical conditions such as glaucoma, stroke, pituitary disease, brain tumors, or other neurological deficits. This examination is performed with the help of a device strapped over the patient' eyes, by flashing intermittent lights in the periphery sight area of the patient's. There are several types of visual field tests. The patient is exposed to a set of moving targets of various light sizes, intensities are shown, and the patient indicates when they become visible in the peripheral vision. The resulting data is used to map the full visual field. The full, normal range of the visual field extends approximately 120° vertically and a nearly 160° horizontally (Bainter, 2018).

– Tonometry test—is often used to detect the presence of glaucoma. This test determines the fluid pressure inside the eye and can reveal if there is an increased fluid pressure in the eyes affecting the patient's vision.

3.3 Technologies Used for Visual Impairments

The usage of mobile screen reader for visual impairments has grown up to 82% in 2014 for 12% in 2009, by visual impairments we mean all people who are completely blind to those who have low vision.

Anyway, the people who are visually impaired are limited when it comes to the reading of textual elements and items on the screen along with some limited ability to enter text. There are a lot of examples of graphical apps that are very hard to access for visual impairments such as drawing apps, video games, maps, or scientific simulations.

Forwards we will talk about the solutions that have been proposed and tested in order to make the access of visual impairments to touchscreens much easier.

3.3.1 Visual Impairment Treatment Methods

The treatment methods for Visual Impairment affections vary depending on several factors: the extent of the condition, the precise cause of the Visual Impairment, but also depends on the age and general state of health of the patient.

In Table 3.1 shown below, we present the current treatment methods for the main visual impairments causes.

Table 3.1 Visual impairments—causes and treatments

Causes	Treatment
Diabetes	Essential for diabetes patients to maintain under strict control their blood sugars, this is the best course of treatment to avoid complications like diabetic retinopathy, where there is little to be done to improve the condition
Cataract	The best treatment for cataract is surgical intervention. Nowadays with the help of the advancement of medical equipment, cataract surgery has become relatively safe and can be performed with minimally invasive procedures. Even, after the surgery, an artificial lens is still required to correct the vision
Myopia, Hypermetropia	Magnification systems are the type of treatment that allows a significant improvement in the patient's sight with the help of proper lens, glasses, and prisms
Glaucoma	In an attempt to improve the Glaucoma patients' condition, medication is prescribed. In addition, surgical procedures and laser techniques can manage this affection
Macular degeneration	As of now, there is no specific treatment for macular degeneration

3.3.2   User Interface

First, we have to emphasize the fact that, nowadays, most of the small touchscreens are commercially available. The problem regarding this kind of touchscreens is that they have a low precision of target acquisition because of the big dimension of the finger compared to the small size of the target. The challenge of using devices through touchscreen for people with visual impairments consists in controlling the device without being able to see what their fingers are touching. Besides this, it is hard for them to make some gestures such as swiping, double or triple tapping or more complex gestures such as L shapes.

Vanderheiden in this regard has made the first research project in 1996. The system proposed in this project had a button at the top of the screen that could activate a spoken overall description of the screen. In addition, the user was allowed to scan through a list on a kiosk by sliding their finger around the screen and hearing each item spoken aloud. After that, they had the possibility to activate the last item they were at by pressing a hardware button.

Kocielinski and Brzostek who have improved the Vanderheiden's system have approached a similar technique. His project has allowed the user to select a new sublist of the main list. In this way, everything could be found faster.

Later, in 2008, Kane implemented new software on an iPhone, which used this time multi-touch gestures than single touch gestures. This software was functioning in the following way: the user holds down a finger on an item and, with another finger, he/she taps to activate the item. In this research, Kane had also included more complex gestures like L gestures to select a musical artist.

In the same year, McGookin created a system, which offers the possibility to search items in the list by swiping left to move up or right to move down. After that, the user can double-tap anywhere on the screen to select the last item he was at.

Lately, commercial screen readers have used most of these technologies in a certain way. Gestures like swiping left or right are largely used by people with visual impairments either to move one element to the left or to the right in a grid of icons, either to move up or down one item in a list. Swiping up and down action is used for moving up or down a heading.

In addition, there have been implemented multi-touch gestures, split tapping, and an amount of taps, which starts an overall description of all the elements on the screen from top to bottom. Among those who adopted these techniques is Apple with Apple's VoiceOver for iOS. They used it in July 2009 to the iPhone 3GS. Regarding Android, this kind of technology has been started on this operating system in October 2009 and it was called Android's TalkBack.

3.3.3   Braille Touchscreen Keyboards

In the case of Braille Keyboards, a key represents each Braille dot so that a Braille keyboard contains six keys. Every key makes up one Braille cell, which represents a character. The technique used by the user for typing is by chording, it means that the person who is using the keyboard presses multiple keys at the same time as a piano.

In the technological field, a Braille soft keyboard is already implemented on iOS 8 in 2012. This system has two modes of operation:

1. Screen away mode: In this mode, the user can type by wrapping three fingers from each hand around the edges to touch the screen.
2. Tabletop mode: In this mode, the user places six of his fingers on the screen.

The studies made using these three methods presented above, a physical Braille keyboard, the Screen away mode and Tabletop mode, showed that the typing rate was at around 20 words per minute, with error rates around 10%.

These types of Braille soft keyboards have also been used to implement educational games for children with visual impairments. The games were called BraillePlay and they give the opportunity to blind children to write Braille characters using vibration feedback. The operation mode of this game implies that the touchscreen is split in six sections, each of these sections representing one of the dots of a Braille character. The user could raise the dot that he wants by tapping one of those sections (Grussenmeyer & Folmer, 2017).

Similar researches have also been made using applications on a computer, an iPod or an iPad. Some examples of such applications are BrailleTouch, BrailleEasy, and AccessBraille (Gómez, Sánchez, López, & Rocha, 2017).

3.3.4 Google Glass as Assistive Technology

Google glass represents a smart gadget that offers the possibility to interact with the world using the Android operating system. These glasses allow you to interact with the web or internet using basic voice or vision commands.

The main advantages of the Google glasses are:

1. You can handle and wear them very easily.
2. You can access documents, images, videos, or maps very fast.
3. You can command them by natural voice language.
4. You can use it through Wi-Fi with android phones.

The biggest challenge of a person who suffers from visual impairments is dealing every day with orientation and navigation issues. In a limited area, such as an apartment, or a room, these kinds of problems are easy to solve but the real problem is when a blind person wants to go outside, in a noisy environment.

In order to solve this problem, an assistive application that is using a Google Glass (GG) has been developed. In this way the recognition of issues outdoors as well as indoor or their navigation will be much easier.

In the paper (Grussenmeyer & Folmer, 2017) two experiments are presented to prove that visual impairments can be independent by using this assistive technology:

the first experiment is about navigation issue and the second one deals with obstacles recognition.

Both the above cases have proved that this application using Google Glasses can help blind people or people who suffer from visual impairments to get to any place or recognize a lot of obstacles faster, easier and without assistance than any other technology (Berger, Vokalova, Maly, & Poulova, 2017).

3.4 Smart System Integrated to Improve Mobility

Care for people with multiple chronic conditions (multimorbidity) requires integrated and patient-centered approaches to adequately meet patient needs. Information and communication technology (ICT) applied in the health care sector (eHealth) constitutes a recognized driver of innovation and improvement in providing tailored and innovative care services to people with complex care needs. Despite the growing investment and interest in eHealth, there are challenges ahead for allowing a wider and more systematic adoption of ICT in the health care sector. This policy brief synthesizes available evidence on the implementation, benefits, and policies related to adopting mobile solutions for people with comorbidity in Europe (Barbabella, Melchiorre, Quattrini, Papa, & Lamura, 2017).

Some devices used for object detection are based on ultrasound, infrared, and LASER technologies, but they are not always effective. Another useful technology is the GPS, but this can't be used inside of buildings and it's not very accurate by itself. A smart cane is a white cane with electronic devices. If it is connected to a smartphone, it can provide vocal information regarding the environment to the person in need. This cane can also use the GPS data.

3.4.1 Useful Technologies

A big problem for people with visual impairments is the fact that they cannot avoid obstacles or recognize people's faces. This is very hard using only audio information, thus is very important to create a device that can do the work for them. Using neural learning techniques can help us with the face recognition part, storing images with friends and family in the database of a Smartphone. The system is much better than a guide dog because it can actually recognize the people in front of it and can send the information to the person in need. The article talks about a new image recognition and navigation system that provides accurate messages in audio form for visually challenged people. The system uses an Android-based mobile phone and some ultrasonic sensors. The sensors can communicate to the Smartphone via Bluetooth. The user can tell the destination and the application can guide the client to walk to the nearest transport station. The ultrasonic sensors send waves into the air and then recognize the objects by the reflected waves. The sensors send data to the Arduino microcontroller which converts the data into speech information (TTS).

Then this information is sending to the Smartphone via Bluetooth (Kumar et al., 2017).

In the paper (Ramadhan, 2018) a wearable smart system is presented to help visually impaired persons (VIPs) walk by themselves through the streets, navigate in public places, and seek assistance. The main components of the system are a microcontroller board, various sensors, cellular communication and GPS modules, and a solar panel. The system employs a set of sensors to track the path and alert the user of obstacles in front of them. The user is alerted by a sound emitted through a buzzer and by vibrations on the wrist, which is helpful when the user has hearing loss or is in a noisy environment. In addition, the system alerts people in the surroundings when the user stumbles over or requires assistance, and the alert, along with the system location, is sent as a phone message to registered mobile phones of family members and caregivers. In addition, the registered phones can be used to retrieve the system location whenever required and activate real-time tracking of the VIP. We tested the system prototype and verified its functionality and effectiveness. The proposed system has more features than other similar systems. We expect it to be a useful tool to improve the quality of life of VIPs.

In the paper (Al-Fahoum, Al-Hmoud, & Al-Fraihat, 2013) a system is proposed that uses three IR sensors and a PIC microcontroller. The sensors perceive the reflective signals and can help the microcontroller to codify the obstacles. This system is very ingenious because the users can get rid of the cane and only wear a hat and a mini stick in which the sensors are placed. Proteus is a software used to simulate a microprocessor, schematic capture, and PCB design. Proteus-VSM can also simulate embedded software and the hardware design of some microcontrollers. This is useful because we can test and modify the system before implementing it. The PIC Microcontroller is a small computer that can store a lot of instructions. Mixed-signal microcontrollers can control non-digital systems. This type of microcontroller can detect a switch triggered and generate the audio sounds and vibrations so it can be very useful for developing a device that can help people in need. PIC operates at +5V and it runs only if its crystal oscillator is used to execute the programming code. IR sensors can be used to acquire details about the environment, such as the nature of the obstacles around. We can place sensors in strategic places so they can scan the area. The objects in the scanning range will be reflected and received by the receiver unit.

3.4.2 Assistive Technologies for Visual Impairment Mobility by IoM and IoMT

Assistive technology is a technology to support people with disabilities and consists in devices and tools designed to improve the functional capabilities of individuals with disabilities (Bouck, 2015).

IoM (internet of mobility) (Frulio et al., 2017) enables the Mobility as a Service (MaaS) (Hietanen, 2014) new transport software and information for all citizens.

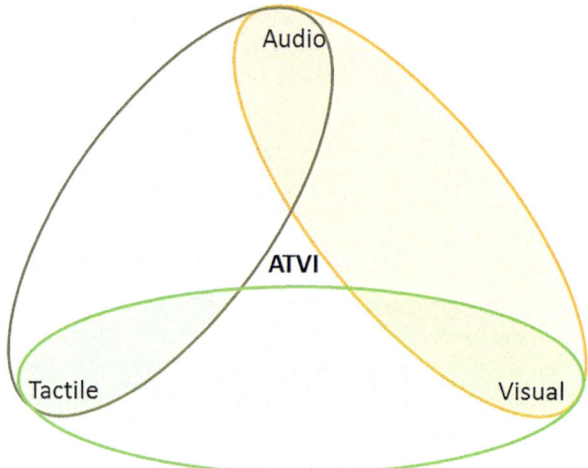

Fig. 3.1 Senses for improving the mobility for people with visual impairment

Internet of Mobile Things (IoMT) is the internet of interconnected devices as mobile phones, trains, and cars, where sensors networks are changing and influencing how people move, communicate, access the distributed information (Nahrstedt, 2014).

Assistive technology for visual impairment (ATVI) involves using the senses such as tactically, smell and hearing (Hersh & Johnson, 2010). The three senses can be used in assistive device all three, taken by two or by one (Fig. 3.1) in order to give rise or strengthen the visual signal.

In general, the technologies that assist people with visual impairments are wearable devices (sensors, actuators and small computers, smartphones) and software apps based on sensors networks (e.g. GPS, maps, cloud services, transport information) generate the internet of mobility and internet of mobile things.

Wearable devices used in assistive technologies for visual impairments use several sensors such as:

- Photoelectric sensors (IR sensors) based on transmitter that sends a light beam (visible or infrared) to an object A, and a receiver that receives the light emitted by the object A;
- Ultrasonic sensors that emit a high-frequency sound beam from transmitter to the object B and detect a reflection of the beam from the object B with its receiver;
- Camera
- Microphone
- Headphone
- Vibration actuators for haptic navigation (Ahlmark, 2016; Kammoun, Jouffrais, Guerreiro, Nicolau, & Jorge, 2012)

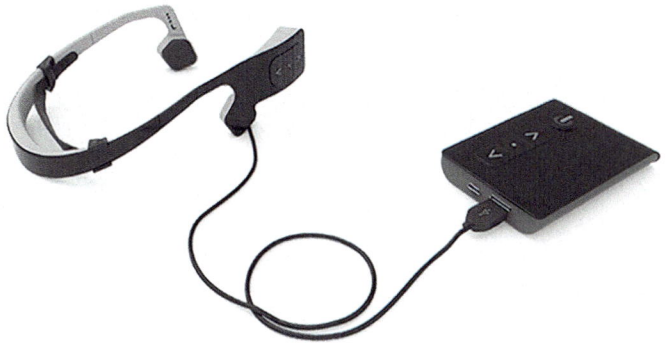

Fig. 3.2 Horus—personal assistant (Munger, Hilkes, Perron, & Sohi, 2017)

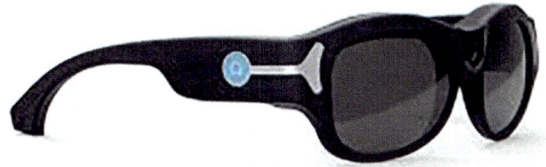

Fig. 3.3 AIRA smart glasses video camera (AIRA, 2018)

The assistive technology for people with visual impairments or blindness, based on augmented reality, uses vision and speech recognition technologies.

Several commercial assistive technologies that allow independent mobility of the people with visual impairment are:

- **Horus** (Fig. 3.2) developed by Eyra is a wearable assistant system with cameras and voice control, which can be worn as a headphone and can be used for mobility assistance by reading text, object identification, and face recognition (Horus, 2018).
- **AIRA** (Fig. 3.3) is a wearable personal assistant based on smart glass video camera for text reading, signing, and helping the wearer in independent mobility (AIRA, 2018).
- **eSIGHT** (Fig. 3.4) is a wearable device with a small camera that streams to a computer and after image processing the results are seen by the user through two Organic-LED screens (To & Régo, 2017).
- **BuzzClip** (iMerciv) is a wearable device for people with visual impairment. The BuzzClip device (Fig. 3.5) uses ultrasound to detect the obstacles that may occur directly in a person's path (BuzzClip, 2018).
- **Sunu Band** (Fig. 3.6) is smart bands that allow people with impairment to walk and travel guiding the wearer way around obstacles. The wearable device uses sonar or echolocation to detect objects up to 16 ft or 5.5 m away and the haptic vibration feedback informs how far away the obstacle is (Sunu, Inc., n.d.).

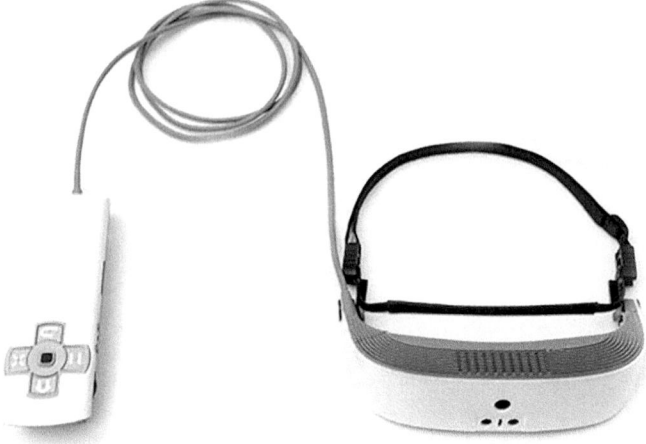

Fig. 3.4 eSIGHT—High-tech smart glasses with camera and OLED display (To & Régo, 2017)

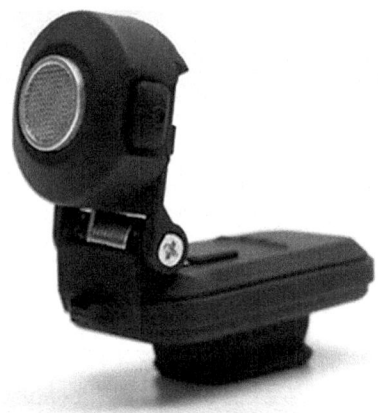

Fig. 3.5 BuzzClip—wearable device for obstacle detection (BuzzClip, 2018)

- **Maptic** (Tucker, 2017)—E. Farrington-Arnas (Fig. 3.7) is a wearable navigation system for people with visual impairments. The system is based on a visual sensor that can be worn like a necklace, and a series of feedback units that can be clipped onto clothing or worn around the wrist. The sensor connects to a voice-controlled iPhone app and the wearer can use GPS directly through a series of vibrations to the left or right side of the body.
- **3D Soundscape (AfterShokz & Microsoft)**, based on bone conducting head-phone, is a device that combines a Windows Phone handset (Lumia) with a bone-conducting headset to deliver a multitude of useful audio cues to the inner ear of the wearer (Fig. 3.8). The device uses smartphone's GPS and

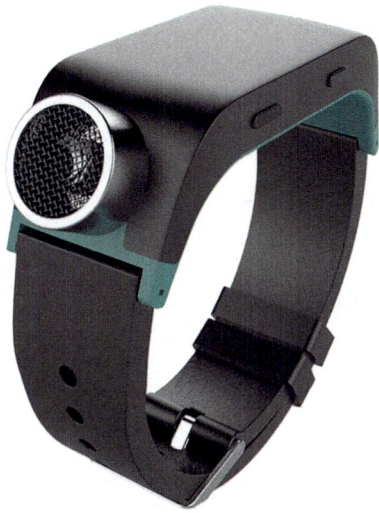

Fig. 3.6 Sunu Band—smart band to avoid obstacles (Sunu Inc., n.d.)

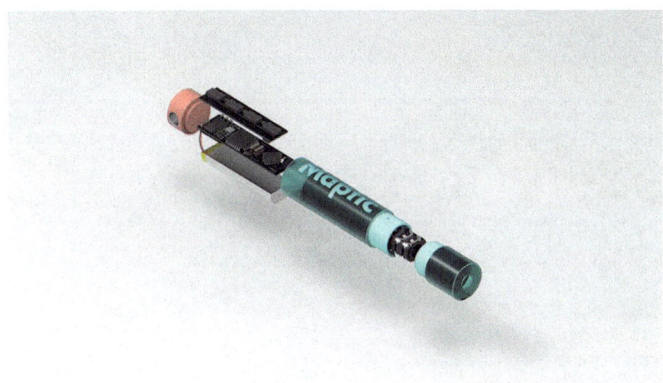

Fig. 3.7 Maptic device—wearable navigation system (Tucker, 2017)

accelerometer sensors while noticing prompts from specially installed Bluetooth and Wi-Fi. Cloud-based location and navigation data from Bing Maps provide contextual information such as transport and points of interest in the location (Shahrestani, 2017).

- **Seeing AI is an app developed by** Microsoft to assist people who are blind and visual impaired (Fig. 3.9). The app is cloud and AI based in order to help through recognizing objects, people, and text (Seeing AI, n.d.).
- **EVA** (Fig. 3.10) is a voice-controlled smart glass for the visually impaired, based on artificial intelligence for recognizing the objects, texts, signs, and verbally describes what it sees ("EVA—Extended Visual Assistant," n.d.).

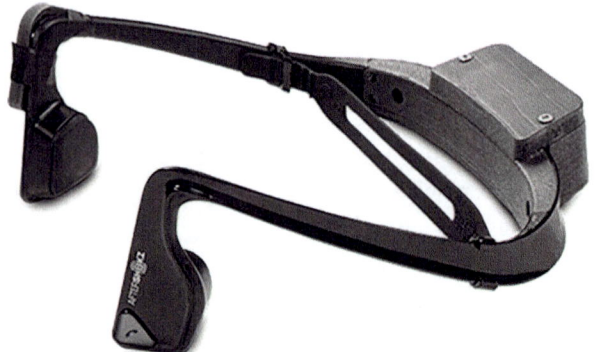

Fig. 3.8 3D Soundscape—bone-conducting headphone for contextual navigation (Lamkin, 2015)

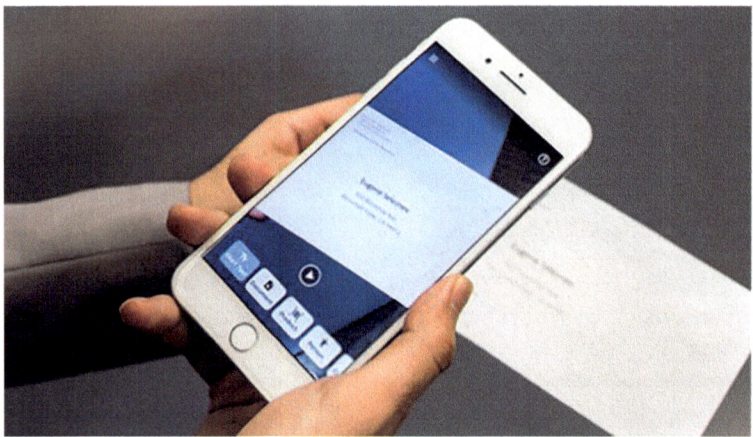

Fig. 3.9 Seeing AI app (Seeing AI, n.d.)

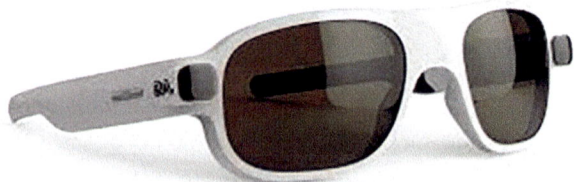

Fig. 3.10 EVA—voice-controlled smart glass ("EVA—Extended Visual Assistant," n.d.)

3.5 Future Challenge in Mobility Improvement for Visual Impairment

In terms of visual impairment domain, among the major problems—low vision or total loss of it—there is still a concern about the mobility of those people. There have been multiple researches and studies to improve the mobility for those people and the conclusions are the following:

- People with visual impairments are facing a major impediment in accessing various areas of health clubs and fitness facilities. AIMFREE (Accessibility Instruments Measuring Fitness and Recreation Environments) is an important tool for increasing awareness of the problems that those people are dealing and it offers some solutions (Rimmer, Riley, Wang, & Rauworth, 2005).
- Partial loss of vision increases crash risk in older drivers. The elderly people suffering from visual processing impairment, eyes diseases and visual dysfunction cause the most vehicle crashes (Rimmer et al., 2005).
- The use of the Alexander Technique (a method of changing movements' habits for improving freedom of movement) did not have a significant impact on the primary outcomes but its results include fewer falls and injurious falls and improved the mobility among past multiple-fallers suggest further investigation of this case (Owsley et al., 1998).

One of the future challenges for improving the mobility of visual impairments patients is related to the improvement of existing solutions:

- Residual Vision Glasses (RVGs)
  These glasses use a head-mounted depth camera in order to present relevant information about the distance of obstacles to the person with visual impairment, and their brightness so that the obstacles closer to the wearer are represented brighter. This allowed finding correlates of obstacle detection and hesitations in walking behavior. The participants of the developed study were able to use the smart glasses to navigate the course, and the mobility performance improved for those visually impaired participants with a greater level of visual impairment. However, the walking speed was lower and hesitations increased with the altered visual representation (Gleeson, Sherrington, Lo, & Keay, 2015).
- The VROOM and OMO tools
  The VROOM (Vision-Related Outcomes in Orientation and Mobility) and OMO (Orientation and Mobility Outcomes) tools are designed to be used in the same discussed domain, but they measure different phenomena, producing a separate score for functional vision and for functional O&M (Orientation and Mobility). Studies conducted in this area are investigating several aspects— avoiding obstacles on a prescribed course, following a white line on a dark floor and locating a contrasting door or a sign on a door (van Rheede et al., 2015). An implementation can be done using image processing from a stereoscopic camera for real-time autonomous system navigation (Mihalcea, Suciu, & Vasilescu, 2018).

- Night-Vision Goggles

  The University of Groningen has been conducting a study which investigated whether the usage of Night-Vision Goggles has improved the life of people suffering from visual impairment. Twenty night-blind subjects with retinitis requested to walk predetermined routes at night with and without NVGs. The number of unintended contacts with obstacles (hits) and the percentage of preferred walking speed (PPWS) en route were assessed in three different situations: a darkened indoor corridor; a moderately lit outdoor residential area; and a well-lit outdoor shopping area. Using NVGs seems to improve nighttime mobility in dark outdoor conditions by decreasing the number of unintended contacts with obstacles and increasing walking speed (Hartong, Jorritsma, Neve, Melis-Dankers, & Kooijman, 2004).

- Braille watches and printers

  Braille, also known as blind language, is used to represent letters, numbers, and punctuation marks for people experiencing visual impairment. In order to ease the life of those people, there have been conceived several solutions in terms of Braille language:

  – SARA device by Freedom Scientific allows people to convert a normal book to a braille edition, connecting to this device PAC Mate™ Braille Display (SARA CE, n.d.).
  – Braille watches allowing people to "read" the exact time by touching the display and feeling the small dots coming above.
  – Braille printer and embosser that render text in braille form.

- Assistive device for orientation and mobility of the visually impaired based on MM wave (millimeter wave) radar technology.

  The operation of this assistive device is based on the FMCW (frequency-modulated continuous wave) radar principle. This means a device transmits and receives radio waves, and then determines the distance and direction of possible obstacles in front of the user based on the received signal properties. The information is then sent to the user using haptic feedback and/or by sound signals. The results indicate important benefits in orientation and mobility registered to people who are the deaf blind, people with low vision and ones living in rural areas (Kiuru et al., 2018). The lowest benefits were encountered to blinds, people living alone and guide dog owners.

References

Ahlmark, D. I. (2016). *Haptic Navigation Aids for the Visually Impaired* (Doctoral dissertation, Luleå tekniska Universitet, 2016).

Al-Fahoum, A. S., Al-Hmoud, H. B., & Al-Fraihat, A. A. (2013). A smart infrared microcontroller-based blind guidance system. *Active and Passive Electronic Components, 2013*, 726480.

Bainter, P. S. (2018). *Visual field test: Learn how the procedure is performed*. Retrieved September 10, 2018, from https://www.medicinenet.com/visual_field_test/article.htm

Barbabella, F., Melchiorre, M. G., Quattrini, S., Papa, R., & Lamura, G. (2017). *How can eHealth improve care for people with multimorbidity in Europe?* Copenhagen: World Health Organization, Regional Office for Europe.

Berger, A., Vokalova, A., Maly, F., & Poulova, P. (2017). Google glass used as assistive technology its utilization for blind and visually impaired people. In *International Conference on Mobile Web and Information Systems* (pp. 70–82). Cham: Springer.

Bouck, E. (2015). *Assistive technology.* Los Angeles, CA: Sage.

Currie, Z., Bhan, A., & Pepper, I. (2000). Reliability of Snellen charts for testing visual acuity for driving: Prospective study and postal questionnaire. *BMJ, 321*(7267), 990–992.

Dandona, L., & Dandona, R. (2006). Revision of visual impairment definitions in the International Statistical Classification of Diseases. *BMC Medicine, 4,* 7.

Elgendy, M., & Lanyi, C. S. (2018). Review on smart solutions for people with visual impairment. In *International Conference on Computers Helping People with Special Needs* (pp. 81–84). Cham: Springer.

EVA. (n.d.). *Extended visual assistant.* Budapest: EVA. Retrieved October 11, 2018, from http://www.eva.vision/

Frulio, F., Sheikhi, E., Rossazza, L., Perfetto, G., Calvachi, A., Picco, G., & Comai, S. (2017). IOM–Internet of Mobility: A wearable device for outdoor data collection. In *International Conference on Smart Objects and Technologies for Social Good* (pp. 88–95). Cham: Springer.

Gleeson, M., Sherrington, C., Lo, S., & Keay, L. (2015). Can the Alexander Technique improve balance and mobility in older adults with visual impairments? A randomized controlled trial. *Clinical Rehabilitation, 29*(3), 244–260.

Gómez, N. L. C., Sánchez, Á. Q., López, E. K. G., & Rocha, M. A. M. (2017). SBK: Smart braille keyboard for learning braille literacy in blind or visually impaired people. In *Proceedings of the 8th Latin American Conference on Human-Computer Interaction* (p. 26). New York, NY: ACM.

Grussenmeyer, W., & Folmer, E. (2017). Accessible touchscreen technology for people with visual impairments: A survey. *ACM Transactions on Accessible Computing (TACCESS), 9*(2), 6.

Hartong, D. T., Jorritsma, F. F., Neve, J. J., Melis-Dankers, B. J., & Kooijman, A. C. (2004). Improved mobility and independence of night-blind people using night-vision goggles. *Investigative Ophthalmology & Visual Science, 45*(6), 1725–1731.

Hersh, M., & Johnson, M. A. (2010). *Assistive technology for visually impaired and blind people.* Berlin: Springer Science & Business Media.

Hietanen, S. (2014). Mobility as a service. The new transport model. *ITS & Transport Management Supplement. Eurotransport, 12*(2), 2–4.

Home - Aira. (2018). Retrieved October 11, 2018, from https://aira.io/

Home - Horus. (2018). Retrieved October 11, 2018, from http://horus.tech

Huang, F. C., Wetzstein, G., Barsky, B., & Raskar, R. (2016). *U.S. Patent No. 14/823,906.* Washington, DC: U.S. Patent and Trademark Office.

iMerciv Inc. (2018). *The all new BuzzClip.* Toronto, ON: iMerciv Inc. Retrieved October 10, 2018, from https://imerciv.com/

Kammoun, S., Jouffrais, C., Guerreiro, T., Nicolau, H., & Jorge, J. (2012). Guiding blind people with haptic feedback. *Frontiers in Accessibility for Pervasive Computing (Pervasive 2012),* 3.

Kerkar, P. (2018). *Visual impairment: Types, causes, symptoms, treatment, diagnosis.* Palm Harbor, FL: PainAssist Inc. Retrieved September 01, 2018, from https://www.epainassist.com/eye-pain/visual-impairment

Kiuru, T., Metso, M., Utriainen, M., Metsävainio, K., Jauhonen, H. M., Rajala, R., . . . Sylberg, J. (2018). Assistive device for orientation and mobility of the visually impaired based on millimeter wave radar technology—Clinical investigation results. *Cogent Engineering, 5,* 1450322.

Kumar, P. M., Gandhi, U., Varatharajan, R., Manogaran, G., Jidhesh, R., & Vadivel, T. (2017). Intelligent face recognition and navigation system using neural learning for smart security in Internet of Things. *Cluster Computing,* 1–12.

Lamkin, P. (2015). *Microsoft's headset for the visually impaired gets voice controls*. London: Wareable Ltd.. Retrieved October 10, 2018, from https://www.wareable.com/wearable-tech/microsoft-bone-conduction-headset-for-the-blind-448

MedlinePlus. (2018). *Vision impairment and blindness*. Bethesda, MD: MedlinePlus. Retrieved October 10, 2018, from https://www.who.int/en/news-room/fact-sheets/detail/blindness-and-visual-impairment

Mihalcea, G., Suciu, G., & Vasilescu, C. (2018). Real-time autonomous system of navigation using a stereoscopic camera. In *2018 International Conference on Communications (COMM)* (pp. 497–500). Washington, DC: IEEE.

Munger, R. J., Hilkes, R. G., Perron, M., & Sohi, N. (2017). *U.S. Patent No. 9,618,748*. Washington, DC: U.S. Patent and Trademark Office.

Nahrstedt, K. (2014). Internet of mobile things: Challenges and opportunities. In *PACT* (pp. 1–2). New York, NY: ACM.

National Eye Institute. (2018). *Facts about retinitis pigmentosa*. Bethesda, MD: National Eye Institute. Retrieved September 04, 2018, from https://nei.nih.gov/health/pigmentosa/pigmentosa_facts

Ounapuu, E. (2016). *VisioPal - Smart solution to the visually impaired and blind*, Tallinn University of Technology, Faculty of Information Technology.

Owsley, C., Ball, K., McGwin, G., Jr., Sloane, M. E., Roenker, D. L., White, M. F., & Overley, E. T. (1998). Visual processing impairment and risk of motor vehicle crash among older adults. *JAMA, 279*(14), 1083–1088.

Ramadhan, A. J. (2018). Wearable smart system for visually impaired people. *Sensors, 18*(3), 843.

Research to Prevent Blindness. (2018). *Uveitis/infectious diseases*. New York, NY: Research to Prevent Blindness. Retrieved September 04, 2018, from https://www.rpbusa.org/rpb/resources-and-advocacy/resources/rpb-vision-resources/infectious-diseases/

Rimmer, J. H., Riley, B., Wang, E., & Rauworth, A. (2005). Accessibility of health clubs for people with mobility disabilities and visual impairments. *American Journal of Public Health, 95*(11), 2022–2028.

SARA CE. (n.d.). Retrieved September 6, 2018, from http://www.envisiontechnology.org/html/visually_impaired.html#SARA

Schwiegerling, J. (2004). *Field guide to visual and ophthalmic optics*. Bellingham WA: SPIE.

Seeing AI. (n.d.). Retrieved October 11, 2018, from https://www.microsoft.com/en-us/seeing-ai

Shahrestani, S. (2017). *Internet of things and smart environments: Assistive technologies for disability, dementia, and aging*. New York, NY: Springer.

Sunu, Inc. (n.d.). *It's your world. Explore it with the Sunu Band*. Somerville, MA: Sunu, Inc. Retrieved October 10, 2018, from https://www.sunu.io/en/index.html

Tanna, P., Strauss, R. W., Fujinami, K., & Michaelides, M. (2017). Stargardt disease: Clinical features, molecular genetics, animal models and therapeutic options. *British Journal of Ophthalmology, 101*(1), 25–30.

To, H., & Régo, N. (2017). *eSight 3: A day will come when all legally blind individuals can get esight at no cost*. Cool Blind Tech. Retrieved October 12, 2018, from https://coolblindtech.com/esight-3-a-day-will-come-when-all-legally-blind-individuals-can-get-esight-at-no-cost/

Tucker, E. (2017). *Maptic is a wearable navigation system for the visually impaired*. London: Dezeen. Retrieved October 10, 2018, from https://www.dezeen.com/2017/08/02/maptic-wearable-guidance-system-visually-impaired-design-products-wearable-technology-graduates

van Rheede, J. J., Wilson, I. R., Qian, R. I., Downes, S. M., Kennard, C., & Hicks, S. L. (2015). Improving mobility performance in low vision with a distance-based representation of the visual scene. *Investigative Ophthalmology & Visual Science, 56*(8), 4802–4809.

Chapter 4
Comprehensive Literature Reviews on Ground Plane Checking for the Visually Impaired

Aylwin Bing Chun Chai, Bee Theng Lau, Zheng Pan, Almon WeiYen Chai, Lil Deverell, Abdullah Al Mahmud, Christopher McCarthy, and Denny Meyer

4.1 Introduction

The World Health Organization (WHO) reported the key fact that approximately 1.3 billion people live with vision impairment globally (WHO, 2018). Approximately 36 million of this population are totally blind. Besides that, WHO estimated that the number of people with vision impairment could become triple due to population growth and ageing. This also indicates that the need for assistive devices will be increased for the group of people with visual impairment to aid in their daily navigation and orientation.

White cane and trained guide dogs are the tools that have been widely used by people with vision impairment for many years. These traditional aids have been shown to assist daily navigation for many in the vision impaired community (Dakopoulos & Bourbakis, 2010). However, these aids are limited in the assistance they provide, particularly in providing full information of the surrounding area to support safe travel. Therefore, electronic assistive technologies have been introduced and developed to further support the daily activities of the vision impaired.

Vision loss can have a profound effect on a person's quality of life and independence. In particular, the ability to travel safely and independently is a well-documented challenge for people with vision impairment, and amongst the most

A. B. C. Chai (✉) · B. T. Lau · Z. Pan · A. W. Chai
Swinburne University of Technology, Sarawak, Malaysia
e-mail: achun@swinburne.edu.my; blau@swinburne.edu.my; pzheng@swinburne.edu.my; achai@swinburne.edu.my

L. Deverell · A. A. Mahmud · C. McCarthy · D. Meyer
Swinburne University of Technology, Melbourne, VIC, Australia
e-mail: ldeverell@swin.edu.au; aalmahmud@swin.edu.au; cdmccarthy@swin.edu.au; dmeyer@swin.edu.au

© Springer Nature Switzerland AG 2020
S. Paiva (ed.), *Technological Trends in Improved Mobility of the Visually Impaired*,
EAI/Springer Innovations in Communication and Computing,
https://doi.org/10.1007/978-3-030-16450-8_4

highly valued functional capabilities to retain (Deverell, Bentley, Ayton, Delany, & Keeffe, 2017). Primary challenges related to safe and independent mobility for people with vision impairment are obstacles and ground plane conditions. While previous literature reviews of low vision assistive technologies have focused mainly on front-on obstacle detection, few have considered technologies that support the detection of ground plane hazards. The ground plane hazards include the staircases, potholes, pits, ramps, ditches, and loose surfaces. Thus, the main focus in this literature review is the assistive devices that carried out the detection on the ground plane hazards.

Domestic space is a complex environment with various obstacles at the surroundings: right, left, top, and bottom. The congestion of such obstacles can cause problems sometimes even for normally sighted people, so what about people with visual impairment? The decision making of the visually impaired often support by the external assistance provided by white canes, trained dogs, humans, or smart electronic devices. Existing devices can detect and recognize objects that present on the floor, but a real risk also comes from the hazards on the floor, for example, drainage, potholes, or staircases.

4.2   Taxonomy of Assistive Technologies

In reviewing the range of assistive technologies available, Dakopoulos and Bourbakis derived a taxonomy for assistive technologies, as shown in Fig. 4.1 (Dakopoulos & Bourbakis, 2010). There are three sub-categories under the category of the vision substitution, which includes electronic travel aids (ETAs), electronic orientation aids (EOAs), and position locator devices (PLDs).

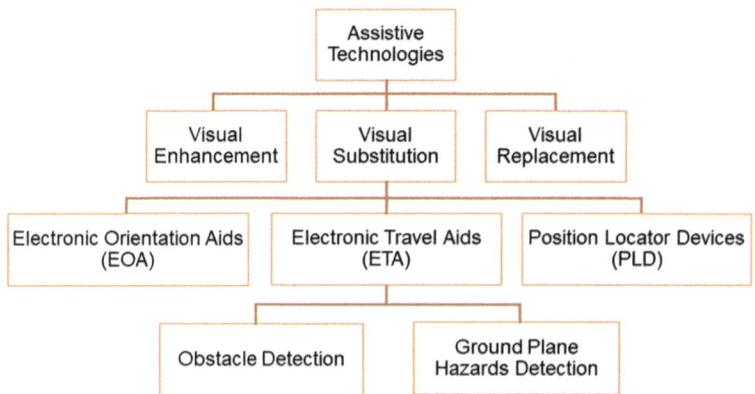

Fig. 4.1 Classification of assistive technologies for the visually impaired (Dakopoulos & Bourbakis, 2010)

Electronic travel aids (ETAs) act as a visual substitution which provides extension towards the perception of the environment outside the reach of the fingertip, tip of the long cane, or handle of the dog guide's harness (Reynolds, Vannest, & Fletcher-Janzen, 2015). ETA provides feedback in the form of auditory sound or tactile vibrations to guide the visually impaired in preventing obstacles and for navigation purposes.

Electronic orientation aids (EOAs) are visual substitution devices that provide orientation for the visually impaired when travelling around (Dakopoulos & Bourbakis, 2010). Position locator devices (PLDs) are devices equipped with technologies like GPS or any navigation services.

The selected articles were divided into two main categories under the electronic travel aids (ETA) which is part of the visual substitution among all the assistive technologies. The two main categories are obstacle detection which is the focus of the current market and the ground plane hazards detection which have little attention in the market.

4.3 Ground Plane Hazards

This section discusses different types of ground plane hazards that will be encountered by the visually impaired. The techniques that have been developed to tackle the different ground plane hazards were discussed in the following section.

According to Deverell et al. (2017), checking the ground plane is one of the travel functions for human and this can be travel difficulties for the people with low or no vision. Deverell developed the VROOM and OMO tools for rating the travel difficulties of the people with low or no vision. The VROOM instrument is a constructivist measure of Vision-Related Outcomes in Orientation and Mobility while the OMO instrument is a constructivist measure of Orientation and Mobility Outcomes (Deverell et al., 2017). These tools allow the researcher to identify the travel difficulties such as getting your bearings, checking ground plane, way finding, recognizing moving parts, and finding things.

Within the travel difficulties suggested by Deverell et al. (2017), checking ground plane would include the ability to recognize steps, ramps, rough ground, or loose surface. This ability is important for the people to prevent falls risk and adjust their position, posture, and balance. Thus, the following sections will look into the smart technologies that help in this travel challenge for the visually impaired.

4.4 Techniques to Detect Obstacles and Ground Plane Hazards

This section discusses assistive devices that have been developed over the past decade, with a primary focus on obstacle detection, staircases or steps detection, ramp, drainage, and loose surface detection. The technologies used in the devices and their limitations are also discussed.

4.4.1 Assistive Device for Obstacle Detection

Range Sensors Based Assistive Technologies

In 2006, Jacquet et al. reviewed existing locomotion supporting low vision assistive devices based on the sensors used and the user interfaces employed (Jacquet, Bellik, & Bourda, 2006). This included devices based on infrared sensing (the Tom Pouce), ultrasonic sensing (the Miniguide, the Polaron, and the UltraCane) and laser telemeters (the Teletact).

The researchers suggested devices utilizing infrared and ultrasonic sensing were, in general, easier to use as compared to laser devices. The very narrow sensing width of laser devise compared with infrared and ultrasonic was the primary factor attributed with this, due to the need for users to scan the environment from side to side when using laser devices. As for the user interfaces, the tactile vibration feedback is preferable for the beginners as it is direct and easier to understand. However, if the user was trained to use the audio output, then the audible feedback was preferred due to its higher precision. From the evaluation, the researchers note that both tactile and audio interfaces need a good spatial representation and proprioception to scan for obstacles in the environment. Also, this would be especially difficult for people who are blind from birth as they do not have the spatial representation abilities (Jacquet et al., 2006).

The Ultracane and the Miniguide represent the two most popular electronic travel aids (ETAs) over the last 10 years. Roentgen et al. carried out a study to evaluate the performance of these two ETAs (Roentgen, Gelderblom, & de Witte, 2012). The mobility performance of these two devices was evaluated based on several criteria such as changes in the travel speed, Percentage of Preferred Walking Speed (PPWS), type and number of mobility incidents made. Results from an indoor mobility course showed that while both ETAs reduced the walking speed of visually impaired participants, both also reduced the total number of the mobility incidents. The authors also reported that there were two another aspect that the users were not very satisfied which are the weight and the safety of the devices.

Lopes et al. proposed the development of a series of electronic mobility aids for the blind (Lopes, Vieira, Lopes, Rosa, & Dias, 2012). The set of devices consists of the MobiFree Cane, MobiFree Sunglasses, and MobiFree Echo. The idea behind the MobiFree concept is to create a network that links all the possible mobility aids to work together through a dedicated Wireless Personal Area Network (WPAN). The MobiFree Cane is an improved long cane that is able to detect the holes and drop-offs at the floor level. Lopes et al. presented the MobiFree Sunglasses and MobiFree Echo in the form of conceptual design in the paper and both are yet to be developed. The MobiFree Cane is equipped with ultrasonic sensors to perform the hole and drop-offs detection. The device keeps track of the distance from the cane to the ground and provides feedback to the user through vibration. Field test results of the MobiFree Cane show it is able to detect drop-offs and holes reliably from one step ahead of the user. However, participants also noted that the cane is heavy.

Bhatlawande et al. proposed an electronic navigation system for detecting obstacles within 5 m range in front, left, and right direction (Bhatlawande, Mukhopadhyay, & Mahadevappa, 2012). The system is made up of spectacles and a waist-belt. These two devices are equipped with five ultrasonic sensor pairs. The system uses ultrasonic sensors to measure the distance from detected obstacles in all frontal direction. This is a basic obstacle detection system and it was unable to detect the ground level obstacles.

Prattico et al. proposed a new hybrid electronic travel aid that is made up of two infrared sensors, one ultrasonic sensor, and four vibration motors (Prattico, Cera, & Petroni, 2013). All the components are located on the waist belt to be worn by the user. The infrared sensors are placed on the left and right of the devices. As the device is a wearable, the researchers implemented a low-pass filter to smooth the output signals from the sensors. The reason for including an ultrasonic sensor is to solve the issue that the infrared sensors cannot intercept a glass or mirror. The users are notified about the presence of the obstacles in front through vibrating motors. The experimental results are not included by the researchers and thus the performance is unknown.

Leduc-Mills et al. proposed a mobility aid that is attachable to the traditional white cane. The mobility aid is called ioCane. The ioCane system consists of an obstacle detection system with three Maxbotic LV series ultrasonic sensors, and a smartphone running a custom Android application (Leduc-Mills, Profita, Bharadwaj, & Cromer, 2013). The first ultrasonic sensor is used to detect overhanging obstacles at head level. The second ultrasonic sensor points at a level slightly above ground to detect low obstacles. The third rear-facing ultrasonic sensor always points to the ground and is used for calibration. The system uses the height value from the sensor to keep track of the change in holding the position of the cane to obtain the exact angle for calculation of the distance to obstacles in real time. When obstacles are detected, the ioCane system uses the mobile phone to provide feedback to the users through chimes and vibrations. The Android app presents the three sensor values and allows to set up the basic information such as the length of the cane and the height of the user.

The testing results showed that ioCane has an improvement in the obstacle avoidance when compared against the traditional white cane. The vibration feedback from the mobile phone is not useful as the vibration is not strong enough if the phone is placed on the pocket or hung around the neck. The ioCane system only focuses on the obstacle detection and is unable to detect the ground state for the visually impaired (Leduc-Mills et al., 2013).

The Walk Safe Cane (WSC) is a navigation aid that helps the visually impaired to detect obstacles in front with the distance and the velocity measurement (Kumar, 2014). Consisting of an Arduino UNO microcontroller, three ultrasonic sensors, and a transmitting module (X-Bee), the detection system is attached to a modified white cane. Additionally, the researchers developed an audible alert system to communicate the presence of obstacles when detected. The alert system consists of three buzzers attached to a bib, each buzzer associated with a corresponding ultrasonic sensor oriented in different directions. The experimental trials were conducted on a group of blindfolded volunteers and the results were promising according to the researcher. However, the researcher did not present any experimental result data and stated that further trials will be conducted.

Ahlmark developed two prototypes of navigation aids that can convey the spatial information non-visually by using a haptic interface: the Virtual White Cane and the LaserNavigator. The authors note the use of a haptic interface allows similar interactions to that of a white cane (Ahlmark, 2016).

The virtual white cane is an additional device added to the existing autonomous powered wheelchair, MICA. The MICA is equipped with a SICK LMS111 laser rangefinder that is able to scan the environment to identify the distance to objects in front of the wheelchair. The virtual white cane is made up of a Novint Falcon haptic interface and a laptop. The laptop is used to collect the range information from the rangefinder and then builds a 3-D model so that the information can be presented to the visually impaired through the haptic interface (Ahlmark, 2016). Field trials with six white cane users showed that experience with the white cane allowed users to quickly adapt to the virtual white cane. However, one participant noted that they were unable to estimate the position of the obstacles that they felt.

The LaserNavigator was developed based on the evaluation from the Virtual White Cane, aiming to complement to the standard white cane by allowing the user to perceive the surrounding environment when necessary (Ahlmark, 2016). Consisting of a laser rangefinder, an ultrasonic sensor, a loudspeaker, and micro-controller, the LaserNavigator simulate a standard white cane as it consists of an automatic length adjustment which varies the length of the detection by moving the device towards or away from the body. For haptic feedback, a small loudspeaker was attached on which the user places the finger rather than the conventional vibration actuator because of its quick response time. In a field trial, participants were able to use the prototype to complete the tasks and demonstrated improvement over repeated trials. However, one participant noted high when using the devices due to its weight and integrating its use together with the white cane.

Bernieri et al. present a smart glove equipped with rangefinders to explore the surroundings and provide vibro-tactile feedback for obstacles. It is designed to be used together with the white cane, enhancing the reliability of the traditional cane (Bernieri, Faramondi, & Pascucci, 2015).

The system consists of HY-SRF05 ultrasonic sensors placed on the backside of the hand, directed up, left, and right. The distance of the object can be calculated from the time of flight of the acoustic waves that propagate at a constant known speed. This allows the user to perceive the obstacles that cannot be discovered using the white cane. Vibro-tactile feedback is delivered through vibration motors. The preliminary results about the usability of this prototype are promising. However, there is still room for improvements such as the comfort of the user needs to be further improved by an accurate ergonomic design of the glove.

Khampachua et al. developed a wrist-mounted wearable device for helping visually impaired to avoid obstacles and move around more efficiently with only a white cane (Khampachua, Wongrajit, Waranusast, & Pattanathaburt, 2016). The device consists of an ultrasonic sensor (HC-SR04), a 1010 microcontroller board, and a smartphone with an accelerometer sensor. The ultrasonic sensor receives commands from the smartphone and sends the distance data back to the phone via a Bluetooth connection. The smartphone will work with the microcontroller board by sending the angles from the accelerometer sensor to the application. There system came with two detection mode, one for obstacles on the ground level and one for obstacles above ground level. The switching between the two modes can be done based on the angle between the arm and torso (vertical axis). The device is tested and showed a satisfactory result on its usability and learning time. However, it can be clearly seen that the device is too heavy as the user need to carry the smartphone on the wrist. This is an issue if the device is used for a longer time.

Vision Sensors Based Assistive Technologies

Miller proposed an Android application that is able to detect and notify the users of the obstacles in front of their path. The detection system is achieved by using the camera of a smartphone (Miller, n.d.).

The smartphone is mounted on the Go Pro Chest Harness and worn by the user. The algorithm starts with the capture of images as the user moves forward. It is followed by extracting the features from the images and making a comparison between the consecutive frames to identify the existence of the obstacles (Miller, n.d.). The presence of the obstacles in front will trigger the vibration mode of the smartphone to alert the user. The walking assistant is controllable by either touch or voice commands depending on the user's preference.

The testing results showed that the detection rate for an obstacle is 42.1% of the time—a low success rate. The researcher suggested that the low performance is caused by the limitations of the field of computer vision, which includes the variance in illuminations, type of road surface, and the shadows under the sunlight. Another issue that must be considered in computer vision is the energy consumption, as suggested by the researcher, the app would drain the smartphone's battery power very quickly.

Headlock is a navigation aid that uses Google Glass to help blind users to cross large open spaces by providing a salient clue as for the landmark such as the doors (Fiannaca, Apostolopoulous, & Folmer, 2014). This navigation aid allows users to scan around the large open space to identify the intended path towards the landmark. When traversing a large open space, the users tend to veer from the intended path as there are no tactile features and a sparsity of visual features along the path. So, Headlock provides audio feedback to the users for correcting the veering from the landmark, e.g. "Left" or "Right". Also, the Headlock provides distance information for the user while moving towards the landmark.

A user study with eight blind participants evaluated the usability and effectiveness of two types of audio feedback (sonification and text-to-speech (TTS)) for guiding a user across an open space to a doorway. Results found TTS to be most effective, though no difference in veering was observed. The study was limited because only doors were used as landmarks. The researchers did not evaluate whether Optical Head-mounted Displays (OHMDs) is a better platform than smartphones for navigation aids (Fiannaca et al., 2014). Also, the researchers did not evaluate the maximum distance at which a landmark can be identified nor how distance affects a cane user's ability to efficiently navigate to a landmark.

Al-Khalifa and Al-Razgan developed Ebsar, a navigation aid that provides indoor guidance for the visually impaired to navigate through various locations within a building (Al-Khalifa & Al-Razgan, 2016). The system first required a sighted person to walk through the building and indicate all point of interests for the system such as restaurant, classroom, restrooms, etc. Next, the printed QR codes indicating its specific locations are placed on the walls. Finally, the Google Glass is used to identify the user's location by detecting the QR codes placed on the walls. The Google Glass microphone is used to capture the user's speech input and its speaker is used to provide audio feedback from the system to the user. The application is well-developed and is suitable for use in common public places such as airports, schools, shopping malls, etc. A user acceptance study of the application by 15 sighted persons and nine blind users were carried out. Users rated the application as satisfactory, noting the application was easy to use. This application is limited to the indoor environment and requires some preparation before the device can be used by the visually impaired.

In 2015, He et al. proposed an ego-motion tracking method which will be used on the wearable blind navigator based on the Google Glass. The motion tracking is designed to cope with the arbitrary body motion and complex environmental dynamics. For achieving ego-motion tracking, the wearable blind navigator based on Google Glass utilizes visual-inertial sensors and Android APIs (He, Li, Guan, & Tan, 2015).

The system hardware consists of a 5 MP CMOS camera and a MEMS inertial measurement unit (IMU). The interaction between the Google Glass and the user is by natural language dialogue using the Android speech recognition. The navigation system can be controlled either by vocal commands or via the touchpad on the Google Glass. The navigation system is designed to track translational and rotational motion. Test results showed a positive outcome towards the effectiveness of visual-inertial fusion with the visual sanity check mechanism for motion tracking.

The tracking accuracy is influenced by a few factors. The first factor is the configuration of the navigator, including the pose and height of the camera, which effects the tracking accuracy of visual features and the computation of global scales. The second factor is the moving speed of the navigator. The achieved processing frequency is around 15 fps on the current version of Google Glass. The navigator is able to track normal walking motion, but large errors occur when the wearer is running or performing the abrupt motion. The third factor is the number of trackable features in the environment (He et al., 2015). The tracking accuracy downgrades to pure inertial tracking when no visual features are detectable, e.g., when the navigator is moving towards a wall.

The major limitation of the proposed ego-motion tracking method for blind navigation is that the tracked trajectory is relative to the starting point, and the scale of a trajectory is not accurate.

The smart cane system is equipped with a face recognition system to detect and identify the faces of the people around the users (Yongsik, Jonghong, Bumhwi, Mallipeddi, & Minho, 2015). The detection result is feedback to the user through vibration on the smart cane. The system hardware consists of a glass-type WIFI camera, a mobile computer, and a cane equipped with a microcontroller, Bluetooth module, and vibration motor. The camera obtained the view in front of the user and the mobile computer performs face recognitions. The detection result is sent to the microcontroller on the cane through Bluetooth communication and is informed through different vibration patterns. The major limitation of the system is the limited number of vibration patterns to indicate the person meet by the user.

Additionally, in 2015, McCarthy et al. evaluated the Augmented Depth visual representation to emphasize the ground obstacles and floor-wall boundaries for promoting safe mobility. This visual representation is achieved by artificially increasing the contrast between obstacles and ground surface via a novel ground plane extraction algorithm (McCarthy, Walker, Lieby, Scott, & Barnes, 2014). The Augmented Depth visual representation has been evaluated through experimental trials with eight normal sighted participants with no health conditions by using different simulated prosthetic vision to determine the usefulness in obstacle avoidance and the advantages over Depth and Intensity. Overall, the results indicate a great performance as the proposed visual representation is able to allow the participants to complete the mobility task with fewer collisions as compared with Depth and Intensity based visual representations.

4.4.2 Assistive Device for Staircases and Steps Detection

In the past few years, many assistive technologies have been introduced for aiding and improving the orientation and mobility of the visually impaired persons (VIPs). Among all the potential hazards faced by the VIPs, stairs or steps are one of the most common structures that are present in urban and living environments. Thus, many devices and algorithms have been developed to help the VIPs to tackle these hazards.

Range Sensors Based Assistive Technologies

Ishiwata et al. proposed a step detection system to support the mobility of the visually impaired. The system is made up of a sensor unit that will be attached to the user's chest and a PC with a battery to be installed in a backpack (Ishiwata, Sekiguchi, Fuchida, & Nakamura, 2013).

The device uses a small laser range sensor to obtain the distance information in the vertical cross-sectional plane in front of the user. The laser range sensor measures the distance to different points in front. Sensor data is with a threshold value to classify it into different segments. The segment is then analysed to identify the pattern of stairs. After the detection, the system provides information on the existence of a step via voice or a beep sound. In experiment trials, the device performed well, with over 95% accuracy for both upstairs and downstairs. The system is yet to be tested in an outdoor environment. For this system, the weight of the sensor unit is about 0.5 kg and the backpack is around 3.4 kg. This is an issue as the device is already quite heavy and might affect the mobility of the user. Besides, the power supply for the device and how long it can be used is not indicated.

Besides, Bouhamed et al. discussed an approach to detect staircases by using an ultrasonic sensor attached to a white cane (Bouhamed, Frikha Eleuch, Kallel, & Sellami Masmoudi, 2012). Their electronic cane is made up of two ultrasonic sensors (for staircase and ground obstacle detection respectively) and a monocular camera for obstacle detection. The researchers selected the "LV-EZ0" ultrasonic sensor for their application. The sensor is able to provide range information of 6–254 in. with 1-in. resolution. The monocular camera selected is "LinkSprite JPEG Color Camera TTL Interface" with a capture range from 10 to 15 m. For the staircase detection, the researchers keep track of the changing reading from the ultrasonic sensor to the ground and use the data to identify the terrain in front such as a floor, and ascending or descending staircases. The experimental results showed that the detection rate of the staircase is estimated to be 89.8%.

Vision Sensors Based Assistive Technologies

Shahrabadi et al. developed a simple algorithm for detecting stairs by using a camera at a distance of 5 m from the stairs. The algorithm starts with capturing of the image and followed by processing the image to identify the edges within a pre-set region of interest (ROI). The candidate step is selected if the edges found within the ROI match with the specific criteria determined by the researchers (Shahrabadi, Rodrigues, & du Buf, 2013). Then, there will be a final validation to further verify that the stair is detected. In the paper, the researchers did not mention whether the algorithm is able to identify the detected stairs as ascending or descending stairs. The researchers stated that the algorithm is unable to avoid false positive and negative detection. This issue is affected by the factors like lighting, low contrast, view angles, and stairs' materials when using the camera for image processing. The researchers did not discuss whether the system is able to detect the staircases if a user faces the staircase within 5 m.

Pérez-Yus et al. developed a wearable navigation assistant device. The wearable device focused mainly on staircases detection to aid the identification and localization of staircases, as well as the numbers of steps and step dimensions (Pérez-Yus,

López-Nicolás, & Guerrero, 2015). The prototype system consists of an RGB-D camera connected to a laptop. The camera is mounted on the chest of the user and pointing downward at an angle of 45° to locate the view in front of the user. The developed algorithm makes use of the colour and depth sensing capabilities of the RGB-D camera to find ground and staircase detection. The algorithm will output whether there is the presence of a staircase, a single step or none. Besides, the algorithm provides full information about the staircase present in front of the user.

Harms et al. proposed a stair detection algorithm to aid people with vision impairment in real time. The prototype is a helmet mounted with a stereo camera rig and Inertia measurement unit (IMU) (Harms, Rehder, Schwarze, & Lauer, 2015). The computation and processing of all the data obtained from the sensors are carried out through a notebook which is carried in a backpack. The IMU is used to determine the global height axis for the running system. The stereo camera rig is used to obtain a pair of rectified grey value images. The images are filtered by a matched filter to detect concave and convex line segments in front of the user. The detected line segments are tracked over time and combined into step segments. The step segments are then merged to stairs for the detection to be completed.

Munoz et al. developed an effective indoor staircase detection algorithm by using an RGB-D camera. The researchers use a Google Project Tango, which includes an RGB-D camera mounted within a tablet (Munoz, Rong, & Tian, 2016). The tablet was mounted on the chest of the user during the prototype development to validate their algorithm. The RGB-D camera is used to capture the environment in front of the user. First of all, the candidate of the stair will be detected in the RGB frames by extracting a set of concurrent parallel lines. After the candidate is detected, the depth information obtained from the RGB-D camera is used to identify the staircase as ascending, descending, or negative (i.e. corridors, bookcases, ladders). Lastly, candidate staircases are validated through a trained support vector machine (SVM) based multi-classifier. The classifier is trained with example images of ascending, descending stairs, and negative examples.

Besides, Cloix et al. developed an assistive system to improve the performance of existing smart assistive devices. In 2015, Cloix et al. suggested that the existing mobility aid devices such as rollator is unable to prevent users from descending stair hazard (Cloix, Bologna, Weiss, Pun, & Hasler, 2015). Thus, the researchers proposed a method to detect descending staircases in real time using a passive stereo camera. The experimental setup consists of the Bumblebee2 stereo camera mounted at a height of 76 cm, on top of a standard three-wheel rollator.

4.4.3 Assistive Device for Potholes Detection

Range Sensors Based Assistive Technologies

Saraf et al. developed an IVR-based intelligent guidance stick for the visually impaired. The device has two main functions which are the obstacle detection and pothole detection. The obstacle detection system consists of three ultrasonic sensors pointed in a different direction and the detection date will be processed by the Arduino Uno Board. The direction and range of incoming obstacle will be detected, and a voice-based instruction will be produced when the obstacle is within the safe zone (Saraf, Shehzad, & Jadhav, 2014). As for the pothole detection system, it is made up of another circuit with an ultrasonic sensor, a buzzer, and the 8051 microcontrollers. In this system, the ultrasonic sensor will keep track of the distance to the ground. When there is a noticeable increase in the distance, the buzzer will sound to alert the user that there is a pothole or a staircase ahead. The intelligent guidance stickan is designed for only one ground state detection which is a pothole. This means that the device is not enough to guide the visually impaired persons to navigate around safely.

Sheth et al. developed a simple, affordable and efficient device to aid the visually impaired, named Smart White Cane. The device is designed with the functions of obstacle detection (low lying, knee level, and above wrist level) and detection of potholes, pits, downfalls, and ascending or descending staircase (Sheth, Rajandekar, Laddha, & Chaudhari, 2014). The system uses ultrasonic sensors for detection plus a sound system and a vibration motor for providing feedback to the user. The system consists of four ultrasonic sensors for detecting an obstacle and identifying the ground floor state. The processed detection information will be feedback through both short pre-recorded messages and vibration according to the risk priority. The performance of the device in detecting the ground state is unknown.

Parikh et al. discussed their development of a new prototype to help the visually impaired to travel independently (Parikh, Shah, Popat, & Narula, 2015). It is a stick which is able to detect obstacles and potholes in the path. The stick is made up of two systems which are obstacles detection and potholes detection. The obstacle detection system uses three ultrasonic sensors for the front, left and right detection. The analogue output signal from the sensors is sent to the microcontroller and converted to a digital signal through an on-chip ADC converter. The microcontroller will calculate the distance from the digital signal. From the calculated distance, if the user is too close to the obstacle, then the microcontroller sends a signal to sound the buzzer and activate the vibrator to provide an alert. As for the pothole detection, the researchers discussed two techniques that were implemented on the stick. Firstly, a pothole can be detected by using the ultrasonic sensor. This can be achieved by the measurement of the distance between the stick and the ground. Once there is an increase in the distance, it can be concluded that the ground state is uneven or a pothole is present. Secondly, the pothole detection is achieved by using the accelerometer. The accelerometer is attached to a stone that hangs on the stick with a thread. Generally, the stone will have a zero to minimal deflection when the stick is on a flat ground. When the stick goes onto the pothole, the stone will have an increased deflection and thus pothole is detected. The severity of the pothole can also be determined from the value of the accelerometer. The limitation of this second method is that the stick needs to go over the pothole in order to detect the pothole.

In 2015, the researchers from BNM Institute of Technology proposed a new system with simplicity and optimum cost after analysing the available solutions (Sourab, Ranganatha Chakravarthy, & D'Souza, 2015). The proposed solution is a jacket with sensors mounted on it for detection. There are five ultrasonic sensors used in the system: one for potholes or stair detection; one for obstacles detection at head level; and the other three for the front, left, and right obstacles detection. In this system, the detection information will be processed by an Arduino Uno microcontroller. Then, the user is notified by specific voice messages through headphones as the output device.

For the potholes detection, the ultrasonic sensors will keep on checking the distance between the user and the ground (Sourab et al., 2015). This distance value will be compared against the reference values for different floor states (pothole, stairs, or normal road). As for the obstacle detection at head level, front left, and right area, the ultrasonic sensors will measure the distance in their corresponding direction and compared against a minimum distance value. If the distance value falls within the minimum reference value, the system will alert the user and ask the user to move towards the direction with maximum distance value.

Vision Sensors Based Assistive Technologies

Rao et al. developed a vision-based approach for potholes and uneven surfaces detection to assist the mobility of blind people. The proposed system targets the scenario after dark which is not achievable by most of the existing system (Rao, Gubbi, Palaniswami, & Wong, 2016).

In the proposed system, a GoPro HERO 4 Silver camera is mounted on a handheld mount. Along with the camera, there is a Ghost Stop's Laser Grid GS1 mounted on top of it to generate a laser grid projection. The camera is used for recording the pattern of the laser projection. The recorded pattern is then analysed to extract the features in order to provide path cues to assist the blind user. According to Rao et al., the existing vision-based systems are capable of aiding the mobility of the blind people but it is expensive to use two cameras and the processing of the video information (Rao et al., 2016). This is because of the need of three frames in order to detect the obstacle. The system requires a laptop for processing the video and carrying a computer in the backpack is reducing the mobility. In contrast, the proposed approach is able to compute the depth and path cues by using just a single video frame rather than stereovision. The experimental results of the proposed approach showed an accuracy of up to 90% in detecting the potholes.

With the satisfied results, the researchers suggested that the team will aim for real-time navigation so that this proposed approach can help in assisting the blind people. The primary limitation of this proposed approach is the projected laser pattern is only visible at night.

4.4.4 Assistive Device for Ramp, Drainage, and Loose Surface Detection

Herghelegiu et al. suggested that the ground plane in front is very important for the visually impaired to navigate around freely and safely (Herghelegiu, Burlacu, & Caraiman, 2016). So, the researchers proposed an algorithm for ground plane detection.

The setup of the proposed system consists of a stereo camera rig which will be worn by the users. In the algorithm, the researchers included the consideration of the orientation of the camera, namely its pitch and roll. According to the researchers, the consideration of the camera orientation is important as the camera is to be worn by the users and the movement while the user navigates around will introduce a variation in the captured images. The proposed algorithm used v-disparity maps to represent the ground plane by a line or a line segment. Then, the algorithm keeps track of the line segment of the detected ground plane in the consecutive frame in order to validate the detected ground plane. The limitation of the algorithm is encountered if the user faces an uphill, downhill or when the camera aligned with the horizontal axis. Also, the performance of the algorithm in real time scenarios is yet to be determined because the testing is only performed by using the synthetic data generated by the virtual environment framework.

Nakashima et al. proposed a method to identify the road surface condition by using the ultrasonic sensor. The recognition of the surface conditions is achieved by using the reflected intensities obtained by the ultrasonic sensor (Nakashima et al., 2016). In the paper, the researchers discussed the improvement of their developed method for the detection of additional road conditions such as puddle, asphalt, soil, and lawn. According to the researchers, the proposed method is able to identify the road surface conditions by using the defined threshold. The defined threshold was determined through the experimental data collected based on the reflected intensities of different road conditions. The effectiveness was confirmed based on the experimental testing. However, the proposed method is yet to be applied on the actual assistive devices for the visually impaired. Another issue would be the effect of the pointing angle of the ultrasonic sensors on the outcome of the detection as the collected data was based on the incident angle of 90°.

4.5 Discussions

Smart technology solutions can help people with visual impairment to recognize steps, ramps, rough ground or loose surfaces like gravel and increase the person's range of preview for these hazards as summarized in Table 4.1.

Throughout the review, the general limitations of the existing devices and techniques are the lack of user testing or proper benchmarking of the detection method and user participation in the overall design. For example, the step detection

Table 4.1 Evaluation of smart technologies for ground plane hazard detection

System name	Sensors used	Coverage/type of usage	Limitations
Step detection system (Ishiwata et al., 2013)	Small laser range sensor	Indoor/research stage	• Heavy weight with sensor unit of 0.5 kg and a backpack of 3.4 kg • Power supply and usable hours are not indicated
Electronic cane (Bouhamed et al., 2012)	Ultrasonic sensors Monocular camera	Staircases/research stage	• Only tested with two raw data sets • Good performance but only for staircases detection
Wearable navigation assistant device (Pérez-Yus et al., 2015)	RGB-D camera	Indoor/research stage	• A staircase detection algorithm • Yet to be tested in real scenarios
Ascending stairs detection device (Harms et al., 2015)	Stereo camera rig Inertia measurement unit	Indoor, outdoor/research stage	• An ascending stairs detection algorithm • False detection at an outdoor environment like pedestrian crosswalks or shadow regions
Assistive system for existing rollator (Cloix et al., 2015)	Bumblebee2 stereo camera	Indoor/research stage	• Detecting only descending stairs
Intelligent guidance stick (Saraf et al., 2014)	Ultrasonic sensors	Outdoor/research stage	• Focus on only obstacles and potholes detection • No result was presented for pothole detection
Smart white cane (Sheth et al., 2014)	Ultrasonic sensors	Indoor, outdoor/deployment stage	• Experimental results are not presented • Performance is an unknown
Blind man stick (Parikh et al., 2015)	Ultrasonic sensors Accelerometer	Indoor, outdoor/deployment stage	• Experimental results are not presented • Performance is an unknown
Simple jacket mobility aid (Sourab et al., 2015)	Ultrasonic sensors	Indoor, outdoor/deployment stage	• The sensors pointing position will vary for different users
Vision-based device (Rao et al., 2016)	GoPro HERO 4 silver camera	Outdoor/research stage	• A pothole and uneven surface detection algorithm • Limited for night time due to the laser beam visibility
Ground plane detection algorithm (Herghelegiu et al., 2016)	Stereo camera rig	Outdoor/research stage	• Performance affected when the users face uphill, downhill or camera alignment with the horizontal axis
Surface condition detection method (Nakashima et al., 2016)	Ultrasonic sensors	Outdoor/research stage	• The method is yet to be applied on the actual assistive device • Data was collected based on the ultrasonic sensor at the incident angle of 90° only

method proposed by Ishiwata et al. (2013) is too heavy for the user and this problem can be prevented by getting opinion through user testing during the construction period. Also, the step detection method is the lack of proper testing in the outdoor environment in order to determine the overall performance. Similarly, the algorithm for staircase detection developed by Pérez-Yus et al. (2015), Harms et al. (2015), and Munoz et al. (2016) are lack of proper testing with the visually impaired to be able to provide real-time detection in daily activities. There is still a lack of consideration for under-foot conditions, and steps/trip hazard perception compared to obstacle avoidance.

Besides, the other limitation of almost all techniques is the assumptions that they make about the environmental conditions. For example, in potholes detection, ultrasonic sensors have been widely used for developing the assistive technologies. Saraf et al. (2014), Sheth et al. (2014), and Parikh et al. (2015) have developed the prototype that is able to aid in obstacles and potholes detection. However, the problem is that the developed devices are yet to be tested by visually. Thus, the techniques, while promising, remain unproven. The use of vision, such as Rao et al.'s (2016) approach for potholes and uneven surface detection using a laser projection, shows promise but is limited by visibility concerns under certain lighting conditions. Another problem with the vision processing algorithm is the need of a laptop and this increases the weight of the device to be carried by the user.

While there has been a recent focus on ramp and ditch detection (e.g., Nakashima et al. (2016)) for the visually impaired, little has been translated to in-the-field use. For ground surface detection, the proposed method to identify the road surface condition is by using the reflected intensities of the ultrasonic sensor from the ground. However, this proposed method is yet to be applied on the actual assistive devices for the visually impaired.

4.6   Recommendations

According to the evaluation and discussion in the previous section, some criteria are suggested while proposing a smart technology solution so that it will be widely adopted and accepted by the visually impaired people.

Firstly, the performance of the assistive devices on its application context must be considered. The assistive devices must be able to meet all the needed functions to help the visually impaired to travel safely and independently. From the reviewed works, 20 out of 30 of the proposed solutions focus only on a single function, and this is not enough to meet the need of helping with the navigation and mobility of the visually impaired people. The two main functions that must be included are the obstacle detection and ground state detection.

Secondly, the simplicity and reliability are also one of the essential considerations. From the works reviewed, 8 out of 30 of the proposed solutions are bulky, and weight is always an important issue that visually impaired people mentioned in the feedback. Besides, many proposed solutions are tested only in the simulated or virtual environment. They are yet to be tested in the real-time application and this might be one of the reasons why these solutions are not adopted and accepted by the visually impaired.

Besides, when designing new assistive technology for the visually impaired, the cost of the proposed solutions must be considered so that the devices are economically accessible by the user. This is important to ensure the developed assistive devices actually reach the visually impaired to improve their quality of life.

References

Ahlmark D. I. (2016). *Haptic navigation aids for the visually impaired.* Thesis, Department of Computer Science, Electrical and Space Engineering, Lulea University of Technology, Lulea, Sweden, pp. 145.

Al-Khalifa, S., & Al-Razgan, M. (2016). Ebsar: Indoor guidance for the visually impaired. *Computers & Electrical Engineering, 54*, 26–39.

Bernieri, G., Faramondi, L., & Pascucci, F. (2015). A low cost smart glove for visually impaired people mobility. In *2015 23rd Mediterranean Conference on Control and Automation (MED).* Washington, DC: IEEE.

Bhatlawande, S., Mukhopadhyay, J., & Mahadevappa, M. (2012). Ultrasonic spectacles and waist-belt for visually impaired and blind person. In *National Conference on Communications (NCC), 2012.* Washington, DC: IEEE.

Bouhamed, S. A., Frikha Eleuch, J., Kallel, I. K., & Sellami Masmoudi, D. (2012). New electronic cane for visually impaired people for obstacle detection and recognition. In *2012 IEEE International Conference on Vehicular Electronics and Safety (ICVES 2012).* Washington, DC: IEEE.

Cloix, S., Bologna, G., Weiss, V., Pun, T., & Hasler, D. (2015). Descending stairs detection with low-power sensors. In *Computer Vision - ECCV 2014 Workshops* (pp. 658–672). New York, NY: Springer.

Dakopoulos, D., & Bourbakis, N. (2010). Wearable obstacle avoidance electronic travel aids for blind: A survey. *IEEE Transactions on Systems, Man, and Cybernetics, Part C (Applications and Reviews), 40*(1), 25–35.

Deverell, L., Bentley, S., Ayton, L., Delany, C., & Keeffe, J. (2017). Effective mobility framework: A tool for designing comprehensive O&M outcomes research. *International Journal of Orientation & Mobility, 7*(1), 74–86.

Fiannaca, A., Apostolopoulous, I., & Folmer, E. (2014). Headlock. In *Proceedings of the 16th International ACM SIGACCESS Conference on Computers & Accessibility - ASSETS '14.* New York, NY: ACM.

Harms, H., Rehder, E., Schwarze, T., & Lauer, M. (2015). Detection of ascending stairs using stereo vision. In *IEEE/RSJ International Conference on Intelligent Robots and Systems (IROS)* (p. 2015). Washington, DC: IEEE.

He, H., Li, Y., Guan, Y., & Tan, J. (2015). Wearable ego-motion tracking for blind navigation in indoor environments. *IEEE Transactions on Automation Science and Engineering, 12*(4), 1181–1190.

Herghelegiu, P., Burlacu, A., & Caraiman, S. (2016). Robust ground plane detection and tracking in stereo sequences using camera orientation. In *20th International Conference on System Theory, Control and Computing (ICSTCC).* Washington, DC: IEEE.

Ishiwata, K., Sekiguchi, M., Fuchida, M., & Nakamura, A. (2013). Basic study on step detection system for the visually impaired. In *2013 IEEE International Conference on Mechatronics and Automation* (pp. 1332–1337). Washington, DC: IEEE.

Jacquet, C., Bellik, Y., & Bourda, Y. (2006). Electronic locomotion aids for the blind: Towards more assistive systems. In *Intelligent paradigms for assistive and preventive healthcare* (pp. 133–163). New York, NY: Springer.

Khampachua, C., Wongrajit, C., Waranusast, R., & Pattanathaburt, P. (2016). Wrist-mounted smartphone-based navigation device for visually impaired people using ultrasonic sensing. In *Fifth ICT International Student Project Conference (ICT-ISPC)*. Washington, DC: IEEE.

Kumar, K. (2014). *Development of walk safe cane for the rehabilitation of blind people*. BTech Thesis, National Institute of Technology, Rourkela.

Leduc-Mills, B., Profita, H., Bharadwaj, S., & Cromer, P. (2013). ioCane: A smart-phone and sensor-augmented mobility aid for the blind. In *Computer science technical reports* (p. 1031). Retrieved from http://scholar.colorado.edu/csci_techreports/1031

Lopes, S., Vieira, J., Lopes, Ó., Rosa, P., & Dias, N. (2012). MobiFree: A set of electronic mobility aids for the blind. *Procedia Computer Science, 14*, 10–19.

McCarthy, C., Walker, J., Lieby, P., Scott, A., & Barnes, N. (2014). Mobility and low contrast trip hazard avoidance using augmented depth. *Journal of Neural Engineering, 12*(1), 016003.

Miller A. (2014). *Walking assistant - A mobile aid for the visually-impaired*. California Polytechnic State University, San Luis Obispo.

Munoz, R., Rong, X., & Tian, Y. (2016). Depth-aware indoor staircase detection and recognition for the visually impaired. In *2016 IEEE International Conference on Multimedia & Expo Workshops (ICMEW)*. Washington, DC: IEEE.

Nakashima, S., Aramaki, S., Kitazono, Y., Mu, S., Tanaka, K., & Serikawa, S. (2016). Road surface condition distinction method using reflection intensities obtained by ultrasonic sensor. In *2016 International Symposium on Computer, Consumer and Control (IS3C)*. Washington, DC: IEEE.

Parikh, A., Shah, D., Popat, K., & Narula, H. (2015). Blind man stick using programmable interrupt controller (PIC). *Procedia Computer Science, 45*, 558–563.

Pérez-Yus, A., López-Nicolás, G., & Guerrero, J. (2015). Detection and modelling of staircases using a wearable depth sensor. In *Computer Vision - ECCV 2014 Workshops* (pp. 449–463). New York, NY: Springer.

Prattico, F., Cera, C., & Petroni, F. (2013). A new hybrid infrared-ultrasonic electronic travel aids for blind people. *Sensors and Actuators A: Physical, 201*, 363–370.

Rao, A., Gubbi, J., Palaniswami, M., & Wong, E. (2016). A vision-based system to detect potholes and uneven surfaces for assisting blind people. In *IEEE International Conference on Communications (ICC)*. Washington, DC: IEEE.

Reynolds, C. R., Vannest, K. J., & Fletcher-Janzen, E. (2015). Encyclopedia of special education: A reference for the education of children, adolescents, and adults with disabilities and other exceptional individuals. *Choice Reviews Online, 52*(07), 52-3423–52-3423.

Roentgen, U., Gelderblom, G., & de Witte, L. (2012). User evaluation of two electronic mobility aids for persons who are visually impaired: A quasi-experimental study using a standardized mobility course. *Assistive Technology, 24*(2), 110–120.

Saraf, M., Shehzad, M., & Jadhav, N. (2014). An IVR based intelligent guidance stick for blind. *International Journal of Current Engineering and Technology, 4*(3), 17.

Shahrabadi, S., Rodrigues, J., & du Buf, J. (2013). Detection of indoor and outdoor stairs. In *Pattern recognition and image analysis* (pp. 847–854). New York, NY: Springer.

Sheth, R., Rajandekar, S., Laddha, S., & Chaudhari, R. (2014). Smart white cane–An elegant and economic walking aid. *AJER, e-ISSN, 03*(10), 84–89.

Sourab, B., Ranganatha Chakravarthy, H. S., & D'Souza, S. (2015). Design and implementation of mobility aid for blind people. In *2015 International Conference on Power and Advanced Control Engineering (ICPACE)*. Washington, DC: IEEE.

WHO. (2018). *Blindness and vision impairment*. Geneva: World Health Organization. Retrieved October 22, 2018, from http://www.who.int/news-room/fact-sheets/detail/blindness-and-visual-impairment

Yongsik, J., Jonghong, K., Bumhwi, K., Mallipeddi, R., & Minho, L. (2015). Smart cane: Face recognition system for blind. In *HAI '15 Proceedings of the 3rd International Conference on Human-Agent Interaction*. New York, NY: ACM. https://doi.org/10.1145/2814940.2814952

Chapter 5
Technologies and Systems to Improve Mobility of Visually Impaired People: A State of the Art

Sara Paiva and Nishu Gupta

5.1   Introduction

The advancement of Information and Communication Technologies and Electronics (ICT&E) has been evident and has targeted exponential growth in recent years. We have witnessed a number of new fields of application in technology such as mobility, transports, and health. The electronics field has also shown considerable progress in the increase of processing capacity of the equipment as well as new hardware devices that often arise to meet new challenges that society is requiring. All these aspects opened doors for the ICT&E area to be applied to visually impaired people (VIP) in order to seek for innovative solutions that can promote the well-being of VIP. Currently, technological solutions for VIP are the subject of plenty of studies by researchers. Many case studies have been published and tested in real-world scenarios with VIP associations around the world. The importance these solutions bring to VIP is undeniable as they contribute to social inclusion and to greater ease in performing various daily tasks. Although the research being done applies to several areas, such as education, communication, etc., in this chapter we will restrict our research to mobility systems and supporting technologies. Mobility itself is a very broad concept and yet, so far, there is no device or application that solves entirely the problems of mobility felt by VIP. Mobility involves the key concept

---
S. Paiva (✉)
ARC4DigiT – Applied Research Center for Digital Transformation, Instituto Politécnico de Viana do Castelo, Viana do Castelo, Portugal
e-mail: sara.paiva@estg.ipvc.pt

N. Gupta
Electronics and Communication Engineering Department, Vaagdevi College of Engineering, Warangal, India
e-mail: gupta_n@vaagdevi.edu.in

© Springer Nature Switzerland AG 2020
S. Paiva (ed.), *Technological Trends in Improved Mobility of the Visually Impaired*,
EAI/Springer Innovations in Communication and Computing,
https://doi.org/10.1007/978-3-030-16450-8_5

of navigation, inside and outside buildings (indoor and outdoor environments) which, in turn, includes the detection of obstacles during the course as well as the development of hardware components. Navigation and pathfinding are the most challenging activity for VIP (Ali & Ali, 2017), who wish to walk without problems in outdoor environments, and to acquire and learn local area topography information specifically (Wang, Wang, Yin, & Zhang, 2010). Additionally, they like to perform most activities in an autonomous way without asking help to other people (Trongwongsa, Chankrachang, Prompoon, & Pattanothai, 2015) but in today's conditions, with the amount of visual information, that is hard to accomplish (Bilgi, Ozturk, & Gulnerman, 2017). This has serious implications in their social and professional life (Shahu & Shinko, 2017).

In this chapter, we present an analysis of several research studies that have been carried out in recent years regarding technologies and systems to improve the mobility of VIP. Our main goal is to provide a synthetic overview of most recent approaches and conclude about future trends.

The chapter is organized as follows: in Sects. 5.2–5.4, several research studies are presented regarding, respectively, outdoor environments, indoor environments, and obstacle detection/avoidance. This last topic makes sense and is a need in both environments but because it has so many specificities and is the subject of several studies dedicated to it, we decided to create a dedicated section. Sect. 5.5 presents a discussion and Sect. 5.6 the conclusions.

5.2 Outdoor Navigation

This section presents several studies that describe different technologies and solutions that are being explored to help VIP in outdoor environments, for several purposes. The scene matching aided navigation is a location information technology which relies on topographic images using image sensors, has a high-accuracy and low-cost (Wang et al., 2010). In order to apply this technique to help VIP in navigation in outdoor environments, the authors propose the methodology shown in Fig. 5.1. The first step is to take local area images, using image acquisition equipment, of the places where navigation is to be provided, and then get feature information by digital image processing. This information goes to a specific database. To use such a system, VIP need to have an appropriate collection device, that processes a real-time obtained image and compares with features stored in the database. The result is prompted to the VIP by voice. To improve the matching accuracy, the authors focused on improving the extraction of reliable features: they used the SIFT algorithm to extract image feature points, the Euclidean distance to have rough match, and then a second exact match by RANSAC algorithm.

Detecting moving objects poses an additional danger to VIP compared to objects that are standing still. Rapid movement of objects represents an additional threat than the obstruction of slower movements, so the use of motion analysis to detect and analyze the faster movement of obstacles becomes a necessary part of the

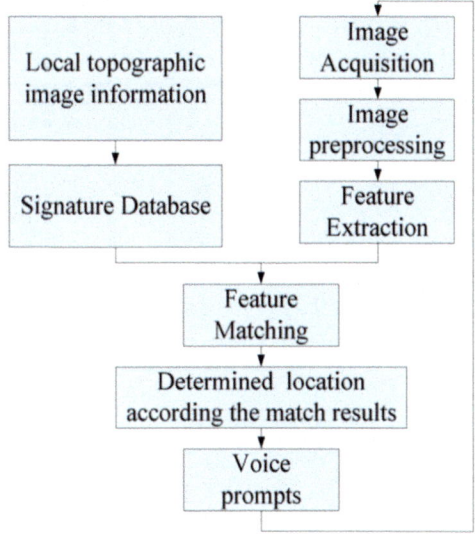

Fig. 5.1 Methodology proposed to use scene matching aided navigation in outdoor environments (adapted from Wang et al., 2010)

navigation system for VIP. To detect and analyze moving objects, authors Zhao, Wang, and Wang (2012) propose an improved algorithm based on LK optical flow, to solve the low detection accuracy and slow speed to fast moving object. In order to validate the improved algorithm, two groups of experiments were done: Optical flow image of a single frame and comparison of the six combined optical flow images from a different scene. The advantage of it is to ensure the feature points completely and stably reproduced. Secondly, it is intuitive to use intensive optical flow. Research was carried out in the Innovation Center of Disabled Rehabilitation in Equipment and Technology.

The system TARSIUS (Masulli et al., 2017) aims to help VIP to understand a visual scene and to allow localization abilities whenever they are outdoor. The authors state the accuracy limitation of GPS as the main prevention for it to be used more widely in mobile apps for the visual impairment segment and propose some low-cost alternatives that include radio-frequency identification (RFID) transponders, near field communication (NFC), Bluetooth low energy (BLE), or iBeacons. To achieve its goal, the TARSIUS system is composed of a mobile app, a web server, and a remote assistance center. Points of interest and dangerous places are marked with tags that allow for a precise location to be computed, dangerous zones to be notified to the user using special warnings, identification of a bus that is coming to a stop, or notification of stops during the bus ride.

The use of 3D audio to provide navigation abilities for VIP was explored by authors in Matsuda and Kondo (2016), with the purpose of giving cues on the direction and distance to the intended location. The architecture, shown in Fig. 5.2, counts on a geomagnetic sensor and a PC. The sensor is responsible for understanding the current direction of the person and the PC to perform a binaural

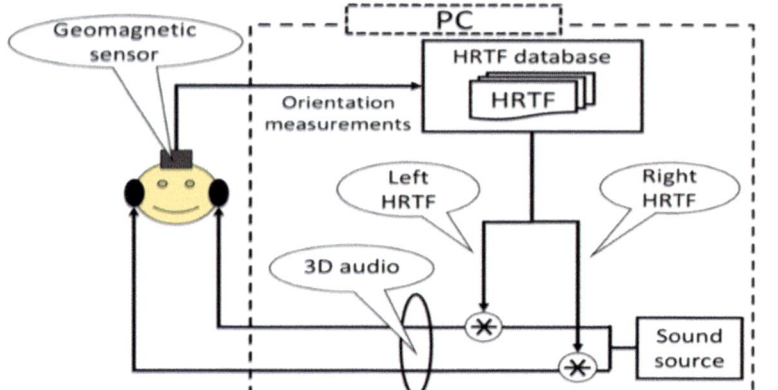

Fig. 5.2 Architecture proposal for outdoor navigation using 3D audio (adapted from Matsuda & Kondo, 2016)

simulation which is the procedure to create a 3D audio whose sound pressure changes depending on the distance.

The practice of sport and physical activity is a universal recommendation to promote health and well-being. Intelligent Transportation Systems are usually not adapted to people with some type of disability such as visual impairment. One study has focused on helping VIP to perform walking and running activities (Mancini, Frontoni, & Zingaretti, 2018) through the use of a vision system that identifies lines and lanes along a given route. The system uses a camera to detect lines and lanes and a haptic device to interact with the user via a processing unit. A representation of the equipment on a user is depicted in Fig. 5.3. The image processing to accurately detect lines and lanes is the main challenge in this system. While having positive results up to a speed of 10 km/h, the authors state that light variation has a big impact on image recognition and further improvements need to be done.

Other authors (Dutta, Barik, Chowdhury, & Gupta, 2018) propose an open, accessible, and extensible navigation system named *Divya-Drishti*, paving the way for a new paradigm for the VIP in navigation and travel. They developed a smartphone-based system to enable VIP to safely and independently navigate around familiar terrains like university campuses. They use a variety of sensors present in common smartphones for this purpose. Particularly, they use the GPS sensor in the smartphone to get the current location of its user. This information is combined with other sensor data to generate approximate user context. They employ an Android-based application that accepts voice commands and generates audible instructions directing further movements based on the current location of its users. The proposed application is practical and provides near accurate location guidance to users in outdoor environments. Also, a wearable low-cost device has been developed for the detection of knee height and hanging obstacles. This device uses ultrasound ranging for identifying obstacles in front and communicates via

Fig. 5.3 Camera, gloves with a haptic device to detect lines and lanes in a walk/jogging activity (adapted from Mancini et al., 2018)

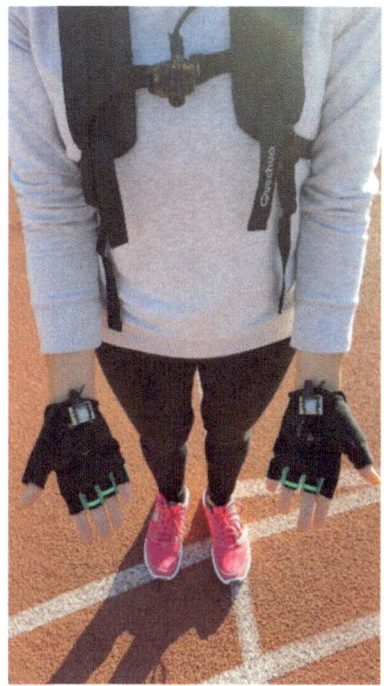

Bluetooth with smartphone-based app, which in turn generates vibrotactile response as a warning to its user.

Another system consists of an Android-based Application (Park, Goh, & So, 2014) that accepts voice commands from the user and generates audio messages giving information regarding the user's orientation, location, etc. For a given target location this application periodically gets the current location of the user and queries the back-end geodata store (either in a cloud or on device cache). The authors developed mobile application accessibility guidelines for people with visual impairment. They investigated various VIP people who were using mobile phones. Their usage patterns and follow-up interviews were analyzed. Moreover, they evaluated and developed systematic guidelines and standards of designing accessible mobile applications through a heuristic walkthrough method.

Raisamo, Nukarinen, Pystynen, Mäkinen, and Kildal (2012) showed that using orientation enquiry for non-visual pedestrian navigation, smartphones with haptic actuator and orientation sensor can be effectively used as a navigation aid. The authors claimed that majority of the users prefer this kind of haptic interaction techniques over tactile icons.

Researchers and scientists (Lanigan, Paulos, Williams, Rossi, & Narasimhan, 2006; Saaid, Ismail, & Noor, 2009; Shiizu, Hirahara, Yanashima, & Magatani, 2007) proposed the application of RFID in navigational system to detect the fall of VIP on the sidewalk by placing RFID at the center of the sidewalk. The experimental works cover antenna polarization, tag performance, tag orientation sensitivity, and tag communication distance for ultra-high frequency (UHF). The project includes development of hardware, software, and integration of both. The limitation of this method is the blind people must walk closely to the border of the sidewalk and use the walking stick to find out their current location.

5.3   Indoor Navigation

In this section, we will present a set of studies that describe different technologies and solutions to help VIP in indoor environments. One example of indoor navigation is within a shopping center in Thailand, with the purpose to allow VIP to go shopping and compare prices by themselves (Trongwongsa et al., 2015). The proposed solution uses proximity-based technology (Estimate iBeacons) based on the low-cost of this technology. The architecture of the system is depicted in Fig. 5.4 and has two main goals: to provide navigation inside the shopping and to detect products. We will focus on the navigation part. To support it, there is a database with maps of the shopping, iBeacons on the shelves. The user has a smartphone that captures iBeacons signals and, based on the maps in the database,

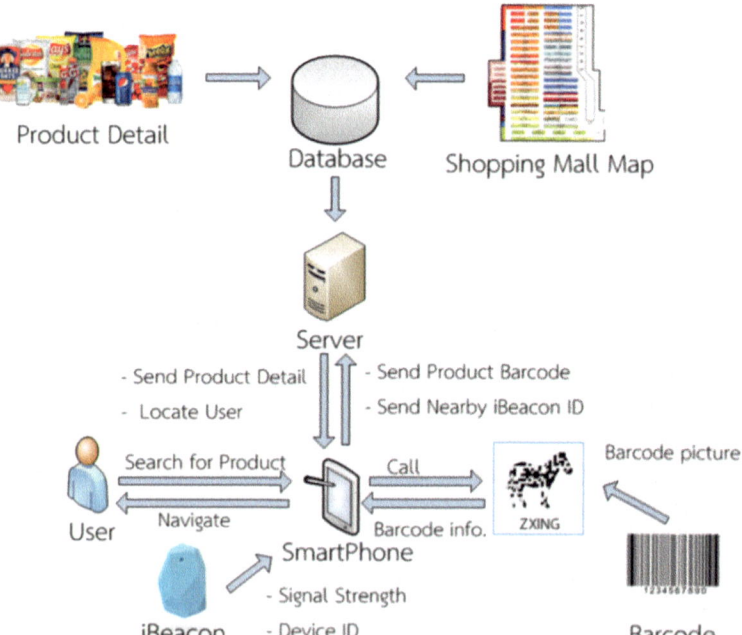

Fig. 5.4 System architecture to provide indoor navigation within a shopping center (adapted from Trongwongsa et al., 2015)

allows the calculation of the shortest path that leads the user to the selected product. The authors made tests with a group of visually impaired people and another group with no visual difficulties. The three tests consisted of successfully reaching shelf one, two, and the cashier register. The average time spent on these tasks by the group with no visual difficulties was 13.1 s. The visually impaired group, before training, spent 17.2 s in the same tasks and, after training, spent 14.6 s.

Another work, that has a similar purpose than the previous one presented, aims to guide VIP toward a target product on a store shelf using audio messages (Hild & Cheng, 2014). The system uses a CCD camera to identify the desired product and then produce all necessary audio messages, so the VIP is guided to the product and grab it. The system always starts with image acquisition. Sparse feature vector matching is used to detect the product inside the image. If the product is detected to be far away, voice messages are given to the user, so he moves toward the product. If the product is undetected, the user is walking away from the product and voice messages are produced to change position and, consequently, the camera orientation so the product is always visible. When the product is detected to be at range, so the user can grab it, the camera direction is kept stable during grasping.

Inspired by the autonomous lane following of self-driving cars, authors Chuang et al. (2018) combine the capabilities of existing navigation solutions for VIP users by proposing an autonomous, trail-following robotic guide dog that would be robust to variances of background textures, illuminations, and interclass trail variations. A deep convolutional neural network (CNN) is trained from both the virtual and real-world environments.

In the Faculty of Civil Engineering in Ayazaga Campus area, in Istanbul, a case study was developed for VIP within the context of the indoor navigation using loud steps (Bilgi et al., 2017), so VIP can freely move in closed areas without help. The architecture of this solution assumes users carry smartphones and Bluetooth beacons transmit their position signals and distance is calculated between the emitter and the receiver (see Fig. 5.5). This is how navigation information is achieved and presented to the user through his smartphone. Although having started in one faculty, the project was then carried out for other 12 faculties and 6 institutes. At the time of publication (2017), the application had been downloaded 130,000 times including more than 20,000 VIP at several institutions in 11 different countries.

Authors Meliones and Sampson (2018) in their work describe the functionality of the application and evaluates candidate indoor location determination technologies, such as wireless local area network (WLAN) and surface-mounted assistive tactile route indications combined with Bluetooth low energy (BLE) beacons and inertial dead-reckoning functionality, to come up with a reliable and highly accurate indoor positioning system adopting the latter solution. The developed concepts, including map matching, a key concept for indoor navigation, apply in a similar way to other indoor guidance use cases involving complex indoor places, such as in hospitals, shopping malls, airports, train stations, public and municipality buildings, office buildings, university buildings, hotel resorts, passenger ships, etc. The presented Android application is effectively a Blind Indoor Guide system for accurate and reliable blind indoor navigation.

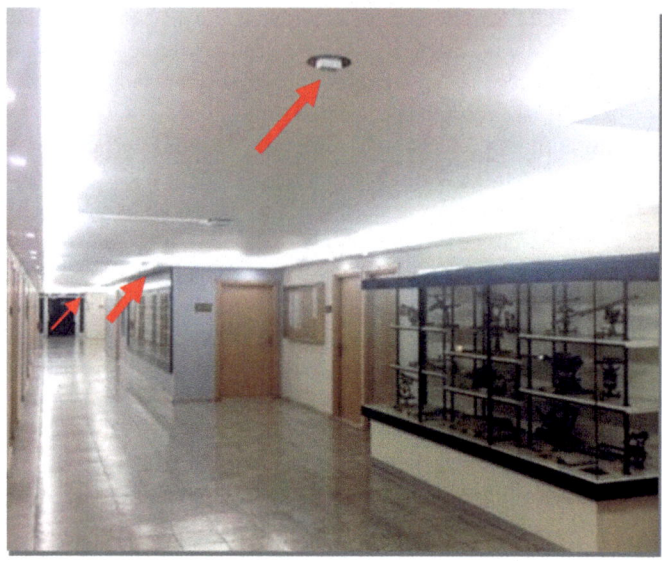

Fig. 5.5 Beacons positioned on the building's corridor to allow positioning to be calculated (adapted from Bilgi et al., 2017)

Authors Zhao et al. (2018) designed Canetroller, a haptic cane controller that simulates white cane interactions, enabling VIP to navigate a virtual environment by transferring their cane skills into the virtual world. It carries three types of feedback: (1) physical resistance generated by a wearable programmable brake mechanism that physically impedes the controller when the virtual cane comes in contact with a virtual object; (2) vibrotactile feedback that simulates the vibrations when a cane hits an object or touches and drags across various surfaces; and (3) spatial 3D auditory feedback simulating the sound of real-world cane interactions. The study performed showed that Canetroller was a promising tool that enabled visually impaired participants to navigate different virtual spaces. Figure 5.6 shows the mechanical parts of Canetroller with usable hardware features.

Authors Sato et al. (2017) have designed and implemented NavCog3, a smartphone-based indoor navigation assistant that has been evaluated in a 21,000 m^2 shopping mall. In addition to turn-by-turn instructions, it provides information on landmarks (e.g., tactile paving) and points of interests nearby. The authors first conducted a controlled study with 10 visually impaired users to assess localization accuracy and the perceived usefulness of semantic features. Later, they conducted another study with 43 participants with visual impairments where they could freely navigate in the shopping mall using NavCog3. It is suggested that NavCog3 can open new opportunities for users with visual impairments to independently find and visit large and complex places with confidence. An overview of this system is shown in Fig. 5.7.

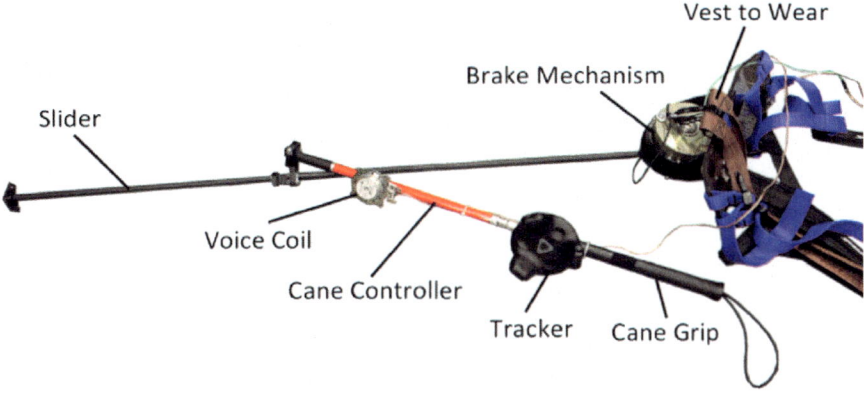

Fig. 5.6 Canetroller with the user interface (adapted from Zhao et al., 2018)

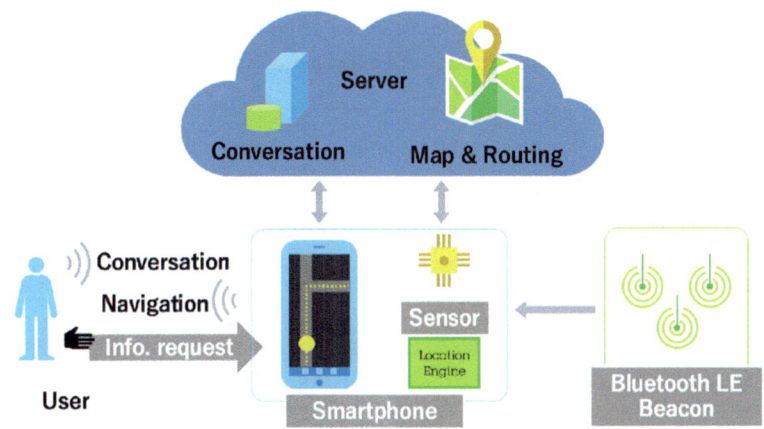

Fig. 5.7 An overview of the NavCog3 system (adapted from Sato et al., 2017)

In Umar et al. (2017), the authors present a method for human detection using a laser scanner with vision or infrared images. An efficient method for multimodal human detection based on a combination of the features and context information is proposed. Any person is detected in the vision/infrared images using a combination of local binary patterns and histogram of oriented gradient features with a neural network in a cascade manner. Next, using coordinates of detected humans from the vision system, the moving trajectory is predicted until the scanner working distance is reached by the individual human. Then the segmentation of data from the laser scanner is further carried out with respect to the predicted trajectory. Finally, human detection in the laser scanner working distance is performed based on modeling of the human legs. The modeling is based on the adaptive breakpoint detection algorithm and proposed improved polylines definition and fitting algorithm. The authors conducted a set of experiments in predefined scenarios, discussed the identified weakness and advantages of the proposed method, and outlined detailed future work, especially for night-time and low-light conditions.

Authors Gomes, Sousa, Cunha, and Morais (2018) present a hybrid indoor positioning system adaptable to the surrounding indoor structure and dealing with different types of signals to increase accuracy. This would allow to lower the deployment costs, since it could be done gradually, beginning with the likely existing Wi-Fi infrastructure to get a fairy accuracy up to a high accuracy using visual tags and NFC tags when necessary and possible.

Another audio-based navigation system (Dunai, Garcia, Lengua, & Peris-Fajarnés, 2012) is '3D CMOS sensor based acoustic object detection and navigation system for blind people' suggested by researchers from the Polytechnic University of Valencia. This system presents us with the prototype of an Electronic Travel Aid for Blind People. The system gains information about its surroundings using an array of 1×64 CMOS Time-of-Flight sensors. The information is converted into binaural signals output to the blind users via the wearable aid. Tests show that it was able to work with precision in the range of 15 m and $64°$ in azimuth which is a significant improvement over the existing Electronic Travel Aids.

5.4 Obstacle Avoidance

Finally, this section presents solutions specifically oriented to obstacle detection and avoidance which is, like we have mentioned before, something that can be applied to both indoor and outdoor environments.

The study presented in Ali and Ali (2017) represents a system for assistive technology based on a depth camera, an earphone, and a computer laptop. In the study, a Kinect camera was used to detect obstacles in front of the person, after processing images using a windowing-based mean average method. The system is intended to replace a guide dog and has a range of 4 m long which can be an advantage over the white cane. The authors are aware that the weight of the equipment is a drawback at this point but the replacement of the laptop for a smartphone would reduce this problem easily in a near future.

Another research intends to propose a system to detect grounded or raised obstacles up to a few meters in front of the subject. As shown in Fig. 5.8, the user carries a white cane with two sensors. Sensor 1 aims to the leg region and sensor 2 to the head. Obstacles in positions such as A and B can be detected by Sensor 1 and notified to the user a few seconds before contact, so he is able to avoid it. Obstacle C can be detected by Sensor 2 which mainly prevents head level injuries. The architecture behind this system includes an Arduino, a GPS receiver (to gather information on user's outdoor location), a GSM module (can be used to make a phone call in case of emergency), an ultrasonic ranging module, a vibration motor, and a buzzer (Shahu & Shinko, 2017).

In Patel, Kumar, Yadav, Desai, and Patil (2017), a wearable device is designed that works with smartphones to give users feedback about bumps and obstacles. But

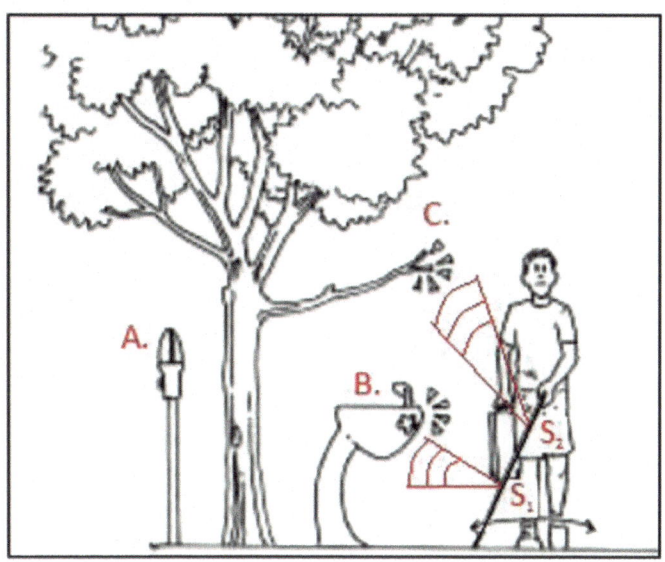

Fig. 5.8 Sensors in white cane and possible obstacles (adapted from Shahu & Shinko, 2017)

a user not only needs to be aware of the obstacles and bumps in his/her surroundings, but also needs to navigate, to know the precise location and nearby landmarks.

Another study with similar technologies is presented in Choi, Yang, Bang, and Kim (2018) where authors propose a system which is made up of the ultrasonic sensor and is interfaced with the microcontroller. The system will allow VIP to freely navigate to their desired destination. It checks for potholes and their depth. The moisture sensor consists of two wire probes which rely on the specific resistance of water to sense its presence when there is a contact. The RF transmitter was interfaced with the microcontroller. It is also user friendly and easy. It is affordable and therefore can be mass produced for use of the VIP. The system has the capacity to detect obstacles that exist on the ground during indoor and outdoor navigation. The smart stick is basically an embedded system integrating the following: pair of ultrasonic sensors to detect obstacles in front of the blind from ground level height to head level height in the range of 40 cm a head Ultrasonic sensors and water sensors take real-time data and send it to the microcontroller. After processing this data, the microcontroller activates the buzzer. The water sensor detects water on the ground, and the battery is used to power the circuits.

An algorithm for obstacle detection is the subject of the research of Jie and Yanbin (2012) who developed an ETA for VIP based on stereo vision. The ETA is composed of two cameras, a portable computer, and an earphone. The algorithm for obstacle detection is based on self-adaptive threshold image segmentation and the steps it is composed of are shown in Fig. 5.9. Experiments made with 75 consecutive frames showed an accuracy of 96% when detecting obstacles.

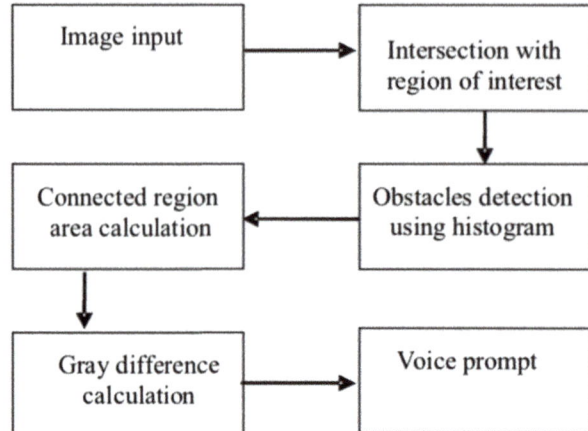

Fig. 5.9 Steps of the algorithm to detect obstacles based on image recognition (adapted from Jie & Yanbin, 2012)

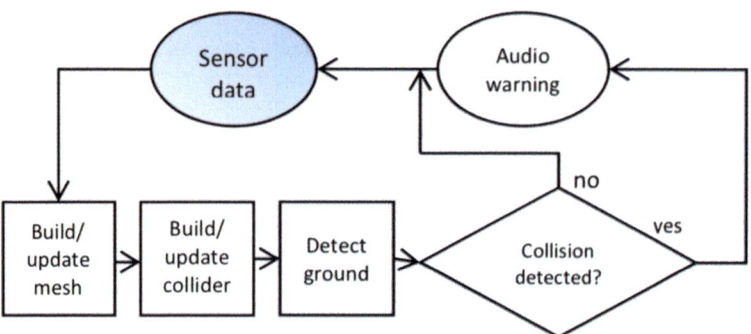

Fig. 5.10 Algorithm for detecting obstacles using 3D reconstruction system (adapted from Jafri et al., 2017)

Google introduced the Google Project Tango Tablet Development Kit (Jafri, Campos, Ali, & Arabnia, 2017), composed by an android device containing a powerful processor and several sensors that include motion tracking camera, 3D depth sensor, accelerometer, ambient light sensor, barometer, compass, GPS, gyroscope, and an integrated infrared based depth sensor. An application was developed, on top on this Kit, to process the depth and motion tracking data gathered from all available sensors. From there, a 3D reconstruction mapping the real-world environment is built. If the user's position is detected to collide with a solid surface, an audio warning is produced. The algorithm is depicted in Fig. 5.10.

The development of new devices that incorporate sensors which can be integrated into objects VIP carry with them along the day is another line of research that currently gathers plenty of investigators. One of such examples is the work described in Cardillo et al. (2018). A white cane is an object all VIP use and, for that reason,

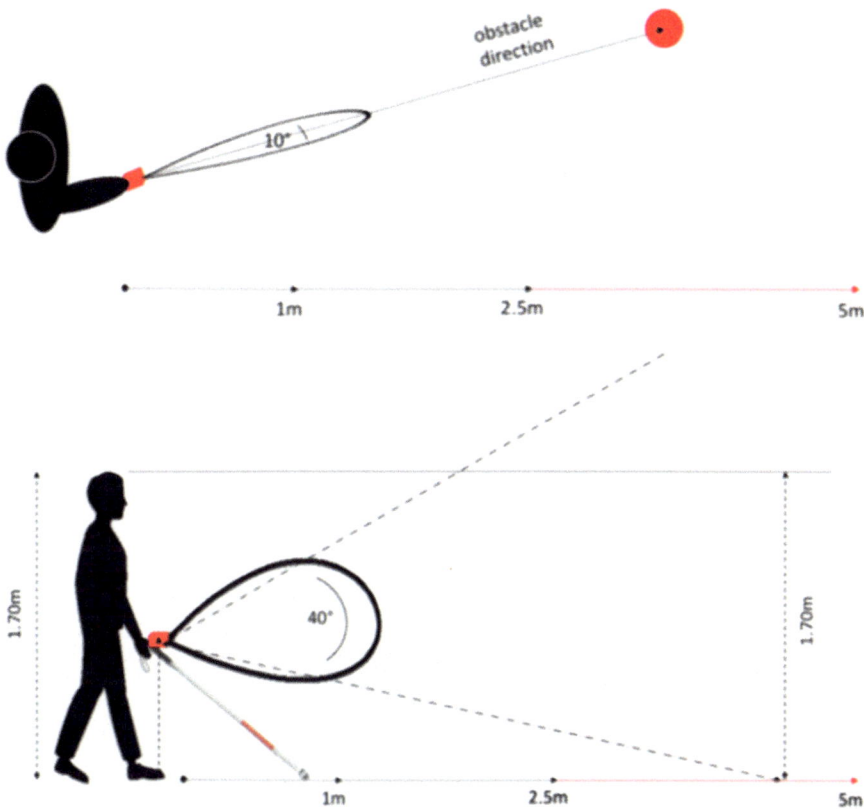

Fig. 5.11 Integration of an electromagnetic sensor (adapted from Cardillo et al., 2018)

can integrate a small device to achieve a given purpose. In this case, the authors propose the integration of an electromagnetic sensor in a white can, so it is possible to detect objects, as shown in Fig. 5.11. The authors emphasize the care that must be taken in the design of the prototype that will be integrated into the white cane, since the final aspect is something that VIP value. The chapter presents a detailed description of the board construction, so obstacle detection is possible within 5 m. As future work, the authors claim to be possible to obtain a small box of about 10 cm of width and weight of a few hundreds of grams.

Developments have also been made in the area of using smartphones as an assistive tool for the VIP. Headsets fitted with smartphones that can detect objects around the user and help them navigate and perceive things around them in detail is the approach of the system proposed in Bai, Liu, Su, and Fu (2017) where users can interact with the system using voice, navigate and inquire about the environment around them. This is one of the major groundbreaking developments in assistive technologies for the VIP as it helps them to live as much like a person without disabilities.

A context-aware smartphone-based visual obstacle detection approach is presented in Gharani and Karimi (2017) to aid VIP in navigating indoor environments. The approach is based on processing two consecutive frames (images), computing optical flow, and tracking certain points to detect obstacles. The frame rate of the video stream is determined using a context-aware data fusion technique for the sensors on smartphones. Through an efficient and novel algorithm, for each consecutive frame, a point dataset on the frames is designed and evaluated to check whether the points belong to an obstacle. In addition to determining the points based on the texture in each frame, the algorithm also considers the heading of user movement to find critical areas on the image plane.

Researchers (Suffoletto, Gharani, Chung, & Karimi, 2018) proposed and developed a complete system to assist VIP for doing their navigational tasks. The system provides the instructions for navigating turn by turn and also could detect obstacles. According to these capabilities, it could be seen that the system tries to integrate both micro and macro navigation systems. In order to make the user aware of the surrounding environment, a wide range of sensors are used. In recent years, sensors of wearable devices have gained considerable attention. The proposed system has different parts and it consists of a microcontroller as a processor, an accelerometer, a footswitch, a speech synthesizer, a hexadecimal keypad, a mode switch, an ultrasonic cane, two ultrasonic sensors, two vibrators, and a power switch. It can detect obstacles in a range of 72° in front of the user which seems to be wide enough. Moreover, it can detect both static and dynamic obstacles at the distance up to 20 ft although detecting both dynamic and static obstacles is a remarkable property, the range of 20 ft could be insufficient.

5.5   Discussion

Throughout the review made on this chapter, we presented several studies that relate to mobility solutions to help VIP both in indoor and outdoor environments, as both have different characteristics.

Regarding outdoor environment activities, several solutions can assist VIP and are the object of study by the scientific community. The navigation/pedestrian orientation in outdoor environments, similar to the one we are accustomed to in cars, is one of the activities that reflects the greater need for solutions and devices that assist the VIP. For this type of scenario, some proposed solutions (a summary can be found in Table 5.1) include image sensors that allow a match of locations, smartphone sensors to conclude about nearby context, the use of 3D audio that allow to provide clues about the current location and distance to a given destination, the use of geo-data and cross-reference functions, geolocation or non-visual navigational aid to support orientation tasks, vision system to identify lines and lanes to support sports activities, LK optical flow to detect moving

Table 5.1 Summary of approaches and equipment for outdoor environment activities

Purpose	Approach	Equipment
General outdoor navigation	Scene matching aided navigation, using image sensors	CCD digital camera
Detecting moving objects	Improved LK Optical Flow	Camera to take the images
Understand a visual scene and obtain localization	Geolocation and use of equipment data	Mobile app, Bluetooth, RFID, NFC, iBeacon
Giving cues on the direction and distance to the intended location	Use of 3D Audio	Geomagnetic sensor and a PC
Perform walking and running activities	Use of a vision system that identifies lines and lanes along a given route	Camera, gloves to receive vibrations
General outdoor navigation	Sensors in the smartphone to generate approximate user context	Android-based application and wearable low-cost device
General outdoor navigation/Get orientation and location	Use of geo-data to cross-reference data	Android-based Application
Orientation	Non-visual navigation aid	Haptic actuator and orientation sensor
Detection of falls on the sidewalk	RFID in navigational system	Antenna, tags, and ultra-high frequency

objects, or antennas and ultra-high frequencies to prevent falls in sidewalks. Several equipments are being used as a support for these technological solutions. Some examples include CCD cameras, orientation sensors, smartphone sensors, antennas, Bluetooth, RFID, NFC or beacons and mobile applications, haptic actuators or gloves to receive vibrations as a way to interact with the VIP.

As far as navigation within buildings is concerned, technologies and solutions are necessarily different (summary in Table 5.2). In terms of purpose, the main one is to navigate and get directions in indoor environments but there are some specific concerns like reaching objects on store shelves and supermarkets or even a large focus on maximum accuracy to allow turn-by-turn message instructions. Approaches for indoor navigation are very wide and include training of deep convolutional neural network, loud steps, map matching using WLAN, sensors and inertial dead-reckoning functionality, multimodal human detection based on a combination of the features and context information, perceived usefulness of semantic features, use of different types of signals to increase accuracy and acoustic object detection. Approaches for helping VIP to reach products in shelves include space maps and optimized route detection and also sparse feature vector algorithm and visual-auditory feedback. On the other hand, technologies that support these indoor navigation solutions and approaches encompass iBeacons, smartphones, hand-held devices and cameras, regarding reaching objects in shelves. For general navigation

Table 5.2 Summary of approaches and equipment for indoor navigation activities

Activity	Approach	Equipment
Reaching objects in shelves	Space maps and optimized route detection	iBeacons, smartphone
Reaching objects in shelves	Sparse feature vector algorithm and visual-auditory feedback	Hand-held, monopod-mounted CCD camera
General indoor navigation	Trained deep convolutional neural network	Trail-following robotic guide dog
General indoor navigation	Loud steps	Beacons and smartphone
General Indoor navigation	Map matching using WLAN and surface-mounted assistive tactile route indications combined with sensors and inertial dead-reckoning functionality	Android application, Smartphone, BLE beacons
General Indoor navigation	Prediction of moving trajectory based on multimodal human detection based on a combination of the features and context information	Laser scanner with vision or infrared images
Turn-by-turn instructions and information on points of interests nearby	Assess localization accuracy and the perceived usefulness of semantic features	Smartphone and server
General Indoor navigation	Use different types of signals to increase accuracy	Wi-Fi infrastructure and/or NFC tags
General Indoor navigation	Acoustic object detection	3D CMOS sensor

equipment include trail-following robotic guide dog, beacons and smartphones, apps, laser scanner with vision or infrared images, Wi-Fi infrastructure and/or NFC tags and 3D CMOS sensor.

Obstacle detection is an important component of navigation systems for the VIP. Table 5.3 shows a summary of the purpose, approaches, and support equipment for some recently proposed solutions. The objectives are varied and can be a general detection of any obstacle that is in front of the user, the detection of the position of the user, and the possibility of colliding with some obstacle that could be near or detection of potholes and their depth. Approaches can include image segmentation, radar, processing, and analysis of frames or images, 3D reconstruction of the real-world environment, ultrasound microcontroller-based system or voice-based systems. Finally, equipment that is typically used includes cameras, smartphones, sensors, white cane, Arduino, GPS receiver or headsets and earphones.

Table 5.3 Summary of approaches and equipment for obstacle detection

Purpose	Approach	Equipment
General obstacle detection	Image segmentation	Cameras, Computer, Earphone
General obstacle detection	Radar	White cane, electromagnetic sensor
General obstacle detection	Processing and analysis of consecutive frames	Context-aware smartphone and wearable device
Detect if the user's position is detected to collide with a solid surface	3D reconstruction mapping the real-world environment	Sensors, Google Tablet Kit
General obstacle detection	Processing of images using a windowing-based mean average method	Kinect depth camera, earphone, and computer laptop
Detect grounded or raised obstacles up to a few meters in front of the subject	Ultrasound microcontroller-based system	An Arduino, a GPS receiver, a GSM module, an ultrasonic ranging module, a vibration motor, and a buzzer
Detect objects around the user and help them navigate and perceive things	Smartphone application controlled by a voice-based user interaction system	Headsets and Smartphone
Check for potholes and their depth	Ultrasonic sensors and water sensors take real-time data and send it to the microcontroller that processes data and activates the buzzer	Ultrasonic sensor interfaced with microcontroller
Detect both static and dynamic obstacles at the distance up to 20 ft	Gather data from sensors and compute user position and obstacles	Sensors, microcontroller, an accelerometer, a footswitch, a speech synthesizer, a hexadecimal keypad, a mode switch, an ultrasonic cane, two ultrasonic sensors, two vibrators, and a power switch
Give users feedback about bumps and obstacles		Wearable device, smartphone

5.6   Conclusions

In this article, we review a set of recent scientific contributions in the area of the mobility of blind people, indoor, outdoor as well as obstacle detection, common to both environments. For each scenario, several articles were reviewed in order to make known their purpose and usefulness to the VIP. We attempt to synthesize the discussed information by presenting a discussion section where we tabulate each scenario, various solutions, their objectives, and approach followed as well as used technologies and equipment. It is observed that whereas much research is going on in the technologies and systems toward imparting assistance and improved mobility to VIP, still we need much more that can provide overall flexibility and independence to them. Most of the proposed techniques are scenario-specific. They focus only on a particular aspect. However, we require an overall well-equipped technique that makes a VIP completely proficient in the use of modern technology which will enhance their overall movement and confidence.

References

Ali, A., & Ali, M. A. (2017). Blind navigation system for visually impaired using windowing-based mean on Microsoft Kinect camera. In *International Conference on Advances in Biomedical Engineering (ICABME)*.

Bai, J., Liu, D., Su, G., & Fu, Z. (2017, April). A cloud and vision-based navigation system used for blind people. In *Proceedings of the 2017 ACM International Conference on Artificial Intelligence, Automation and Control Technologies* (p. 22). New York, NY: ACM.

Bilgi, S., Ozturk, O., & Gulnerman, A. G. (2017). Navigation system for blind, hearing and visually impaired people in ITU Ayazaga campus. In *Proceedings of the IEEE International Conference on Computing, Networking and Informatics, ICCNI 2017*. https://doi.org/10.1109/ICCNI.2017.8123814

Cardillo, E., Di Mattia, V., Manfredi, G., Russo, P., De Leo, A., Caddemi, A., & Cerri, G. (2018). An electromagnetic sensor prototype to assist visually impaired and blind people in autonomous walking. *IEEE Sensors Journal*. https://doi.org/10.1109/JSEN.2018.2795046

Choi, D. S., Yang, T. H., Bang, W. C., & Kim, S. Y. (2018). Design of a multi-functional module for visually impaired persons. *International Journal of Precision Engineering and Manufacturing, 19*(11), 1745–1751.

Chuang, T. K., Lin, N. C., Chen, J. S., Hung, C. H., Huang, Y. W., Tengl, C., & Wang, H. C. (2018). Deep trail-following robotic guide dog in pedestrian environments for people who are blind and visually impaired-learning from virtual and real worlds. In *Proceedings of the 2018 IEEE International Conference on Robotics and Automation (ICRA)* (pp. 1–7).

Dunai, L., Garcia, B. D., Lengua, I., & Peris-Fajarnés, G. (2012, October). 3D CMOS sensor based acoustic object detection and navigation system for blind people. In *IECON 2012-38th Annual Conference on IEEE Industrial Electronics Society* (pp. 4208–4215).

Dutta, S., Barik, M. S., Chowdhury, C., & Gupta, D. (2018, January). Divya-Dristi: A smartphone based campus navigation system for the visually impaired. In *2018 Fifth IEEE International Conference on Emerging Applications of Information Technology (EAIT)* (pp. 1–3).

Gharani, P., & Karimi, H. A. (2017). Context-aware obstacle detection for navigation by visually impaired. *Image and Vision Computing, 64*, 103–115.

Gomes, J. P., Sousa, J. P., Cunha, C. R., & Morais, E. P. (2018, June). An indoor navigation architecture using variable data sources for blind and visually impaired persons. In *2018 13th IEEE Iberian Conference on Information Systems and Technologies (CISTI)* (pp. 1–5).

Hild, M., & Cheng, F. (2014). Grasping guidance for visually impaired persons based on computed visual-auditory feedback. In *Computer Vision Theory and Applications (VISAPP)* (pp. 75–82).

Jafri, R., Campos, R. L., Ali, S. A., & Arabnia, H. R. (2017). Visual and infrared sensor data-based obstacle detection for the visually impaired using the Google project Tango Tablet Development Kit and the Unity Engine. *Access, 6*, 443–454. https://doi.org/10.1109/ACCESS.2017.2766579

Jie, Y., & Yanbin, S. (2012). Obstacle detection of a novel travel aid for visual impaired people. In *4th International Conference on Intelligent Human-Machine Systems and Cybernetics, IHMSC* (pp. 362–364).

Lanigan, P. E., Paulos, A. M., Williams, A. W., Rossi, D., & Narasimhan, P. (2006, October). Trinetra: Assistive technologies for grocery shopping for the blind. In *ISWC* (pp. 147–148).

Mancini, A., Frontoni, E., & Zingaretti, P. (2018). Mechatronic system to help visually impaired users during walking and running. *IEEE Transactions on Intelligent Transportation Systems.* https://doi.org/10.1109/TITS.2017.2780621

Masulli, F., Rovetta, S., Cabri, A., Traverso, C., Capris, E., & Torretta, S. (2017). An assistive mobile system supporting blind and visual impaired people when are outdoor. In *3rd International Forum on Research and Technologies for Society and Industry* (pp. 1–6).

Matsuda, K., & Kondo, K. (2016). Towards an accurate route guidance system for the visually impaired using 3D audio. In *IEEE 5th Global Conference on Consumer Electronics* (pp. 433–434).

Meliones, A., & Sampson, D. (2018). Blind MuseumTourer: A system for self-guided tours in museums and blind indoor navigation. *Technologies, 6*(1), 4.

Park, K., Goh, T., & So, H. J. (2014, December). Toward accessible mobile application design: Developing mobile application accessibility guidelines for people with visual impairment. In *Proceedings of HCI Korea* (pp. 31–38). Seoul, Korea: Hanbit Media, Inc.

Patel, S., Kumar, A., Yadav, P., Desai, J., & Patil, D. (2017, March). Smartphone-based obstacle detection for visually impaired people. In *2017 IEEE International Conference on Innovations in Information, Embedded and Communication Systems (ICIIECS)* (pp. 1–3).

Raisamo, R., Nukarinen, T., Pystynen, J., Mäkinen, E., & Kildal, J. (2012). Orientation inquiry: A new haptic interaction technique for non-visual pedestrian navigation. In *Proceedings of Eurohaptics* (pp. 139–144).

Saaid, M. F., Ismail, I., & Noor, M. Z. H. (2009, March). Radio frequency identification walking stick (RFIWS): A device for the blind. In *5th IEEE International Colloquium on Signal Processing & Its Applications (CSPA 2009)* (pp. 250–253).

Sato, D., Oh, U., Naito, K., Takagi, H., Kitani, K., & Asakawa, C. (2017, October). Navcog3: An evaluation of a smartphone-based blind indoor navigation assistant with semantic features in a large-scale environment. In *Proceedings of the 19th International ACM SIGACCESS Conference on Computers and Accessibility* (pp. 270–279).

Shahu, D., & Shinko, I. (2017). A low-cost mobility monitoring system for visually impaired users. In *International Conference on Smart Systems and Technologies (SST)* (pp. 235–238).

Shiizu, Y., Hirahara, Y., Yanashima, K., & Magatani, K. (2007, August). The development of a white cane which navigates the visually impaired. In *29th Annual International Conference of the IEEE Engineering in Medicine and Biology Society (EMBS 2007)* (pp. 5005–5008).

Suffoletto, B., Gharani, P., Chung, T., & Karimi, H. (2018). Using phone sensors and an artificial neural network to detect gait changes during drinking episodes in the natural environment. *Gait & Posture, 60*, 116–121.

Trongwongsa, T., Chankrachang, K., Prompoon, N., & Pattanothai, C. (2015). Shopping navigation system for visual impaired people based on proximity-based technology. In *Proceedings of the 2015 12th International Joint Conference on Computer Science and Software Engineering, JCSSE 2015.* https://doi.org/10.1109/JCSSE.2015.7219807

Umar, B. U., Agajo, J., Aliyu, A., Kolo, J. G., Owolabi, O. S., & Olaniyi, O. M. (2017, November). Human detection using speeded-up robust features and support vector machine from aerial images. In *3rd IEEE International Conference on Electro-Technology for National Development (NIGERCON), 2017* (pp. 577–586).

Wang, X., Wang, L., Yin, J., & Zhang, C. (2010). Research on local image navigation method for visual-impaired person. In *Proceedings - 5th International Conference on Frontier of Computer Science and Technology, FCST 2010.* https://doi.org/10.1109/FCST.2010.96

Zhao, Y., Bennett, C. L., Benko, H., Cutrell, E., Holz, C., Morris, M. R., & Sinclair, M. (2018, April). Enabling people with visual impairments to navigate virtual reality with a haptic and auditory cane simulation. In *Proceedings of the 2018 ACM CHI Conference on Human Factors in Computing Systems* (p. 116).

Zhao, G., Wang, X., & Wang, L. (2012). Motion analysis and research of local navigation system for visual-impaired person based on improved LK optical flow. In *Proceedings - 5th International Conference on Intelligent Networks and Intelligent Systems, ICINIS 2012.* https://doi.org/10.1109/ICINIS.2012.80

Part II
Navigation Systems Proposals

Chapter 6
Cloud Video Guidance as "Deus ex Machina" for the Visually Impaired

Thanasis Loukopoulos, Maria Koziri, Natalia Panagou, Panos K. Papadopoulos, and Dimitris K. Iakovidis

6.1 Introduction

As estimated by the World Health Organization, more than one billion people suffer from some sort of vision impairment (WHO: World Health Organization, 2018). Visually impaired people face difficulties in accomplishing everyday tasks, particularly when interacting in an open environment, away from their leaving places. Issues like obstacle avoidance, navigation, and social interaction which are done effortlessly by the majority, for the visually impaired pose significant difficulties. Furthermore, more than 80% of the cases concern vision impairment resulting from diseases that are usually triggered in high ages, e.g., cataract, macular degeneration, etc. Thus, a holistic approach to assistive technologies for the visually impaired is needed, whereby independent solutions to particular aspects of the problem will be combined together with other solutions, e.g., for the elderly people, in order to form a *personalized assistive ecosystem*.

In order to materialize the above holistic vision, a modular, open-ended system architecture is needed with components that can be dynamically added/subtracted depending on the situation. Cloud computing can play this role ideally, since most providers offer a variety of virtualization options that can be used to abstract hardware and computer programs. We envision that the assistance per se will be offered in the form of a customizable workflow that runs in the Cloud (Liu, Zhang,

T. Loukopoulos · P. K. Papadopoulos · D. K. Iakovidis (✉)
Department of Computer Science and Biomedical Informatics, University of Thessaly, Lamia, Greece
e-mail: luke@uth.gr; ppadopoulos@uth.gr; diakovidis@uth.gr

M. Koziri · N. Panagou
Department of Computer Science, University of Thessaly, Lamia, Greece
e-mail: mkoziri@uth.gr; npanagou@uth.gr

© Springer Nature Switzerland AG 2020 127
S. Paiva (ed.), *Technological Trends in Improved Mobility of the Visually Impaired*,
EAI/Springer Innovations in Communication and Computing,
https://doi.org/10.1007/978-3-030-16450-8_6

Lin, & Qin, 2014). The application workflow will be fed by the various (mainly portable) sensors the visually impaired person will carry and results from processing will be sent back to some mobile smart device. The workflow itself might invoke various services (Rao & Su, 2004) to complete specified tasks.

As an example consider the case where a visually impaired person wants to visit an archeological site. By using a camera and a mobile smart device a variety of options can be made available. Using the camera's feed the application workflow might be set so as to invoke obstacle detection and provide acoustic guidance to avoid them. Alternatively, the video feed could be delivered to a specified social group involving friends and relatives that would like to actively participate by providing speech feedback. Using GPS positioning and/or orientation information and relating it to the archaeological site, the application workflow might be able to provide tourist guide narration involving the history of the visited site, or navigational information such as guidance toward the nearest exit, or a particular POI (Place of Interest). Lastly, in much the same way common people build memoires from their visits by capturing photos, the assistive application will be able to build an optical and acoustical album of the visit. By contrast, such rich options will not be needed if a visually impaired person wants to visit her local store to buy everyday supplies.

This chapter is largely based on preliminary results from the ENORASI project that has been recently spawned under EU and Greek funding. The aim of the project is to develop an assistive tool for the visually impaired, the core of which will rely on video processing and artificial intelligence techniques. The primary goal of ENORASI is to make the options discussed in the motivating example (visit of an archaeological site) feasible in a practical way. Furthermore, the resulting system should follow a modular design to enable customization ease, extensibility as well as the integration of subcomponents produced by different vendors. In this chapter, we focus on describing the intended system architecture and identifying related research challenges, without delving on the details of particular application components. While assistive technologies for the visually impaired have gained significant traction lately, e.g., in the form of smart glasses (Lee & Hui, 2018), to the best of our knowledge most existing efforts focus on providing the desired functionality using rather monolithic system designs. Our contributions include the following:

- We propose a modular Cloud-based system architecture that can be used to implement various assistive applications for the visually impaired people;
- We identify engineering challenges that must be tackled in order to effectively deploy the proposed application and capitalize on its extensibility and maintainability potential;
- We outline research directions to optimize the end system performance.

The rest of the chapter is organized as follows. Section 6.2 presents the related work. Section 6.3 illustrates the system architecture. Section 6.4 provides details on the application workflow. Section 6.5 discusses data capturing issues with a particular focus on video. Section 6.6 identifies optimization potentials concerning the cross-layer system deployment between Cloud and network Edges. Finally, Sect. 6.7 concludes the chapter.

6.2   Related Work

Visually impaired people face difficulties when they have to navigate through unfamiliar environments. For the purpose of enhancing those people's quality of life by being able to navigate into the place of their choice independently, extensive research has focused on developing assistive systems. An assistive system is a device that is able to help individuals with certain disabilities to enjoy everyday activities while ensuring their normal integration into society. Traditional assistive means, like white canes, guide dogs, or screen readers proved to be insufficient to satisfactorily assist visually impaired individuals. Such assistive means cannot provide a comprehensive picture of the environment, as is the case with white canes, or can be demanding to train and maintain, as is the case with guide dogs.

In the context of assistive technologies for visually impaired people, a variety of systems concerning spatial orientation and navigation have been introduced. An extensive review of such systems can be found in Fernandes, Costa, Filipe, Paredes, and Barroso (2017). In Vorapatratorn and Nambunmee (2014) the authors proposed an obstacle detection device based on ultrasonic sensors that can be used as a walking assistant. In Guerreiro, Ahmetovic, Kitani, and Asakawa (2017), a smartphone application system offering turn-by-turn navigation while simultaneously informing the user about points of interest is proposed. The stated goal was to create a mental representation of the route for the visually impaired. Similarly, in Kim, Bessho, Kobayashi, Koshizuka, and Sakamura (2016) a smartphone-based system utilizing Bluetooth technology was developed in order to provide navigational guidance in large train stations.

A wearable, camera-based system was proposed in Wang et al. (2017) with the aim of accomplishing object detection and notification, while in Brilhault, Kammoun, Gutierrez, Truillet, and Jouffrais (2011) a system for improving positioning of the user in city environments was proposed. The system used information fusion from GPS and visual data to achieve its stated goal. In Lee and Medioni (2016), a wearable system, based on RGB-D camera for indoor navigation is presented, while a system for validating user location through object recognition was proposed in Fernandes, Costa, Paredes, Filipe, and Barroso (2014). Guidance through voice instructions was described by Šimunovi, Aneli, and Pavlinuši (2012), while a cloud-based system, with object recognition and detection, able to interact via voice with the user is proposed in Bai, Liu, Su, and Fu (2017).

Apart from spatial orientation and navigation, visually impaired individuals need also to be able to detect and discriminate objects in their environment. Object recognition and detection can be achieved through computer vision. Various such systems are described in Sosa-Garcia and Odone (2017). Concerning visual recognition, in Chincha and Tian (2011), a system able to assist blind people to detect missing items is proposed. Object recognition is achieved through a wearable camera and a database which holds a variety of images of user's personal items, captured from different angles. Also, in Winlock, Christiansen, and Belongie (2010), a system able to assist blind people while shopping in a grocery store, detecting items in shopping list is introduced. Finally, in the context of object detection, in Mekhalfi, Melgani, Bazi, and Alajlan (2015), a real-time, camera-based scheme is introduced to detect multiple objects in an indoor environment.

6.3 Generic System Architecture

Even if the systems described in Sect. 6.2 share some goals with the targeted ENORASI platform, they differ in scope as they are usually standalone system architectures making interoperability a tough challenge. In the sequel, we present the proposed open-ended Cloud-based system architecture.

6.3.1 Overview

The primary goal of the proposed architecture is to improve system's maintainability and extensibility. In order to realize the target, the system follows a modular design which is graphically depicted in Fig. 6.1. On the end-user side, various data streams are generated including video, audio commands, GPS positioning, etc. The stream-generating process is governed by a smart mobile application acting as the system's client side. Streams are sent to the relevant monitoring spouts which are responsible among others for adapting the sampling rate (wherever applicable). It should be noted that although the primary focus of the design concerns data generated by the visually impaired person and the carried sensors, nothing precludes the system to incorporate data streams from other sources. The visionary goal will be to fully make the proposed system interoperate in a smart city environment. For instance, information concerning weather, public transportation availability, ongoing road or pedestrian road works, etc., when translated in suitable acoustic descriptions can significantly enhance the system's impact.

At the core of the system lies the main Cloud application in the form of a workflow. The workflow takes as input information fed by related spouts and implements the main logical flow of the desired application functionality. In doing so, the main parts of the desired functionalities are obtained by invoking separate software modules implemented as Cloud services. We consider image processing, speech processing, and navigation/guidance services as key system components to implement the targeted assistive technology, i.e., aiding the mobility of visually impaired people. In practice, these services might be further split down. For instance, the image processing service might be comprised of obstacle detection, object recognition, depth estimation, etc. Navigation/guidance services

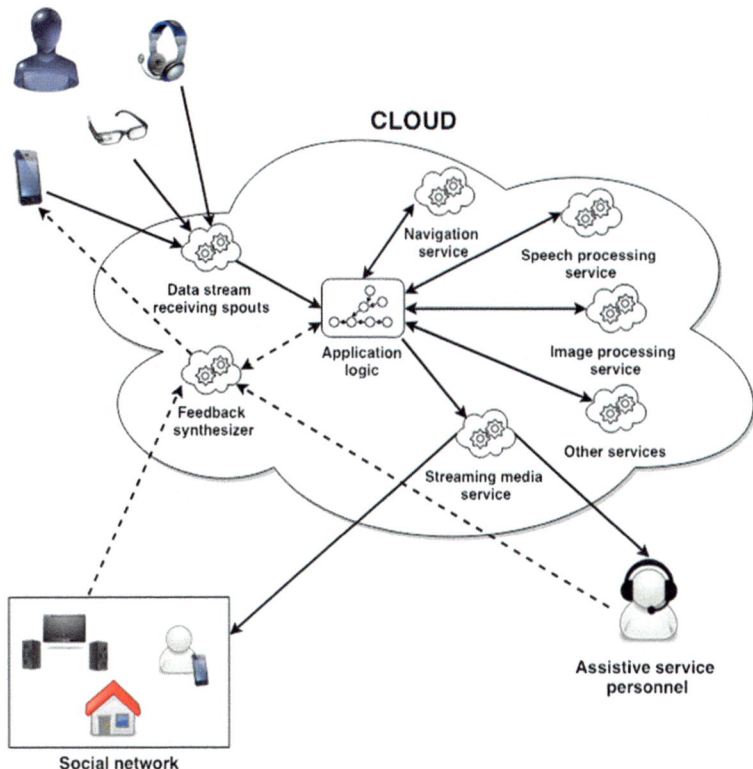

CLOUD

Navigation service

Speech processing service

Data stream receiving spouts

Application logic

Image processing service

Feedback synthesizer

Other services

Streaming media service

Assistive service personnel

Social network

Fig. 6.1 System architecture overview

may be automated, providing directions based on GPS data and/or inferred by an intelligent system, exploiting different resources within the Cloud (e.g., mobile processing units and servers). They may also be non-automated, facilitating real-time interaction between humans, e.g., in case of a difficult situation, where the automated services are insufficient to guide the visually impaired user to resolve it.

The output of the workflow to the visually impaired users primarily consists of audio but other signaling feedback is also possible (e.g., vibration). It also includes parameter adaptation to the client side software in order to optimize performance. For instance, the quality of the video feed could be tuned to aid in accurate obstacle recognition once an obstacle is detected. Depending on the desired functionality, the application might choose to forward the client video and audio streams to a set of interested parties that might include persons belonging in the social network of the client or even specialized human assistants tasked with providing guidance or touring services. Feedback from these sources also comes in the form of audio and is directed to a feedback synthesizer module together with the output of main application logic.

The task of the feedback synthesizer is to prioritize system output in the presence of multiple options. For instance, assuming a visit to an archaeological site is followed by a friend network, it is straightforward to assume that human interaction should take priority over, e.g., automatically generated tourist guide information. Nevertheless, in case a threatening obstacle is detected obstacle avoidance is prioritized.

6.3.2 Resource Sharing and Customization

The system is targeted for scalability and practicality. It is expected that the various subscribed users will have different functionality demands. This means that the application logic should be customizable in an easy way. We envision that a basic workflow application template exists, that is tunable according to user needs through easily accessed menu options. Services will be described as virtualized resources that must support a fixed Application Programming Interface (API) for interoperability.

Different application logics might refer to the same or different service implementations in order to accomplish the same task. This is shown in Fig. 6.2 whereby three different application logics exist in the system (presumably depicting three

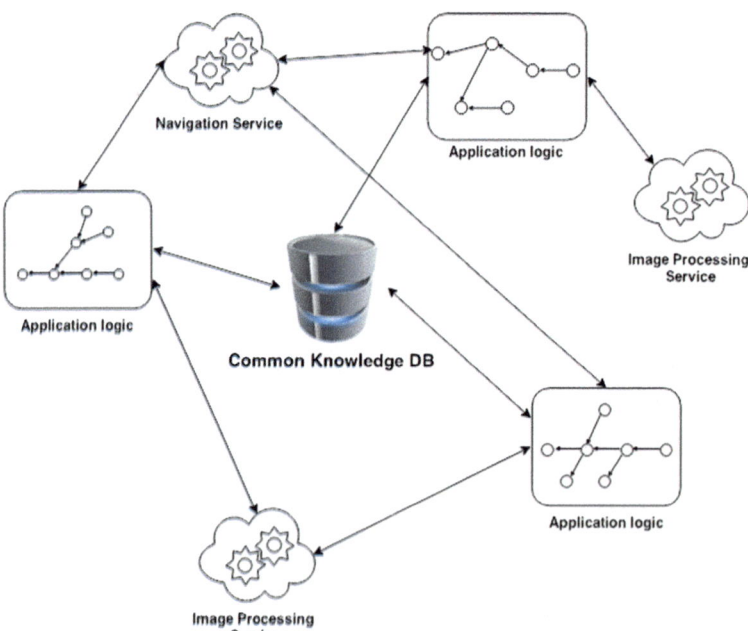

Fig. 6.2 Resource sharing and workflow tuning among different end-users

different end-user requirements). All applications use the same navigation service but two different image processing services.

In order to make the system agile and facilitate object and feature discovery as well as content generation, a common knowledge database is kept and used by all application logics. For instance, the contents of the database involve entries of the form:

```
<id, object_type, user, location, timestamp, Blob>
```

that are used to maintain information about identified objects of interest. Such information can be used to streamline processing when other users are in proximity to the location coordinates. Other information that can be useful to improve system performance involves commands issued with interacting modules, user preference changes according to location, navigational paths, etc. It should be noted that at the current stage of the ENORASI project the contents of the common knowledge database as well as services' APIs have not been finalized yet.

6.4 Application Workflow

The application logic is captured as a workflow. Workflows can be represented by means of a directed acyclic graph (DAG), whereby graph nodes represent processing entities and links represent precedence constraints due to the fact that the pointed node by the link should wait for output by the source node. As discussed in the previous section, our aim is not to provide a standalone application to be used by everybody. Instead, a more flexible, personalized approach should be the goal. For this reason, we envision that the system offers an application template that can be instantiated using on-demand components. The particular instance specifications will be determined through the use of existing *building blocks*.

The building blocks themselves capture necessary *happens_before* precedence constraints among the potential workflow nodes and the relevant services. For instance:

```
<obstacleDetection> happens_before <objectRecognition>
```

This is of utmost importance in order to enable common users to form their own requirements. Such requirements should be given by speech interpreted menus, or ideally in free language form. Therefore, in the example relationship, the user will only have to specify that she wishes to include obstacle detection and object recognition features. The system will generate the workflow with the necessary constraint in presence. Assuming service A and service B are unrelated, the code generation will produce the following workflow for them (given as fork-join threads):

```
fork thread A
fork thread B
join_all
```

whereas in case a precedence constraint exists, the pseudocode will involve consecutive fork-joins as follows:

```
fork thread A
join A
fork thread B
join B
```

In the system, all pairwise service precedence constraints will be manifested and updated upon system extension with additional services. In common user mode, the system will use the default constraint manifestation file. Potential system programmers might be able to use their own manifestation files to enable more agile workflow building. Clearly, such manifestations should not include cyclic dependencies and a set of rules must apply to avoid unwanted behaviors, e.g., launching a DoS attack.

Of particular interest are cases where a processing node in the workflow is optional or might change behavior depending on input. Consider for instance the speech command recognition subcomponent. Since a command might be of the form: `stop/pause module X` in principle, all the related services will have a precedence constraint with speech command recognition. Nevertheless, although this design is logically accurate, it is inefficient in practice since all the modules will have to wait for the output of a single module that might never come (the user did not issue a command) or that affects only one module and not the rest. To tackle the situation, depending processing nodes might be replicated accounting for two states (one whereby no input will be signaled and another one where input command will be sent). The command receive state will pause execution, while the other will execute normally. A sink node for the two states will be enforced so as to evaluate whether command execution took place or not, selecting the output among the output of the two states accordingly. Another approach is to buffer such events and add an artificial buffering processing node as the source node of the workflow. Since the buffered elements are already processed output destined to particular services, the root node processing overhead is minimized.

The system design should be able to incorporate state of the art workflow generation and scheduling techniques and fine-tune them for the specific application domain. A survey on this issue has been performed by Wu, Wu, & Tan (2015).

A final note concerns implementation issues on the workflow processing nodes. As described in Fig. 6.1, the primary and most computing demanding functionalities will be implemented by means of external services. Thus, respective workflow nodes will have to call the related service, passing valid parameters and parsing the results according to API specifications. Other workflow nodes are expected to perform more lightweight functions, e.g., flaw control, synchronization points, lightweight result filtering, etc. Such nodes might be implemented by means of RESTful services (Pautasso, Zimmermann, & Leymann, 2008) developed over containerized resources. In case parallelization is needed, the system might take advantage of the massive parallelization offered by micro services, e.g., AWS Lambda. While a one on one service-container assignment completely decouples logical from physical execution levels, other policies that assign more than one process per container might also bear merits, especially in case of services exchanging data. The final decision on the implementation details will be taken after the set of supported services together with their dependencies and expected computational loads are finalized. In any case different deployment strategies will be considered, according to related literature suggestions (see Ko et al. (2011) for a relevant survey).

6.5 Data Capturing

Though not integral with the application logic, data capturing is bound to affect system performance since low-quality data streams will act as poor input to the higher decision modules. Clearly, for the intended system purpose, the most important and load burdening data stream is the video stream. The other streams described in the architectural design of Fig. 6.1, i.e., audio and positioning information, are very light weighted by comparison, thus, do not require particular effort to integrate. For this reason, we present in this section an overview of the video capturing subcomponent. Similar design ideas are applicable for other heavy load streams that may be incorporated in the future.

6.5.1 Overview of Video Coding in the Proposed System

Video coding is the process of compressing an initially raw video stream, e.g., in YUV format. The compression process takes advantage of spatial (intra-picture) and temporal (inter-picture) similarity existing in a video sequence in order to reduce the number of bits necessary to represent the original signal, usually with some loss. This is of paramount importance since transmitting raw sequences is impractical even with the highest available network speeds. As an example, the transmission of a raw RGB sequence of 8-bit color and 1920×1080 resolution captured at 24 fps requires a network bandwidth of 1.19 Gbps, whereas a compressed sequence usually requires between 2 and 3 orders of magnitude less bandwidth, depending on the encoding standard used and the settings.

Currently, the most popular video coding standard is the H.264/AVC (Wiegand, Sullivan, Bjontegaard, & Luthra, 2003) which has been adopted by most hardware vendors, e.g., in smart mobile devices, TV sets, etc. Based on H.264/AVC, Google developed the VP8 and later on the VP9 standard in 2013 (Mukherjee et al., 2013) to be used by YouTube. As H.264/AVC is showing its age (the standard was developed to fulfill the requirements for Blue Ray disks) the MPEG group developed its successor, termed High Efficiency Video Coding (HEVC) also referred to as H.265 in 2012 (Sullivan, Ohm, Han, & Wiegand, 2012). Both HEVC and VP9 were shown to achieve a better compression ratio for the same video quality compared to H.264/AVC (Chi et al., 2012). Bit savings can well reach 50% when comparing HEVC to H.264/AVC which is particularly important for transmitting

4K sequences. Since the wide adoption of HEVC was initially hindered by royalties' complications, AOMedia was formed in 2015 by blue-chip companies of the high-tech industry with the aim of launching a royalty-free video coding standard to succeed VP9 and HEVC. The efforts culminated with the launch of AV1 standard in Spring 2018 (AV1, 2018). Simultaneously, the MPEG group is developing a next-generation video coding standard termed Versatile Video Coding (VVC) (2018) with the goal of offering at least 50% better compression rate compared to HEVC and AV1.

The existence of such a plethora of video coding standards dictates an *agile system design for the ENORASI project that can cope with at least the main candidate standards.* Depending on network conditions, but also on the characteristics of end devices whereby the initial video sequence must be streamed, transcoding of the input stream into different standards, resolutions, and bitrates might be necessary. Efficient transcoding schemes have been proposed in the literature that take advantage of the encoded motion vectors to reduce coding time in the targeted standard (Franche & Coulombe, 2015), while large-scale transcoding of social network videos is discussed in Koziri et al. (2017). The question of whether to rely on proprietary video coding software, Transcoding as a Service (TaaS) providers (Koziri et al., 2018) or develop home-made solutions based on open software e.g., ffmpeg (FFmpeg, 2018), depends on financial considerations and the desired scale of deployment. In any case, the system should be in principle able to integrate any of the three available options. It should be noted however that the initial deployment of the ENORASI system will be based on open software whereby performance optimizations will be made at a research level.

6.5.2 Smart Middleware and Video Codec Optimizations

One of the key system components involves automatic obstacle detection. In order to achieve this, the video from the portable camera should be fetched for processing by the related software either at the Cloud, Fog, or Edge points (Roman, Lopez, & Mambo, 2018). Regardless of hardware details, the arriving feed must be of high quality to enable smooth obstacle identification and possibly recognition. Since it is well documented that the newer video coding standards incur notoriously high encoding times to achieve the required compression efficiency (Topiwala, Krishnan, & Dai, 2018), the technological challenges posed for the live feed subsystem are high. This is especially true in an open-ended system design whereby no guarantees are given as to the compression efficiency and quality of the camera's output (in the extreme case the used camera might output uncompressed video).

The above necessitates the existence of smart compression software throughout the application development layers, i.e., Cloud, Edge, and the possibly intermittent Fog layer. Regardless of the layer, such software must be able to automatically select appropriate video coding parameters depending on the available hardware and network conditions. This is crucial since default settings are less likely to produce the required online performance. Key concepts that should be explored are the following: (a) encoding mode, (b) quantization parameter (QP), (c) motion estimation parameters, (d) scaling, and (e) parallelization modes.

Encoding mode. Reference configurations for H.264/AVC and HEVC can be found in Bossen (2011). Of particular interest are Low Delay (LD) and Random Access (RA) modes. The first is commonly applied for teleconferencing applications and targets at reducing coding time. It usually involves a GOP (Group of Pictures) structure in the form of an initial I (Intra-predicted) frame followed by P frames (Inter-predicted from predecessor frames). The second one (RA) aims at improving compression thus, it usually involves bi-predicted inter-coded B frames that use as a reference both preceding and succeeding frames. Depending on the available hardware, mode decision should be made with the aim of achieving real-time performance. As an extreme measure for speeding up the encoding process (in case of hardware limitations) an all Intra coding mode could be selected, whereby the encoding time is significantly reduced at the expense of compression efficiency, leaving the RA compression to be performed at the Fog or Cloud levels.

Quantization parameter. The value of QP plays an important role in the outcome. Typically, higher QP values favor a smaller encoding time and larger compression rate at the expense of video quality. Depending on the infrastructure layer, a fixed QP of rather medium value can be selected in combination with single pass encoding to favor coding time with acceptable quality loss. Alternatively, if hardware permits, multi-pass encoding can be used with adaptive QP, for instance in order to optimize quality for a targeted bitrate output.

Motion estimation parameters. Since motion estimation is the most time-consuming task during the encoding process, the main governing parameters of it such as: the search algorithm, the number of frames in reference list, size of search area, variable block size split depth, etc., are candidates for fine-tuning in order to speed up the compression time if necessary.

Scaling. In case of hardware restrictions, scaling down the resolution of a video sequence before compressing it should also be examined, bearing the trade-off between coding time and video quality.

Parallelism. Depending on the available hardware, finer or coarser grained parallelization might be possible. At a fine level, SIMD instructions to speed up vector operators might be available at a CPU level, e.g., AVX2 (Lemmetti, Koivula, Viitanen, Vanne, & Hämäläinen, 2016) or using GPUs (Xiao, Li, Xu, Shi, & Wu, 2015). At a coarser grained, a frame might be split into independent areas, e.g., slice or tile partitioning (Koziri, Papadopoulos, & Loukopoulos, 2018; Papadopoulos, Koziri, & Loukopoulos, 2018) that can be coded by independent threads. Another approach is to use wavefront parallelism (Chi et al., 2012) whereby for each row of blocks a frame is split into, a separate thread is created that encodes the blocks of the row. In HEVC dependencies exist among blocks. Namely, in order to commence the encoding process of a block, the coding of the previous, upper and upper right blocks should have finished. Figure 6.3 portrays examples of tile and wavefront parallelization. It should also be noted that using tiles allows the encoding and transmission of a region of interest (tile) at a higher quality than the rest. This

a

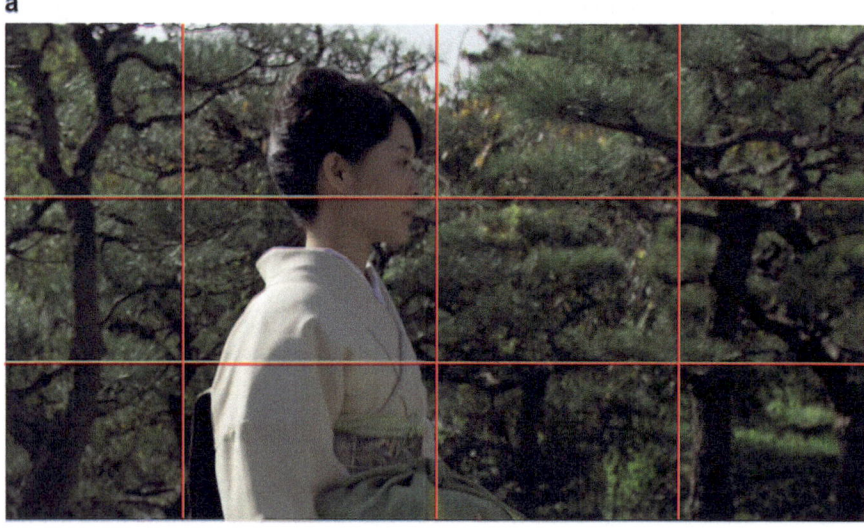

b

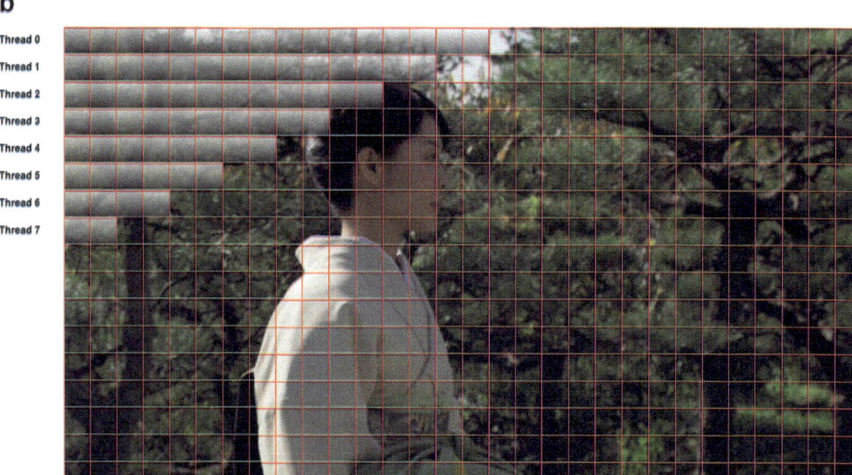

Fig. 6.3 Examples of tile and wavefront parallelism. The image belongs to the HEVC/H.265 common test sequence "Kimono". (**a**) An example 3 × 4 partitioning into independent tiles. (**b**) An example wavefront parallelism with eight threads. Each rectangle depicts a 64 × 64 pixel block. Shaded rectangles show the blocks where coding has finished. Notice, that the upper and upper right block dependencies limit the rate at which a thread can commence encoding

can prove particularly useful in object detection and recognition tasks. Finally, parallelization options also involve per frame and per GOP levels (Fouladi et al., 2017; Franche & Coulombe, 2012). At a GOP level, GOPs starting with an I frame can be trivially parallelized while at a frame level, block encoding can commence once inter-frame block dependencies are satisfied.

While as part of the ongoing research, producing more efficient video coding techniques is of high interest, regarding the ENORASI project and the corresponding system design, it is crucial to be able to seamlessly incorporate any underlying video codec. For this reason, we envision the *smart compression software as essentially a driving middleware between the application logic and the video codec itself.* Its role will be to select encoding parameters on the underlying codec so as to achieve the required performance. In doing so, the smart compression component will rely on machine learning techniques and sophisticated estimations concerning the effects of the five previously described encoding aspects on particular codec/hardware combinations.

6.6   Cross-Layer System Deployment and Optimizations

With the proliferation of Big Data created by IoT systems, the need to ease the burden of main datacenters by shifting part of the computations toward micro-datacenters resting at network Edges was recognized. A general survey on Edge computing can be found in Roman et al. (2018). Particularly in data stream processing applications, the premise is that by shifting some processing bolts of the application workflow toward Edges: (a) network overhead will be reduced since the streams will not have to travel in the backbone network, and (b) application response time will be improved due to reduced propagation delays (among others). A survey on stream processing at Edges can be found in Assuncao, Silva Veith, and Buyya (2018).

Of particular importance is to decide which computations to fulfill at the main datacenter and which at the Edge. This is also termed as the operator placement problem. A mathematical programming approach was followed in Block, Beckett, Lange, Arnold, and Kounev (2017) where the authors developed an ILP algorithm in order to optimize application availability and response time. The algorithm was shown to achieve good solution quality at the expense of high running time. Placing workflow bolts was also the aim of Li, Tang, and Xu (2015). The proposed scheme was based on using support vector regression in order to predict response time changes that might occur due to bolt relocation. Producing a set of Pareto optimal solutions with multi-objective optimization criteria involving delay and energy performance metrics was the scope of Loukopoulos et al. (2018). The aforementioned schemes assume for the biggest part a centralized decision taking scheme. Distributed algorithms for the problem were also proposed in the literature in, e.g., Tziritas, Loukopoulos, Khan, and Xu (2015). Finally, on a system level, automatic deployment of application components between Cloud and Edge so as to minimize response time was the target of Peng, Hosseini, Hong, Farivar, and Campbell (2015).

Similar in scope are the works related to server consolidation and virtual machine migrations. In Beloglazov, Abawajy, and Buyya (2012) the problem of server consolidation with the aim of minimizing energy consumption without affecting

SLAs was tackled. Through simulation experiments, the proposed bin packing heuristic was found to outperform among other DVFS alternatives. In Tziritas et al. (2017) the problem was attacked from the standpoint of migrating services between Cloud and Edge in an online distributed fashion assuming general underlying application graphs.

Related are also works on elasticity. The premise is to dynamically allocate computational and network resources to tackle predicted load peaks while releasing the resources during off-peak periods. Example works on the category with a focus on stream processing Cloud applications include for instance (Lolos, Konstantinou, Kantere, & Koziris, 2017) where the authors proposed a reinforcement learning approach to estimate load and amount of resources necessary to tackle them.

The aforementioned aspects of *Cloud—Edge interoperability should be taken into account in order to build the ENORASI system for scalability*. Parts of stream processing can be performed at the mobile devices of the visually impaired users. This creates the chance of reducing traffic and save battery, particularly in the case of video stream processing. For instance, one can argue that fast object detection methods based on depth (assuming a camera with such capability) are better suited for the Edge level, leaving the heaviest task of object recognition for the Cloud level. Depending on the required functionality the application logic will be able to capture the optimization potential by reducing the amount of video traffic required from the source, limiting it only in cases of potential obstacles.

In a similar manner, the deployment of data capturing middleware in multiple layers Edge, Cloud, and the intermediate Fog layer offers unique potential for cross-layer optimizations. For instance, parts of stream filtering and enhancement can be delegated to the bottom level layers leaving the Cloud arriving streams free from noise and erroneous values. As far as the video coding process is concerned, cross-layer parameter orchestration has the potential of overcoming any deficiencies of the standalone approach described in Sect. 6.5.2.

Overall, it is imperative for the system design to account for efficient distributed deployment involving Cloud and Edge nodes with elasticity.

Last but not least, given the fact that a set of formally described application logic workflows will exist, *the potential for building specific purpose scheduling software cannot be overlooked.* Such software should have the goal of optimizing system performance as a whole, by judiciously perform resource allocation to the executing workflows. As a point of further consideration, the incorporation of *dynamic service selection* in the application workflow could be investigated with the aim of tackling potential performance bottlenecks (in case a particular service fails to respond in a timely manner another one supporting the API will be selected).

6.7 Conclusions

In this chapter, we proposed an open-ended flexible architectural design to build a holistic assistive system for the visually impaired. The architecture is based on combining the processing power offered by Cloud computing with the flexibility offered by services computing. We presented the general system overview and delved on aspects of high interest that can directly affect user perceived performance such as: workflow generation and processing, video coding middleware, Edge-Cloud deployment, and judicious resource allocation.

The modular Cloud platform advocated in the chapter enables navigation/guidance of the visually impaired through efficient video content delivery. Video streams are efficiently transcoded and transmitted to support data analysis for automated navigation services, but also non-automated services offered by remotely located human agents, such as professional assistants or friends. In that sense, it can play the role of "Deus ex Machina" to assist the visually impaired users who would urgently need assistance for mobility.

Acknowledgments This research has been co-financed by the European Union and Greek national funds through the Operational Program Competitiveness, Entrepreneurship and Innovation, under the call RESEARCH-CREATE-INNOVATE (project code: T1EDK-02070).

References

Assuncao, M. D., Silva Veith, A., & Buyya, R. (2018). Distributed data stream processing and edge computing: A survey on resource elasticity and future directions. *Journal of Network and Computer Applications., 103*, 1–17.

AV1. (2018). Bitstream & decoding process specification. Retrieved from https://aomedia.org/av1-bitstream-and-decoding-process-specification/

Bai, J., Liu, D., Su, G., & Fu, Z. (2017). A cloud and vision-based navigation system used for blind people. In *Proceedings of the ACM International Conference on Artificial Intelligence, Automation and Control Technologies* (p. 22).

Beloglazov, A., Abawajy, J., & Buyya, R. (2012). Energy-aware resource allocation heuristics for efficient management of data centers for cloud computing. *Journal of Future Generation Computing Systems, 28*, 755–768.

Block, H., Beckett, J., Lange, K. D., Arnold, J. A., & Kounev, S. (2017). Analysis of the influences on server power consumption and energy efficiency for CPU-intensive workloads. In *Proceedings of the ACM/SPEC International Conference on Performance Engineering* (pp. 223–234).

Bossen, F. (2011). Common test conditions and software reference configurations. In *Joint Collaborative Team on Video Coding (JCT-VC) of ITU-T SG16 WP3 and ISO/IEC JTC1/SC29/WG11, 5th meeting*.

Brilhault, A., Kammoun, S., Gutierrez, O., Truillet, P., & Jouffrais, C. (2011). Fusion of artificial vision and GPS to improve blind pedestrian positioning. In *IFIP International Conference on New Technologies, Mobility Security (NTMS)* (pp. 1–5). IEEE.

Chi, C. C., Alvarez-Mesa, M., Juurlink, B., Clare, G., Henry, F., Pateux, S., & Schierl, T. (2012). Parallel scalability and efficiency of HEVC parallelization approaches. *IEEE Transactions on Circuits and Systems for Video Technology, 22*, 1827–1838.

Chincha, R., & Tian, Y. L. (2011). Finding objects for blind people based on SURF features. In *Proceedings of the IEEE International Conference on Bioinformatics and Biomedicine Workshop* (pp. 526–527).

Fernandes, H., Costa, P., Filipe, V., Paredes, H., & Barroso, J. (2017). A review of assistive spatial orientation and navigation technologies for the visually impaired. In *Universal Access in the Information Society* (pp. 1–14).

Fernandes, H., Costa, P., Paredes, H., Filipe, V., & Barroso, J. (2014). Integrating computer vision object recognition with location based services for the blind. In *International Conference Universal Access Human Computer Interaction* (pp. 493–500). Basel: Springer.

FFmpeg. (2018). Retrieved form https://www.ffmpeg.org/

Fouladi, S., Wahby, R. S., Shacklett, B., Balasubramaniam, K., Zeng, W., Bhalerao, R., ... Winstein, K. (2017). Encoding, fast and slow: Low-latency video processing using thousands of tiny threads. In *2017 Symposium on Networked Systems Design and Implementation (NSDI)* (pp. 363–376).

Franche, J. F., & Coulombe, S. (2012). A multi-frame and multi-slice H. 264 parallel video encoding approach with simultaneous encoding of prediction frames. In *Consumer Electronics, Communications and Networks (CECNet), 2012 2nd International Conference* (pp. 3034–3038). IEEE.

Franche, J. F., & Coulombe, S. (2015). Fast H.264 to HEVC transcoder based on post-order traversal of quadtree structure. In *Proceedings of the IEEE International Conference on Image Processing* (pp. 477–481).

Guerreiro, J., Ahmetovic, D., Kitani, K.M., Asakawa, C. (2017). Virtual navigation for blind people: Building sequential representations of the real-world. In *Proceedings of the International ACM SIGACCESS Conference on Computers and Accessibility* (pp. 280–289).

Kim, J. E., Bessho, M., Kobayashi, S., Koshizuka, N., & Sakamura, K. (2016). Navigating visually impaired travelers in a large train station using smartphone and bluetooth low energy. In *Proceedings of the ACM/SIGAPP Symposium On Applied Computing* (pp. 604–611)

Ko, A. J., Abraham, R., Beckwith, L., Blackwell, A., Burnett, M., Erwig, M., et al. (2011). The state of the art in end-user software engineering. *ACM Computing Surveys, 43*(3), 21.

Koziri, M. G., Papadopoulos, P. K., & Loukopoulos, T. (2018). Combining tile parallelism with slice partitioning in video coding. In *Proceedings of the SPIE Conferences Optics and Electronics*.

Koziri, M. G., Papadopoulos, P. K., Tziritas, N., Dadaliaris, A. N., Loukopoulos, T., & Stamoulis, G. (2017). I: On planning the adoption of new video standards in social media networks: A general framework and its application to HEVC. *Social Network Analysis and Mining, 7*, 1–32.

Koziri, M. G., Papadopoulos, P. K., Tziritas, N., Loukopoulos, T., Khan, S. U., & Zomaya, A. Y. (2018). Efficient cloud provisioning for video transcoding: Review, open challenges and future opportunities. *IEEE Internet Computing (IC), 22*, 46–55.

Lee, L. H., & Hui, P. (2018). Interaction methods for smart glasses: A survey. *IEEE Access, 6*, 28712–28732.

Lee, Y. H., & Medioni, G. (2016). RGB-D camera based wearable navigation system for the visually impaired. *Computer Vision and Image Understanding, 149*, 3–20.

Lemmetti, A., Koivula, A., Viitanen, M., Vanne, J., & Hämäläinen, T. D. (2016). AVX2-optimized Kvazaar HEVC intra encoder. In *IEEE International Conference on Image Processing (ICIP)* (pp. 549–553).

Li, T., Tang, J., & Xu, J.. (2015). A predictive scheduling framework for fast and distributed stream data processing. In *IEEE International Conference on Big Data* (pp. 333–338).

Liu, L., Zhang, M., Lin, Y., & Qin, L. (2014). A survey on workflow management and scheduling in cloud computing. In *2014 IEEE/ACM International Symposium on Cluster, Cloud and Grid Computing (CCGrid)* (pp. 837–846).

Lolos, K., Konstantinou, I., Kantere, V., & Koziris, N. (2017). Elastic management of cloud applications using adaptive reinforcement learning. In *IEEE International Conference on Big Data* (pp. 203–212).

Loukopoulos, T., Tziritas, N., Koziri, M., Stamoulis, G. I., Khan, S. U., Xu, C. Z., & Zomaya, A. Y. (2018). Data stream processing at network edges. In *Proceedings of the IEEE Workshop on Parallel/Distributed Computing and Optimization*.

Mekhalfi, M. L., Melgani, F., Bazi, Y., & Alajlan, N. (2015). A compressive sensing approach to describe indoor scenes for blind people. *IEEE Transactions on Circuits and Systems for Video Technology., 25*, 1246–1257.

Mukherjee, D., Bankoski, J., Grange, A., Han, J., Koleszar, J., Wilkins, P., ... Bultje, R. (2013). The latest open-source video codec VP9-an overview and preliminary results. In *IEEE Picture Coding Symposium (PCS)* (pp. 390–393).

Papadopoulos, P. K., Koziri, M. G., & Loukopoulos, T. (2018). A fast heuristic for tile partitioning and processor assignment in HEVC. In *Proceedings of the IEEE International Conference on Image Processing.*

Pautasso, C., Zimmermann, O., & Leymann F. (2008). RESTful web services vs. "Big" web services: Making the right architectural decision. In *Proceedings of the International Conference on World Wide Web* (pp. 805–814).

Peng, B., Hosseini, M., Hong, Z., Farivar, R., & Campbell, R. (2015). R-storm: Resource-aware scheduling in storm. In *Proceedings of the ACM Annual Middleware Conference* (pp. 149–161).

Rao, J., & Su, X. (2004). A survey of automated web service composition methods. In *International Workshop on Semantic Web Services and Web Process Composition* (Vol. 3387, pp. 43–54).

Roman, R., Lopez, J., & Mambo, M. (2018). Mobile edge computing, fog et al.: A survey and analysis of security threats and challenges. *Future Generation Computer Systems, 78,* 680–698.

Šimunovi, L., Aneli, V., & Pavlinuši, I. (2012). Blind people guidance system. In *International Conference, Central European Conference Information Intelligent Systems.*

Sosa-Garcia, J., & Odone, F. (2017). "Hands on" visual recognition for visually impaired users. *ACM Transactions on Accessible Computing, 10*(8), 1–30.

Sullivan, G. J., Ohm, J. R., Han, W. J., & Wiegand, T. (2012). Overview of the high efficiency video coding (HEVC) standard. *IEEE Transactions on Circuits and Systems for Video Technology, 22,* 1649–1668.

Topiwala, P., Krishnan, M., & Dai, W. (2018).. Performance comparison of VVC, AV1 and HEVC on 8-bit and 10-bit content. In *Applications of Digital Image Processing XLI International Society for Optics and Photonics* (Vol. 10752, p. 107520).

Tziritas, N., Khan, S. U., Loukopoulos, T., Lalis, S., Xu, C. Z., Li, K., & Zomaya, A. Y. (2017). Online inter-datacenter service migrations. *IEEE Transactions on Cloud Computing*https://doi.org/10.1109/TCC.2017.2680439

Tziritas, N., Loukopoulos, T., Khan, S. U., & Xu, C. Z. (2015). Distributed algorithms for the operator placement problem. *IEEE Transactions on Computational Social Systems, 2,* 182–196.

Vorapatratorn, S., & Nambunmee, K. (2014). iSonar: An obstacle warning device for the totally blind. *Journal of Assistive, Rehabilitative & Therapeutic Technologies, 2,* 23114.

VVC. (2018). Versatile Video Coding. Retrieved from https://jvet.hhi.fraunhofer.de/

Wang, H. C., Katzschmann, R. K., Teng, S., Araki, B., Giarré, L., & Rus, D. (2017). Enabling independent navigation for visually impaired people through a wearable vision-based feedback system. In *2017 IEEE International Conference on Robotics and Automation (ICRA)* (pp. 6533–6540). IEEE.

WHO: World Health Organization. (2018). Blindness and visual impairment. Retrieved from https://www.who.int/en/news-room/fact-sheets/detail/blindness-and-visual-impairment

Wiegand, T., Sullivan, G. J., Bjontegaard, G., & Luthra, A. (2003). Overview of the H. 264/AVC video coding standard. *IEEE Transactions on Circuits and Systems for Video Technology., 13,* 560–576.

Winlock, T., Christiansen, E., & Belongie, S. (2010). Toward real-time grocery detection for the visually impaired. In *2010 IEEE Computer Society Conference on Computer Vision and Pattern Recognition Workshops (CVPRW)* (pp. 49–56).

Wu, F., Wu, Q., & Tan, Y. (2015). Workflow scheduling in Cloud: A survey. *The Journal of Supercomputing, 71*(9), 3373–3418.

Xiao, W., Li, B., Xu, J., Shi, G., & Wu, F. (2015). HEVC encoding optimization using multicore CPUs and GPUs. *IEEE Transactions on Circuits and Systems for Video Technology, 25,* 1830–1843.

Chapter 7
Virtual Vision Architecture for VIP in Ubiquitous Computing

Soubraylu Sivakumar, Ratnavel Rajalakshmi, Kolla Bhanu Prakash, Baskaran Rajesh Kanna, and Chinnasamy Karthikeyan

7.1 Introduction

The number of visually impaired people is increasing rapidly. The assistive technology that helps those people does not provide enough convenience and utility. One of the major problems with such people is indoor navigation within buildings and in outdoor environment. The cost of the equipment used in aiding these people is expensive. It is difficult to take all the aiding devices with them all the time. Smartphones provide better support and assistance to the VIP because they all have the ability to run many applications for a different purpose in a single device.

It is difficult for the disabled people to navigate in a new place. Although GPS provides a better navigation system along with the smartphone, GPS signal is not available inside buildings and in low coverage area. This has become one of the major problems for VIP in the detection of the obstacle. The obstacle may be in the form of moving object (living object or nonliving object) and stationary or non-movable object. It is a challenging task to provide better navigation with the available technology.

Smartphone has specially designed capabilities to assist the VIP through a simple and clear means of communication. This assistive communication is done through the voice command. Voice and Haptic technology are one of the communication

S. Sivakumar (✉) · K. B. Prakash · C. Karthikeyan
Computer Science Engineering, Koneru Lakshmaiah Education Foundation, Guntur, Andhra Pradesh, India
e-mail: drkbp@kluniversity.in

R. Rajalakshmi · B. R. Kanna
Computing Science Engineering, Vellore Institute of Technology, Chennai, India
e-mail: rajalakshmi.r@vit.ac.in; rajeshkanna.b@vit.ac.in

© Springer Nature Switzerland AG 2020
S. Paiva (ed.), *Technological Trends in Improved Mobility of the Visually Impaired*,
EAI/Springer Innovations in Communication and Computing,
https://doi.org/10.1007/978-3-030-16450-8_7

methods to the VIP. The SRE system is used to convert voice to text and text to voice. The voice from the VIP is recorded and converted to a respective text command by the SER. The converted text is given to the IMS for processing. The response from the IMS is converted into voice response by the SER and given to the ANS. Internally, the IMS gives another response to ANS for haptic action through LRA. The LRA gives a vibrating sensation for the VIP. Through the voice command, the VIP can access the web server for paying the electricity bill, to book tickets, to gather current event information, etc.

A smart cane is a better assistance to the VIP in determining the obstacle along the navigation path. It conforms to the existence and non-existence of an object. Our Obstacle Detection System has a cane to which a Mobile Kinect is attached. Six ultrasonic transducers tied to the belt of the VIP and PIR sensor is tied to the shirt button of the VIP. Three ultrasonic transducers cover the head side and remaining three cover the tail side of the VIP. The combination of Mobile Kinect and three ultrasonic sensors in the head or front portion gives a better degree of obstacle detection during the day time, while PIR along with the ultrasonic transducer gives obstacle detection during night time at the indoor environment. The three ultrasonic transducers at the back or tail portion give less degree of obstacle detection during day and night time.

The rest of this chapter is organized as follows: in the next section the literature review of similar solutions and related work are presented. In Sect. 7.3, the overall architecture of the entire system is described in detail. The integration of various architecture and the methods are analyzed in detail in Sect. 7.4. The proposed methods are explained lucidly and evaluated in Sect. 7.5. Finally, the conclusion and future directions of this research work are included.

7.2   Related Work

The authors (Lee, Kim, Lee, & Shin, 2013) have used Zigbee modules to find the position of the VIP. They have built a grid-based map to support the visually impaired to reach home safely. The ultrasonic sensor is used to detect the obstacle. This system is called as Smart Backpack which helps the user for the free outdoor walking of the user. Chung, Kim, and Rhee (2014) have used two sensors for finding the obstacles and to prevent the falls using ultrasonic sensor and gyrosensor respectively. The AVR microcontroller is built inside the handgrip of the cane along with the battery. This controller and mobile phone are paired using Bluetooth V2.0 protocol. The information about the VIP is informed to the conservator in real time through this smartphone.

Li, Pundlik, and Luo (2013) used the mobile phone camera to reveal the discerning scene details to the user. They provide motion-based stabilizing on IOS mobile to defeat the jitter effects. This implementation is more sensitive than the Gyrosensor and provides improved in performance to humans in calculating the distance details more precisely. The authors (Ghidini, Almeida, Manssour, & Silveira, 2016) have used the smartphone to open the electronic calendar through voice. Smartphone provides a better interaction capability for the visually impaired by this. Other application also can be opened and accessed through the voice. Because of this, they can have better support in their day to day life.

Prudtipongpun, Buakeaw, Rattanapongsen, and Sivaraksa (2015) have given a method to navigate the VIP along their indoor building in a convenient way. They have used IndoorAtlas to store the navigation path of the user. The map is stored on the IndoorAtlas database. The rooms are considered as a node in a graph. Dijkstra's algorithm is used to navigate through the shortest path between the rooms. The NavEye architecture is proposed by AlAbri, AlWesti, AlMaawali, and AlShidhani (2014). It consists of mobile applications and a smart cane. The VIP interacts with the phone through voice and cane is used to find any obstacle in the path. Both are synchronized through Bluetooth. The QR code reader is employed to determine the current location of the VIP.

The authors (Zhou, Yang, & Yan, 2016) use an obstacle detection system which finds the objects at a distance of 10 ft using the Ultrasonic sensor. The system gives a voice announcement about the obstacle detected. The announcement is given to the VIP through the mobile phone. It also detects the traffic light signal along the road. They have given a name as Virtual Eye to their architecture. The authors (Ramani & Tank, 2014) use the Geo codes (i.e., latitude and longitude) information of the building elements like rooms, stairs and corridors which are stored in the Google Cloud using Google Maps. The shortest path Dijkstra's algorithm is used to determine the path between the building elements. To access the map, the Google API is used.

The Internet consists of web sites, web document and web pages. It contains a collection of texts, audios, images, videos, etc. Mining the text and extracting the features from it is a difficult task. Mining using conventional approach does not give a better result for text across multilingual. The authors (Prakash & Dorai Rangaswamy, 2016a) have given an effective method in the identification and extraction of biological datasets from multilingual web documents. The proposed method does not need domain knowledge or a list of document categories; it is purely data-driven. Prakash and Dorai Rangaswamy (2016b) have introduced the classification method for content extraction along with data reduction from multilingual web document. It is a pixel-based approach developed based on the complexity of different Indian web page.

Prakash and RajaRaman (2016) have given a neural network approach for multilingual web pages for extracting the content based on the attribute generation. The author given a pixel-based content extraction approach for a bilingual web document, the attributes are generated by reducing the pixel matrix. They have selected five attributes for their study. In this paper (Rajalakshmi & Aravindan, 2011), the authors have proposed a method for websites classification. It is based on the extraction of features from URLs. The Naïve Bayes classifier is applied on the extracted features. Rajalakshmi and Aravindan (2013) have proposed an approach for web page classification. In this method, n-gram character is extracted from URLs alone and classification is done by Maximum Entropy Classifiers and Support Vector Machines.

The authors (Karthikeyan & Ramadoss, 2016) have used Structural Similarity Index Measure and Edge-Based Similarity Measure to assess the performance of similarity measures. They also used the medical image fusion technique for their comparison. Karthikeyan and Ramadoss (2015) have used medical fusion technique to combine two or more images to improve the quality of medical diagnosis. The MRI and CT are used as two image modalities. The authors (Karthikeyan & Ramadoss, 2014) have proposed a new medical fusion method named as Dual Tree Complex Wavelet Transform (DTCWT). This method eliminates the two disadvantages of Discrete Wavelet Transform such as deficiency of shift invariance and bad directional selectivity. In this paper, the Karthikeyan (Karthikeyan, Ramadoss, & Baskar, 2011) has used a segmentation algorithm with ANN for CT scanned images to find and solve various lung diseases. They compared all the DWT, NSCT, FDCT and ended up that DTCWT used with multimodality image fusion will give better results.

7.3 Architecture

7.3.1 Head Obstacle Detection System and Tail Obstacle Detection System

The architectural diagram of Virtual Vision is shown in Fig. 7.1. The component used in the HOD and TOD subsystems is shown in Fig. 7.2. This system consists of two main components: (1) environment information acquisition and analysis and (2) information organization and representation. The first component aims at capturing the environment data by using various sensors like Mobile Kinect, Ultrasonic Sensor and PIR Sensor in order to determine the predefined obstacles for VIPs, while the second is used to represent the presence of an obstacle through vibrating sensor and through voice over headset.

Mobile Kinect (MK)

Xbox 360 is a Kinect (Machida, Cao, Murao, & Hashimoto, 2012), which consists of Microsoft built hardware and software. The hardware includes a camera, infrared projector and a microchip which generates a grid. The grid is used to locate the nearby object in three-dimension space. It includes Multi-array microphone, depth sensor and RGB camera. This setup gives voice recognition, facial recognition and full-body motion capture. The microphone enables to guide acoustic source localization and noise suppression facilities. The depth sensor has a monochrome CMOS element with an infrared laser projector; in any ambient light conditions it captures video data.

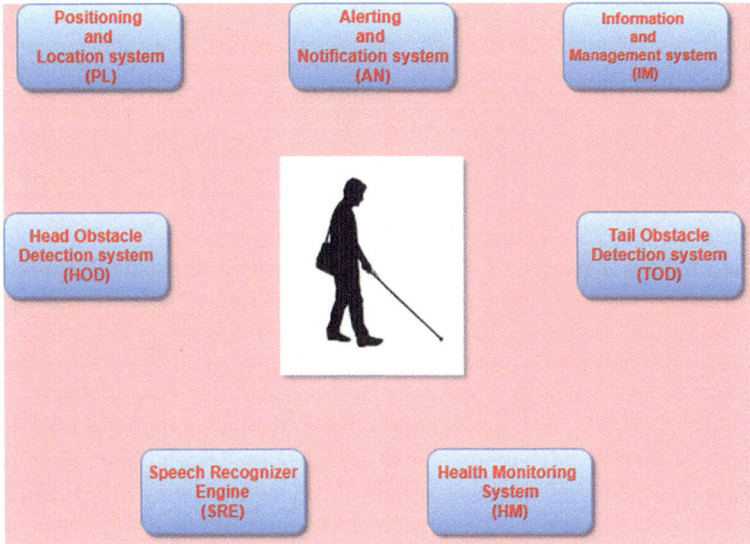

Fig. 7.1 Architecture diagram of the virtual vision system

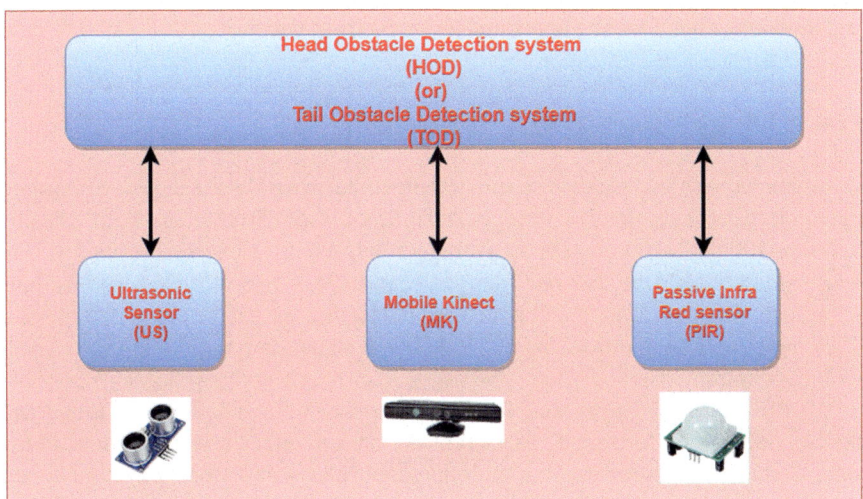

Fig. 7.2 Components used in the HOD and TOD subsystem

The sensing range is calibrated by Kinect software to adjust for the physical environment for the players involved in games. The Kinect is capable of tracking two dynamic players by extracting the feature of 20 joints per player to a maximum of six people. Depending on resolution, the sensor outputs a video at a frame rate of 9–30 Hz. The RGB default video stream with a Bayer color filter uses VGA resolution 640 × 480 pixels up to 1280 × 1024 pixels. When the sensor is used with Xbox software it has a practical ranging limit of 120–350 cm distance. The motorized pivot should tilt the sensor element either down or up at an angle of 27°, it should have an angular view field of 43° vertical and 57° horizontal.

Ultrasonic Sensor (US)

Ultrasonic sensors (Sivakumar, Kamatchi, Sangeetha, Subha, & Ramachandran, 2017) are used in a variety of applications both indoors and outdoors around the world. Usually these sensors are made with piezoelectric crystals and use high frequency sound waves to vibrate at a desired frequency to convert the energy into invisible sound energy and sound energy into electric energy. US emit sound waves; the sound waves hit the target and reflect back to the source. Certain variables, such as changes in humidity and atmospheric temperature and target surface angle, and roughness of the reflective surface, can affect the normal function of this sensor.

There are two types of ultrasonic sensors: (1) Ranging Measurement: Distance of an Obstacle object (moving or stationary) is measured via time difference between transmitted and received acoustic sound from the objects. Distance change between the obstacle and the sensing element is endlessly calculated and updated. (2) Proximity Detection: An object passing through a specific range will be detected and an output signal will be generated based on the proximity.

Passive Infrared Sensor (PIR)

It is made up of a pyroelectric sensing element that observes the degree of infrared radiation. The literal detection range of the PIR sensor (Sivakumar et al., 2018) is between 500 and 1200 cm. On an average it detects any movement around within approximately 1000 cm distance from its location. It is used in various applications or projects where an individual has entered or left the area can be easily determined. They are simple to interface, have a wide range of lens and require minimal effort with flat control.

All PIR have a three-pin, one for power supply of 5 V, another for ground and the last one will be for signal. These pins are present either at the bottom or in the side. Connecting and interfacing the microcontroller with PIR is very simple and easy. The output of the PIR sensor is in digital form. The high signal in the output pin detects the motion. The output of the PIR will be low, i.e., warm, until there is a motion in the sensor range. To meet a specific end goal, for capacity fitting, the sensor needs a warm-up. This time is called settling time which may be around 10–60 s.

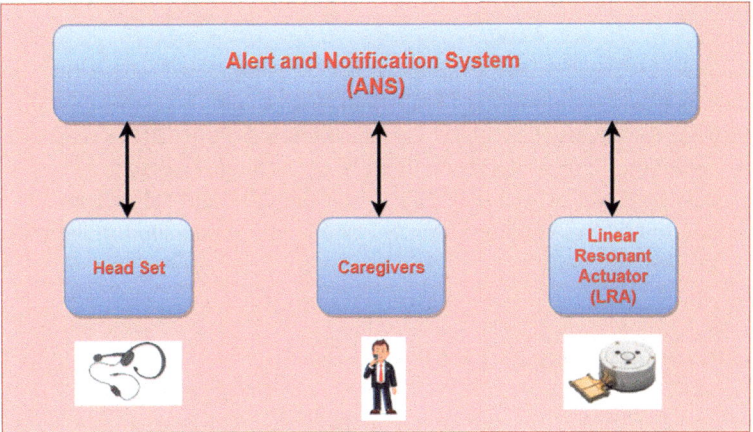

Fig. 7.3 Components used in the ANS subsystem

7.3.2 Alert and Notification System

This system must provide protection to VIP. An alert tells about someone that certain things have happened. A notification tells about the importance of an alert and that it needs immediate attention for a solution to be provided. There are certain needs for this system to be considered. They are speed, multi-channel notification delivery, map view, easy-to-use experience, interactive and geo-fencing. It is the first step to be prepared before critical events. The alert and notification can be given through SMS to caregivers, voice message and vibration to VIPs, and Phone call to doctors and caregivers. Figure 7.3 shows the component used in ANS subsystem.

Headset

The microphone combined with headphone is the headset. It comes with a single earpiece (mono) or a double earpiece (stereo). They provide the functionality equivalent to a telephone handset. The headset is used in many call centers, mobile phones and telephone-intensive jobs. The other name for single ear set is also called as monaural headsets. This headset frees up one ear, allowing the person to interact with others and according to the environment. The microphone design comes with either noise-canceling or omnidirectional type. The first type uses the bi-directional microphone as elements. It has a receptive field only in two angles, back and front of the microphone. The above design picks up sound from the close proximity of the user.

Caregivers

VIP requires guidance for their everyday tasks to be completed successfully. In order to be in touch with community, friends and their leisure time pursuits, they need support from caregivers (Chaudary, Paajala, Keino, & Pulli, 2016). The caregivers may be relatives, family members, friends or employed persons. They have to continuously monitor "where they go", "what they do" and "How they are". They may be monitored physically or virtually (mobile phones) to support them in all the aspects.

Linear Resonant Actuators (LRA)

LRAs (Kato & Hirata, 2017) are simple, popular and widely used in various haptic applications like touchscreen, wearable and handheld devices. They are alternatives to Eccentric Rotating Mass (ERM) vibration motors. It provides faster response time, longer life in usage and better performance characteristics when compared to ERMs. With less power, they vibrate at a more steady frequency and deliver a better quality haptic experience. When the reminiscent frequency is applied to the voice coil, it vibrates with a detectable force. When the AC input is changed, the amplitude and frequency of LRA can be adjusted easily.

7.3.3   Health Monitoring System

The IoT along with sensors enables the Telemedicine to reach remote areas like villages and rural areas. The hospitals and doctors can monitor in-house patients by using Information and Communication Engineering. Successful health management of a patient includes monitoring health-related parameters such as body temperature, heart rate, diastolic and systolic blood pressure, blood sugar and body mass index. By providing these facilities, the quality of life is improved for VIPs by creating a low-cost health care self-monitoring system. The GPRS and GSM facilities of microcontrollers help to transmit the biomedical information to the hospitals, doctors, caregivers, relatives, friends and parents in the form of SMS, Email and pre-recorded voice calls. Health suggestions from the doctors can be conveyed to VIPs through a phone call or through a voice message. Figure 7.4 shows the components used in HMS.

Body Temperature Measurement

To read the body temperature of VIP, LM35 is used as Sensor (Sivakumar, Jennifer, Marrison, Seetha, & Sathish Saravanan, 2017). The temperature is usually measured in "Fahrenheit" or "Centigrade". This sensor provides an output only in

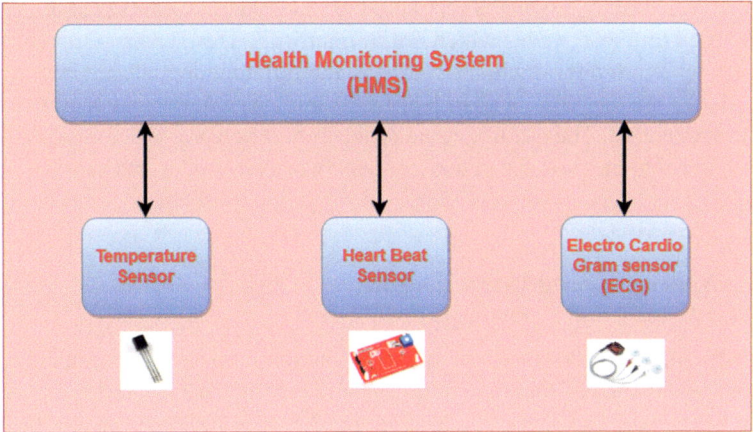

Fig. 7.4 Components used in the HMS subsystem

degree Centigrade. It does not require any external trimming or calibration to give distinctive accuracies at room temperature. It is a three pin sensor similar to that of the transistor device. The pins are numbered as, PIN1 is connected to V_{cc} power supply of +5 V, PIN2 is used to collect the Output signal which is connected to ADC chip and last PIN3 is connected to Ground. At 0 °C the sensor has an output of 0 V, if the temperature of the body is 1 °C the output of the sensor will be +10 mV.

Heartbeat Sensor

Sunrom Model 1157 is used as a heartbeat sensor (Rodríguez, Goñi, & Illarramendi, 2003). It is based on the rule of photo plethysmography. The blood flows via any organ of the body. Any change in mass of blood directly causes a variation in the light intensity through that organ. Since the heart pumps the blood, the flow of blood volume is directly related to the pulse rate of the human heart.

The heartbeat sensor contains a LED and a photodiode. When a tissue is illuminated by a light emitted from the led, it either transmits or reflects the light. Some part of the light is absorbed by the blood and remaining part is reflected toward the light detector. The amount of light captured by the detector depends on the blood volume in the tissue. The detector output is an electrical signal which is used to measure the heartbeat rate.

ECG Sensor

Sunrom AD8232 is used as ECG sensor (Rodríguez et al., 2003). The pulsating electrical waves propagate toward the skin from the heart are recorded by the sensor. The electricity amount is very small; the electrodes connected to the skin can reliably pick up those waves which are in microvolt. This sensor setup comprises at least four electrodes which are placed at the different appendages according to standard terminology (RL = right leg; LL = left leg; RA = right arm; LA = left arm) or at the chest. The electrodes are typically wet sensors, which needs a special conductive gel to increase the conductivity between electrodes and skin.

7.3.4 Speech Recognition Engine

The SRE (McTear, 2004) system is a very complex system, implemented in the form of a wide range of speech synthesize and language analysis technologies. This system has to work not only in real time but they also have to consider the needs and behavior of the user for whom they are working. It includes the following components (1) Automatic Speech Recognition (ASR), (2) Natural Language Understanding (NLU), (3) Natural Language Generation (NLG), (4) Dialogue Management and Control (DMC) and (5) Text-To-Speech synthesis (TTS). The components used in the SRE subsystem are shown in Fig. 7.5.

Automatic Speech Recognition

It takes the acoustic input from the user, treat it as a noisy version of the speech, substituting all possible word sequences to the speech and computing the probability, and chooses the maximum probability sequences (Huang, Acero, &

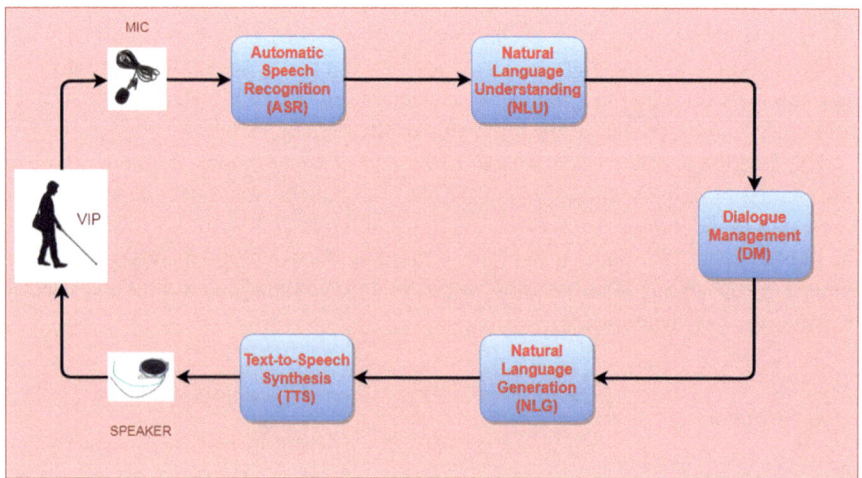

Fig. 7.5 Components used in the SRE subsystem

Hon, 2001). To implement this, a set of models for computing these probabilities, an effective method to parameterizing the audio signal into a feature vector, and an optimized search algorithm are needed because of the huge amount of word sequences.

Natural Language Understanding

The main objective of the NLU component is to scan the ASR result and generate an equivalent semantic representation of the probabilistic output. A classic-based parsing approach used in NLU is a CFG-based grammar which provides enhanced semantic information. In a robust approach, in which each word is linked with some semantic construct is known as keyword spotting or pattern-matching (Jackson, Konopka, & Hartwell, 1991). An alternative approach is to parse input with possibly modified CFG, but extend the parsing algorithm with robustness techniques (Gazdar & Mellish, 1990; Kasper & Reininger, 1999; Van Noord, Bouma, Koeling, & Nederhof, 1999).

Natural Language Generation

The NLG takes the semantic representation from the system and generates a textual equivalent. The simplest approach is to map between a discrete set of communicative acts and their realizations. An alternative suggestion to this method is to use the template which may contain a slot for values. The spoken dialogue on the whole is a disclosure model, the new utterance semantics must be integrated into the system, so that it may be used for the future realization of the utterances. The communicative act can be realized in various ways, by using different anaphoric grammatical construction or by selecting between full utterances and elliptical constructions.

Dialogue Management and Control

It is known as the executive controller of the system. It holds the current state of the dialogue and makes a decision that influences the system behavior. The major task of the DMC is split into three groups: (1) Contextual interpretation, (2) Domain knowledge management and (3) Action selection. Contextual interpretation is used for making guesses and interpreting the various examples of ellipses and anaphora to be used in the system. Domain knowledge management includes various models, methods and mechanisms for reasoning about the domain and the method and way of accessing external information sources, such as a graphical information system (GIS) or SQL database. The third main task is to make the decisions on what the dialogue system should do next.

Text-to-Speech Synthesis

It is mainly divided into two subproblems—the mapping from a text to a phonetic string using prosodic markup, and then converting the string into an audio signal. The first problem has been addressed with both data-driven (Van Den Bosch & Daelemans, 1993) and knowledge-driven (Carlson & Granström, 1986) approaches. To the second problem, there are three common approaches: formant synthesis, unit selection and diphone synthesis. A formant synthesizer uses the features of the acoustic signal providing a very flexible model. Unit selection is based on concatenation. Instead of using phoneme transitions, the largest chunks are found from the database and concatenated. In diphone synthesis, a few phoneme transitions are recorded in the database, and the synthesized speech is concatenated with it. During the post-processing of the signal, prosodic features are added to deliver a meaningful text.

7.3.5   *Positioning and Location System*

This system helps to track and locate the VIP through the GPS unit present in the mobile phone. The mobile phone used in the system is Samsung Galaxy J6. From the current location of the VIP, the caregivers can instruct them on how to reach their destination. The camera helps to take a snapshot of their location and also to read the door number, nameplates, signboards, etc. The motion status of the VIP whether they are walking or standing can be monitored through the accelerometer and through the gyroscope. The fingerprint scanner app is used for authentication purpose. It is used to scan and extract the fingerprint of the VIP. Figure 7.6 shows the components used in the PLS subsystem.

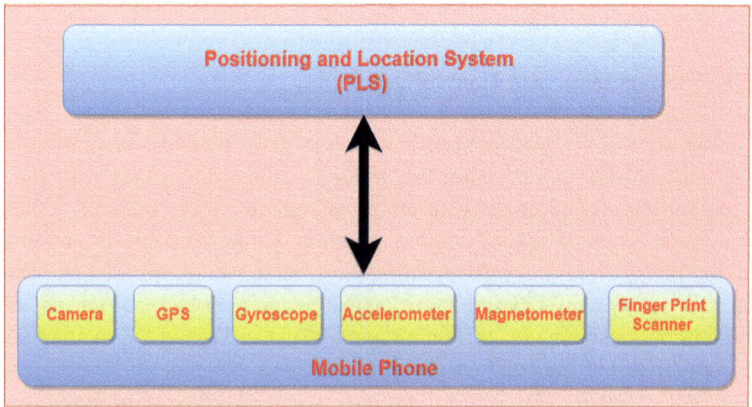

Fig. 7.6 Components used in the PLS subsystem

Camera

The smartphone having a camera has versatile applications. A camera takes a snapshot of a picture and records an event. It is used to capture the locations and views in 3D space. Any image shown in the 3D view is created by one of the cameras. The videos taken from the camera are used for archive purpose.

GPS

It stands for Global Positioning System (Sivakumar, Arun, Lokeshvarma, & Krishnakumar, 2015). GPS units in phone help to locate which region of the earth you are walking or standing by a ping with the satellite. This unit helps to find your location, even when your phone losses the signal. All the calculating and communicating part of the GPS may drain your battery. The GPS helps to determine the shortest path to the destination and helps in tracking the VIPs using Google Maps.

Gyroscope

It is a device that measures or maintains rotational motion (Varadan & Varadan, 2000). A new small device named Micro Electro Mechanical System (MEMS) measures angular velocity. The angular velocities are measured by revolutions per second (RPS) or degrees per second ($°/s$) as a unit. It also provides position information with higher accuracy.

Accelerometer

It is used to measure the acceleration which may be caused due to tilting action or gravity of movement (Varadan & Varadan, 2000). It also senses the mobile angle. It adjusts/changes the screen of the mobile phone to be viewed properly; when VIP changes the orientation from landscape/horizontal to portrait/vertical and vice versa. When the device is facing downwards, it mutes the mobile phone so that the music which is being played or the incoming call is put on hold.

Magnetometer

This creates a miniature Hall-effect by utilizing the modern solid state technology. It detects the magnetic field effect along the three axes X, Y and Z. This sensor raises a voltage which is directly relative to the sign of the magnetic field along the three axes. The sensor senses the voltage which is equivalent to the magnetic field intensity and is converted to a digital signal. It is enclosed along with another sensor, i.e., accelerometer in a small electronic chip.

Finger Print Scanner

It is a type of biometric technology that authenticates an individual to gain or lose an access to a physical facility or computer system based on the fingerprint (Gao, Hu, Cao, & Li, 2014). It uses both software and hardware to identify an individual. The scanner first records the fingerprint of the individual by scanning and storing it in the database. The user requiring access places the finger on the scanner hardware. The scanner takes a copy of the fingerprint. It compares and matches with the already stored image in the database. If the match is positive, the individual will be given access. Otherwise, access to the facility will be denied.

7.4 Materials and Methods

7.4.1 Asymmetric Encryption

It is also known as public key cryptography. It encrypts the plain text using two keys. The two keys are called as private key and public key. The private key is also called the secret key. This method ensures that a third person does not misuse the key. With the help of the secret key, anyone can decrypt the message very easily. For this reason, the public key is made available freely so that anyone can send a message easily. The secret key is kept unknown from the third person. A plain text that is encrypted in the sender using a public key can only be decrypted using a secret key at the receiver side, while vice versa is also true. The public key is available to everyone through the internet. The most popular public key algorithm includes RSA, ElGamal, Elliptic curve method, DSA and PKCS.

RSA Algorithm: This algorithm is asymmetric public key cryptography algorithm (Tahir, 2015). It works well on two different keys, i.e. Private Key and Public Key. The main idea behind RSA is factorizing the large integer which is difficult. The public key consists of two large prime numbers. It is a multiplication of those two numbers. The secret key is also derived from those numbers. The private key is compromised only after factorizing the prime numbers. When the length of the key is doubled or tripled, the effectiveness of encryption gains exponentially. Therefore, the effectiveness of the algorithm totally lies on the key size. RSA keys length can generally be 1024 or 2048 bits long. This algorithm has the following three steps:

1. Key Generation: Both the secret and public keys are generated to be used in the encryption process and decryption as well. The key generation steps are shown below:

- Choose two numbers m and n as two large prime numbers.
- Calculate the modulus number p as $m \times n$.
- Calculate the Euler function $\varphi(p) = (m - 1) \times (n - 1)$.
- Randomly select an integer number e as a public key. It should meet the constraints as Greater Common Divisor $GCD(e, \varphi(p)) = 1, 1 < e < \varphi(p)$.
- The private key d can be computed such that $d \times e = 1(\mod \varphi(p))$.

2. Encryption: It is the procedure of converting the data into a class that has become very difficult to read without prior knowledge (a key). In this algorithm the cipher text is generated from the plaintext using the below Eq. (7.1).

$$C = M^e \mod p \qquad (7.1)$$

3. Decryption: It is the reverse process of encryption. It includes the process of converting the encrypted data back into a readable form. In this algorithm the plain text is generated from the cipher text using the below Eq. (7.2).

$$M = C^d \mod p \qquad (7.2)$$

7.4.2 Selenium Architecture

Selenium web driver (Ramya, Sindhura, & Vidya Sagar, 2017; Sivakumar, Kasthuri, Nivetha, Shabana, & Veluchamy, 2017) is a browser model that takes instructions from the program and transmits them to a web browser. Selenium web driver architecture is shown in Fig. 7.7. It has a web browser-specific driver that operates the browser by communicating with it. The web driver supports PHP, Perl, Java, Ruby, C#. It is a set of tools which automatically controls the browser. Every browser has different logic of performing actions like clicking a button, opening a hyperlink, etc. Most of the browsers are open source and some are not. In open

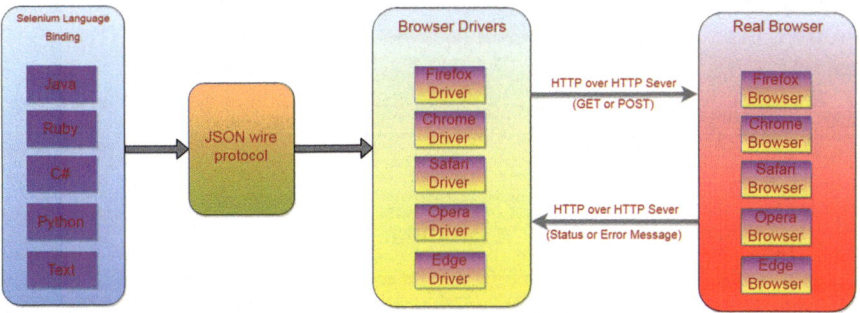

Fig. 7.7 Selenium web driver architecture

source, the code can be seen and edited. The programmer cannot see the code to do automation for controlling the various components in the browser.

The automation is done by the Selenium web driver. It makes it possible for the program developer to communicate with web browsers through web driver. For every browser, Selenium provides a driver through which communication to browser takes place.

When the automation coding script is executed, the succeeding steps are done internally:

- The HTTP request is made in the client side using an automation script and sent to respective browser driver for each specific Selenium commands or instructions.
- A HTTP server sends the HTTP request to the browser-specific driver.
- HTTP server decides the steps to be performed based on the commands which are performed on the browser.
- Execution status about the browser action is sent back to HTTP server which is in turn sent back to automation source script.

There are four components of Selenium Architecture:

- JSON Wire Protocol above HTTP,
- Selenium Client Library,
- Browsers and
- Browser Drivers.

JSON WIRE PROTOCOL above HTTP Client: JSON stands for JavaScript Object Notation. It is applied to transmit data between a client and a server over the web. It is a REST API that transfers and controls the information between two HTTP servers. Each Browser Driver (such as ChromeDriver, FirefoxDriver, etc.) possesses its own HTTP server.

Selenium Language Bindings/Client Libraries: Selenium holds and supports many programming languages such as Java, Ruby, Python, etc., The Developers have formulated language bindings to support many languages.

Browser Drivers: Each browser has its own distinguished web browser driver. The drivers communicate with the web browser without disclosing the inner logic operation of the browser. The browser will execute the command received by the browser driver and the response will be return back in the form of HTTP response packet.

Browsers: It supports multiple browsers such as Chrome, Firefox, Safari, IE, etc. It can also support different versions of browsers.

7.4.3 Distance Calculation Methods

The image stored in Google cloud is also used to measure the distance of the object from the MK. There three methods used in measuring the distance of an object. It is given below.

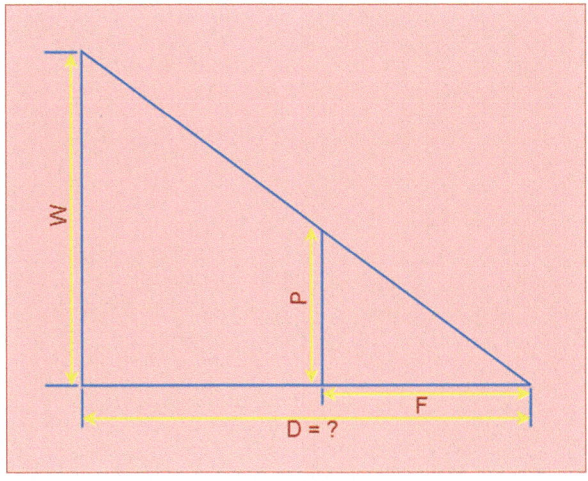

Fig. 7.8 Distance measured using triangle similarity

Method 1

The concept of triangle similarity can be used to measure the distance of a known object using Eq. (7.3). Let us take the width of the object as 'W', the distance of the object from our camera be 'D', when a picture of the object is taken using the camera, let the width of the picture in pixels be 'P' and the focal length of the camera be 'F'. Figure 7.8 shows the triangle similarity between the above-said parameters.

By triangle inequality,

$$\frac{W}{P} = \frac{D}{F} \tag{7.3}$$

$$D = \frac{W \cdot F}{P}$$

For example, the width of the object is 15, the image width of the object in pixel is 3 and the focal length of the camera is 5. Figure 7.9 shows the distance calculation using triangle similarity. The distance of the object with the above-given values is calculated in Eq. (7.4).

$$\mathbf{D} = \frac{\cancel{15}^{\,5} * 5}{\cancel{3}^{\,1}}$$

$$= \mathbf{25 \ feet} \tag{7.4}$$

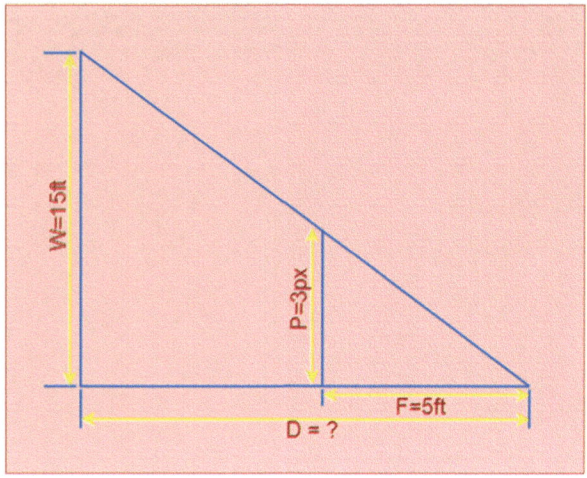

Fig. 7.9 Example of distance calculation using triangle similarity

Method 2

In this method, approximated or actual width/height of the real object is used. Two more parameters are considered in measuring the distance of the object in this method. One of the parameters is sensor size of the camera 'S' and another parameter is image size in the camera 'I'. Equation (7.5) is used in finding the distance of an object in this method. Table 7.1 shows how the equation influenced by the various parameter.

$$\text{Distance to object (mm)} = \frac{\text{Focal length (mm)} \times \text{real height (mm)} \times \text{image height (mm)}}{\text{object height (mm)} \times \text{sensor height (mm)}}$$
$$= \frac{F \times W \times S}{I \times S}$$

$$(7.5)$$

Method 3

The ultrasonic sensor is triggered to transmit a signal to detect the obstacle by using ODS and then it waits for receiving the ECHO signal from the obstacle. The ODS learns the time difference between the sending ECHO signals and receiving the reflected signal. The speed of sound is around 34,000 cm/s. The distance of the obstacle is calculated by using the given Formula (7.6) in the Ultrasonic Sensor.

$$\text{Distance} = \frac{\text{(Travel time)}}{2} \times \text{Speed of sound} \qquad (7.6)$$

Table 7.1 Various parameters influencing the distance calculation

Sl. No.	Parameter varied	Position of parameter in equation	Relating to distance	Influence in distance
1	Focal length	Numerator	If the first object has been zoomed to the size of the second object, then first object is far-off	Increase
2	Real height of the obstacle or object	Numerator	The distance increases as if two objects or obstacles of different original heights appear the equal height in the image, height image will be far away	Increase
3	Real image height	Numerator	In an image, an object alone is cropped then the uncropped image which has the object will be farther away	Increase
4	Increase object height in pixel	Denominator	Two images are similar but they differ in pixel. The pixel in the object in an image is more, then it is closer	Decrease
5	Increase Sensor Size	Denominator	Two different camera capture an image which of equal size in both cameras. The camera with wide lens will have the object further away than the object captured in lone lens	Decrease

The Universal gas constant is shown in Eq. (7.7) is defined as

$$\mathbf{R_u = k * N_A}$$

$$= 1.381 * 10^{-23} * 6.022 * 10^{+23} \left[\frac{\mathbf{J}}{\mathbf{K}} * \frac{1}{\mathbf{mol}} \right]$$

$$= 8.316382 \left[\mathbf{J/K} * \frac{1}{\mathbf{mol}} \right] \tag{7.7}$$

where

k = Boltzmann's constant = 1.381×10^{-23} J/K
N_A = Avagadro Number = 6.022×10^{23} 1/mol
Molecular weight of Air M_{gas} = 28.9647 g/mol

The individual gas constant R for a gas can be calculated from the universal gas constant, R_u and gas molecular weight, M_{gas} is shown in Eq. (7.8). The R_u value from Eq. (7.7) is substituted in Eq. (7.8).

$$R = \frac{R_u}{M_{gas}} \tag{7.8}$$

$$R = \frac{8.316382}{28.9647} \left[\frac{\text{J/K mol}}{\text{g/mol}} \right]$$

$$= 0.2871212 \left[\frac{\text{J}}{\text{K} * \cancel{\text{mol}}} * \frac{\cancel{\text{mol}}}{\text{g}} \right]$$

$$= 0.2871212 \ [\text{J/K gram}]$$

$$= 287.1212 \ [\text{J/kg K}] \tag{7.9}$$

According to newton speed of sound is shown in Eq. (7.10),

$$V = \sqrt{\frac{P}{D}} \tag{7.10}$$

where P is the pressure and D is the density.

After the corrections by Laplace the speed of sound is shown in Eq. (7.11), it became as

$$V = \sqrt{\frac{\gamma P}{D}} \tag{7.11}$$

where γ is the Adiabatic constant.

The specific heat ratio of gas is shown in Eq. (7.12) as the ratio of the specific heat at constant pressure, C_p, to the specific heat at constant volume, C_v. It is sometimes referred to as the isentropic expansion factor or the adiabatic index or the adiabatic exponent or the isentropic constant or the heat capacity ratio.

$$\gamma = \frac{C_p}{C_v} \tag{7.12}$$

where

C_v is the specific heat for gas in a constant volume process (kJ/kg K)
C_p is the specific heat for gas in a constant pressure process (kJ/kg K)

After carrying several experiments it was found that sound speed is independent of pressure and density. The density is directly proportional to pressure as shown in Eq. (7.13),

$$\frac{P}{D} = \text{Constant} \tag{7.13}$$

Equation (7.14) shows Ideal gas law,

$$PV = nRT$$

$$PV = \frac{m \times R_u \times T}{M_{gas}}$$

(7.14)

where

M is given mass,
M_{gas} is the molecular mass of gas and
R_u is universal gas constant.

$$\frac{m}{V} = \frac{P \times M}{R_u \times T}$$

$$D = \frac{P \times M}{R_u \times T}$$

(7.15)

Substitute Eq. (7.15) in Eq. (7.11), the speed of sound equation (7.16) is obtained as

$$V = \sqrt{\frac{\gamma P}{\left[\dfrac{PM_{gas}}{R_u T}\right]}}$$

$$V = \sqrt{\frac{(\gamma \cancel{P}) * (R_u T)}{\cancel{P} M_{gas}}}$$

$$V = \sqrt{\frac{\gamma * R_u * T}{M_{gas}}}$$

(7.16)

Substitute Eq. (7.8) in above equation, it becomes as Eq. (7.17)

$$V = \sqrt{\gamma \times R \times T}$$

(7.17)

Substitute Eq. (7.9) and the value $\gamma = 1.4$ in above equation, the final Eq. (7.18) for speed of sound depends on the temperature is given below

$$V = \sqrt{1.4 \times 287.12 \times T}$$

(7.18)

7.5   Results and Discussion

7.5.1   Proposed Method 1

Information Management System

The interaction of IMS with other module is shown in Fig. 7.10. The entire sensor in each of the subsystem is controlled by the Raspberry Pi. In turn, the Raspberry Pi is monitored and controlled by the IMS. The IMS has an internet dongle to make communication with the Raspberry Pi. The IMS is Intel core i7 processor with Ubuntu 16.04 operating system installed. It has a RAM capacity of 8G and 1 TB hard disk. It retrieves all the sensor data from the Ubidots cloud server. The retrieved data are stored in the MySQL database (Sivakumar, Thirumalai Raj, & Sanjay, 2016) for permanent storage. This module is used as an offline module. It is placed in the resident of the VIPs.

HMS (Baig & Gholamhosseini, 2013) is used to retrieve the information like body temperature, heartbeat rate and ECG sensor values. The sensor values are sent to the IMS for further processing. A threshold value is stored in the IMS for each sensor. The sensor value retrieved from the cloud is compared with the threshold value. If the value is not exceeding the predefined threshold value, the IMS sends normal messages through Email and SMS, and it remains silent. The doctor and the caretakers make a note of the current status of VIPs from this message. If the values are exceeding the predefined threshold value, the IMS will send emergency message through SMS, email and sometimes voice message to VIPs. The caretakers and the doctors also will be intimated about the current situation.

Web Interaction Workflow

The workflow of the web interaction performed by the VIP and the web server is illustrated in Fig. 7.11. The AMS subsystem has a MIC through which the VIP provides command to the IMS. The IMS pass on the voice command to the SRE. The first component of the SRE is ASR which filters the noise and calculates

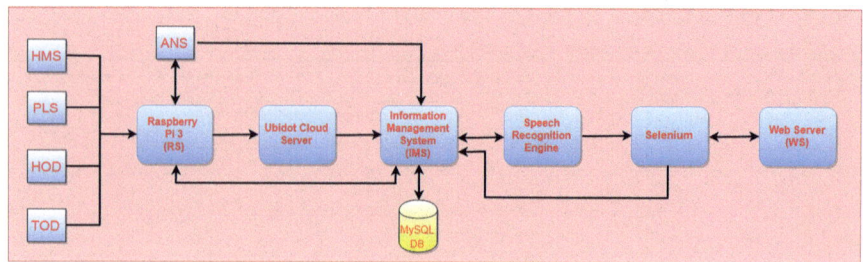

Fig. 7.10 Interaction of IMS with other module

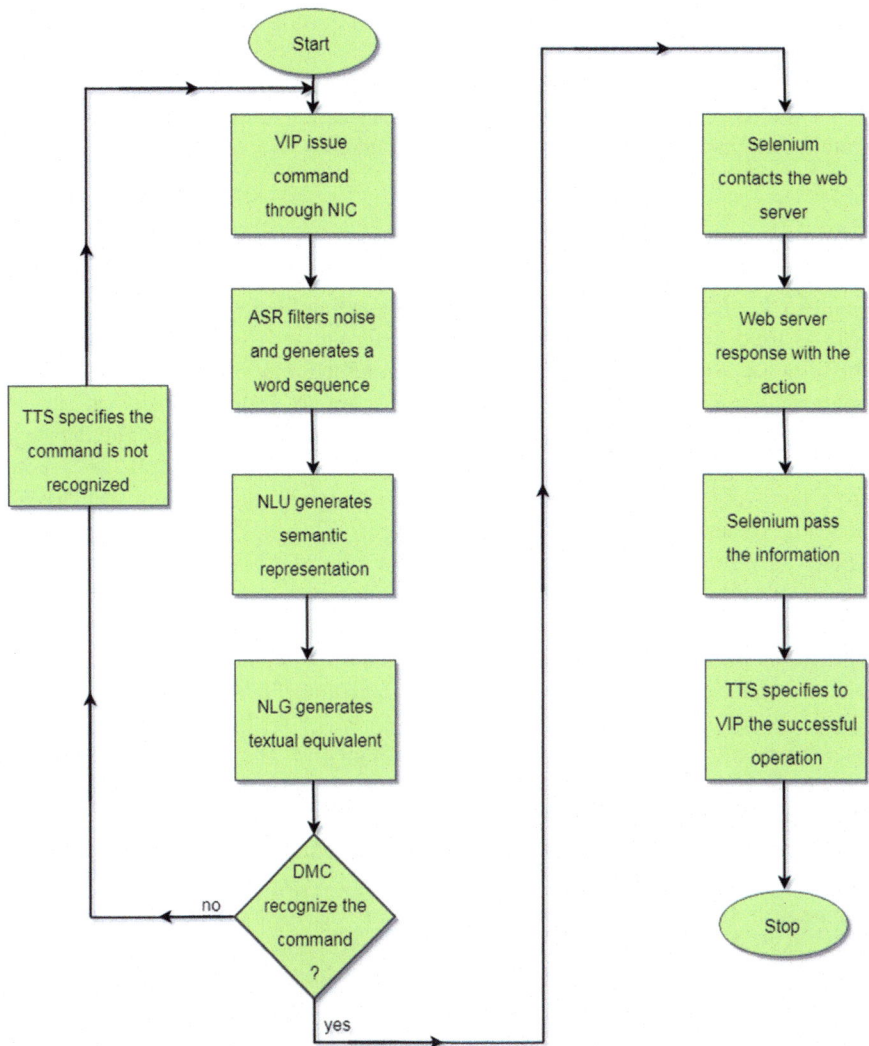

Fig. 7.11 Workflow of IMS subsystem

the maximum possible word sequence. The NLU is the second component which generates the semantic representation. The SRE has a third component as NLG, which generates the textual equivalent. If the DMC recognize the command, then the word or command equivalent is given to the Selenium. If the DMC does not recognize the command, then the TTS issues a voice message conveying that command is not recognized.

Web server is contacted by the Selenium for various action or retrieval of information from it. The retrieved information is passed on to the DMC of SRE for further processing. The SRE TTS component converts the successful web action into speech which is recognized by the VIPs. The VIPs know what must be given next as a command to accompany his/her final task. A sequence of speech to text and text to speech is used to satisfy the necessary action of the VIPs, i.e., booking a train ticket, paying electricity bill, hotel booking, etc.

Web Interaction Illustration

Figure 7.12 shows the sequence diagram representing the login activity of the VIP. IMS is used to navigate the user (VIP) to different web server with the help of the browser. We have provided a simple web interaction of VIP with the electricity payment server for paying the electricity bills online. IMS is capable of storing all web server URLs in its database including electricity web server. The database is under the controller of IMS. For this purpose, the following package is used from java "org.openqa.selenium.WebElement", "org.openqa.selenium.WebDriver" and "org.openqa.selenium.firefox.FirefoxDriver". When VIP gives the command as "*Electricity Bill Payment*", the voice from the mic of ANS is given to the IMS. The IMS gives the URL of the server to the Selenium. The Selenium opens the URL in the browser through *get( )* and *navigate( )* method. The login page is opened in the browser and the VIP is intimated about the successful operation of the login page through headset of ANS. Selenium finds the location of login and password textbox through *findElement(By.name())* method. The VIP issues the username and password for the login page through mic. The *SendKeys( )* method is used by Selenium web driver for autocompletion of the text. The ANS specifies the successful operation of login through autocompletion operation.

The submit element is identified and the form is submitted by the *click()* method of *webElement* class. The successful login message is sent to the VIP. The *QuickPay* submenu is chosen by the VIP. A new subform is loaded into the page which contains dropdown box (region of consumer), two textbox (one for consumer no. and another one for capatcha) and a submit button in the form. The dropdown box list content is specified to the VIP through headset. The VIP had chosen his own region from the box. The text in the capatcha image is automatically recognized by the IMS. Once all the form fields are filled, the subform is submitted by the VIP through the voice command. On successful completion, the payment gateway will be opened, through that the VIP can give payment option and the name of the bank. The login page of the bank will be opened, which contains username and password field.

Two-Step Authentications

For the authentication of the bank, a two-step procedure (Chen & Goh, 2015) is used. First-step authentication is done by the predefined voice password and second is done by biometric finger (Sivakumar et al., 2017). A set of predefined password is

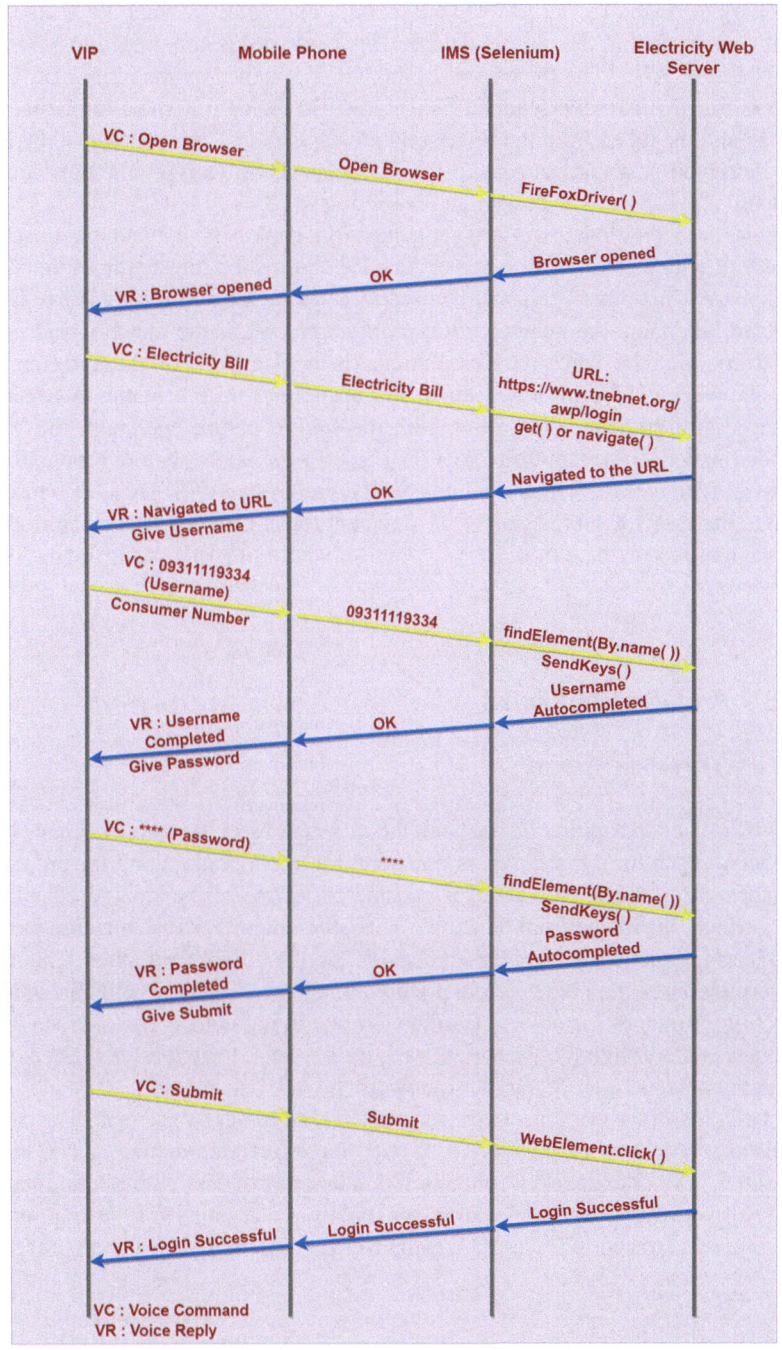

Fig. 7.12 Sequence diagram representing the login activity of VIP

chosen by the IMS. This predefined password is encrypted by using RSA algorithm and it is decrypted at the mobile device. This password is announced to VIP using the headset of ANS. The fingerprint of the VIP is scanned by the mobile device. A token is formed from the scanned fingerprint. The voice password (predefined) of the VIP and the token from the fingerprint are appended. This is encrypted by RSA. The encrypted password is sent to the IMS. The IMS decrypts the concatenated password and separates the token and voice password.

Figure 7.13 shows the two-step authentication, bank payment and logout activity of the VIP with electricity web server. The IMS stores the fingerprint of the VIP in its database. This fingerprint will be used to generate a token for comparison. The extracted token and the generated token are compared. If the match is successful, then it goes for the voice password comparison. If anyone of the authentication fails, the VIP will be informed about the unsuccessful authentication operation. On successful authentication along with the submit button operation, the VIP is provided with the payment form. An OTP (Eldefrawy, Alghathbar, & Khan, 2011) is sent to the VIP mobile, which is automatically read by the ANS. The OTP details are given to the IMS for submission of the payment form. On completion, the webpage will navigate to the electricity board website, where the VIP has to logout of the web server.

7.5.2 Proposed Method 2

Obstacle Detection System

The MK is used to capture the image of the moving object. It sends the image to the Raspberry pi. In turn, the image is transferred to the Google cloud for processing and storing the image. The cloud is considered as one of the storage places. The IMS retrieves the image from the cloud. Then, the image processing technique (i.e., Deep learning method) called object classification methods are applied. The object is determined based on the previously stored image in the IMS. The IMS contains a collection of images for object classification like living objects (i.e., human being, cat, dogs, etc. non-living objects (i.e., cars, trucks, auto, lorry, bus, bicycle, etc. and Stationary objects (table, chair, desk, flowerpot, wall, banner, etc.).

A two dataset for our object classification is used in our experiment. The cat and dog dataset[1] contains a collection of 25,000 images for training and 12,500 images for testing. The Cars dataset[2] contains 196 categories of cars with a total image of 16,185. It is divided into 8144 training or trailing images and 8041 testing images. The code was written in Python 3.6 using Keras 1.1.0 library for image processing

---

[1]https://www.microsoft.com/en-us/download/details.aspx?id=54765

[2]https://ai.stanford.edu/~jkrause/cars/car_dataset.html

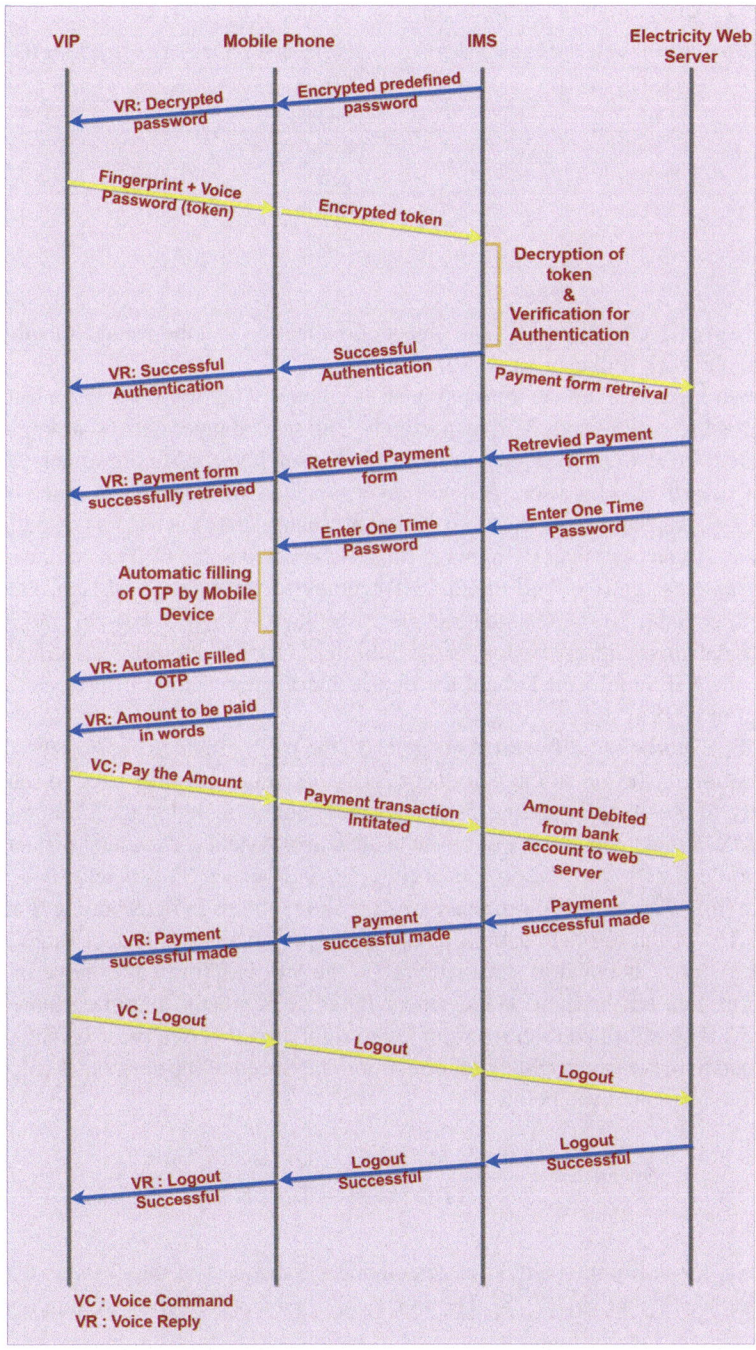

Fig. 7.13 Sequence diagram representing two step authentication, payment and logout activity of VIP

Table 7.2 Arrangements of Ultrasonic Sensor on the belt of VIP

Sl. No.	Obstacle detection system	Position of US in belt	User ID
1	HOD	Left	US01
2	HOD	Middle	US02
3	HOD	Right	US03
4	TOD	Left	US04
5	TOD	Middle	US05
6	TOD	Right	US06

on the top of TensorFlow 1.8. The object classification is done using Convolutional Neural Network (Fukushima, 1980) (CNN).[3]

A two layer of 2D convolutional layer is created. The first layer has a filter size and kernel size of 32 and (3, 3) respectively. The second layer with 64 as kernel size is created. In between the Convolutional and Flatten layer, a MaxPooling layer with a pool size of (2, 2) is used. A dense layer is added with an output space of 500. In a fully connected layer, Softmax (Zang & Zhang, 2011) is used as an activation function. Adam optimizer (Kingma & Ba, 2015) is used in the CNN model, with loss as binary cross entropy and metric as Accuracy for first dataset (Elson, Douceur, Howell, & Saul, 2007). Cars dataset (Krause, Stark, Deng, & Fei-Fei, 2013) uses categorical cross entropy for loss in the optimizer. Once the object is identified using CNN, the VIP is informed about the object that is approaching it through the mic present in ANS system.

In the experiment, different ID is given to the 6 US. Table 7.2 shows the ID and the position of the US in the belt of the VIP. Ultrasonic sensor is used to sense the distance of the obstacle at time T_1. The sensed value is stored in the Ubidots cloud. The IMS initiates the respective obstacle detection system for the next distance and direction estimation of the objects at time T_2. The sensor ID is determined by the IMS at time T_1 and T_2. A variable named '*control*' helps in determining the speed (Eq. 7.19) of the obstacle using the two distances obtain at different times. If the sensor ID at T_1 is equal to sensor ID at T_2, the VIP is informed to move in either direction, i.e., left or right. If the sensor ID at T_1 is greater than the sensor ID at T_2, the VIP is informed to move from left to right direction otherwise he/she will be informed to move from right to left direction. The Speed of the obstacle is calculated using the formula given below:

$$\text{Speed} = \frac{(\text{Distance at time } T_2 - \text{Distance at time } T_1)}{(\text{Time at } T_2 - \text{Time at } T_1)} \tag{7.19}$$

Table 7.3 shows the method of calculating the distance of the obstacle from the centigrade using the Eq. (7.18). The workflow of Object Detection System is shown

---

[3] https://github.com/ankitrhode/Dogs-vs-Cats-Image-Classification

Table 7.3 Calculation of the distance from a degree centigrade

Temperature	Centigrade	Kelvin	Speed of sound (m/s)	Travel time (s)	Distance (m)
Heat	45 °C	318	357.53	0.04	7.15
Normal	21 °C	294	343.77	0.08	13.75
Cold	−1 °C	272	330.65	0.065	10.75

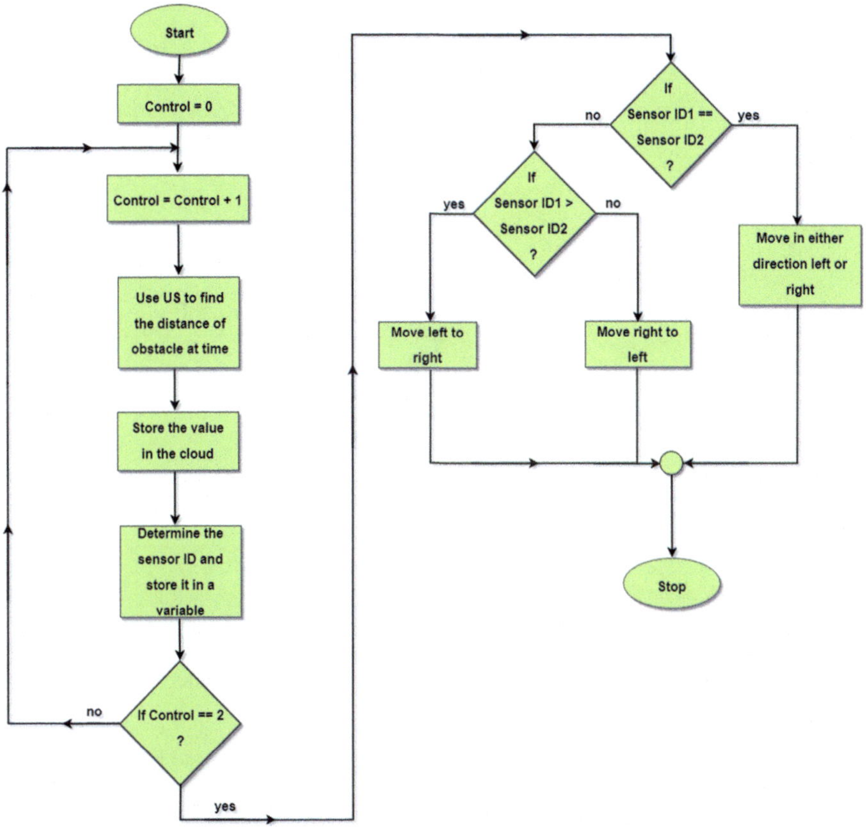

Fig. 7.14 Workflow of object detection system

in Fig. 7.14. The person is informed to move in the direction in which the accident can be avoided. The information is conveyed to the VIP person through the ANS and SER subsystem. This ANS uses the LRA to alert the VIP; to in which direction he/she has to move to avoid obstacle collision. The SER make use of the last three components (DM, NLG and TTS) to deliver the required audio signal through the headset to VIP. Based on the voice and vibration, the VIP will move in a direction to avoid collision. The different ways in which the VIP may collide with the obstacle

Table 7.4 Calculation of speed based on distance at different time interval

Case No.	Distance (D_1) at T_1 (cm)	Distance (D_2) at T_2 (cm)	$D_2 - D_1$ (cm)	Time T_1 (s)	Time T_2 (s)	$T_2 - T_1$ (s)	Speed (cm/s)
1	13	10	3	39,572	39,643	71	42.25
2	16	14	2	42,214	42,260	46	43.47
3	17	16	1	31,352	31,439	87	11.49

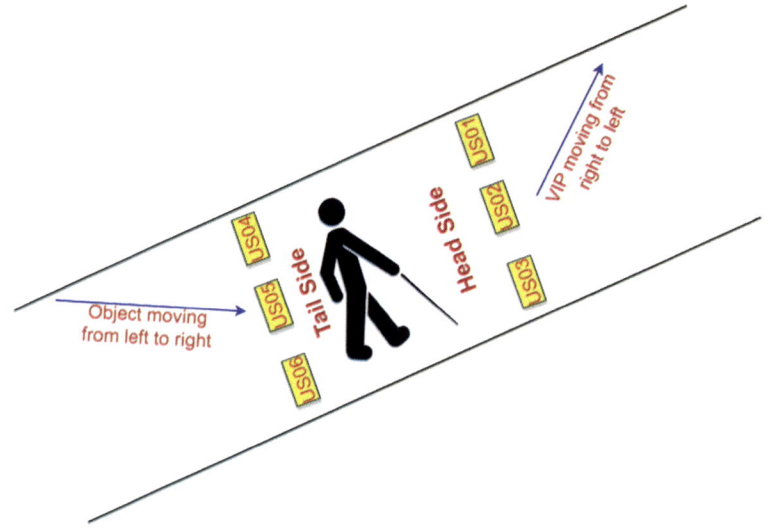

Fig. 7.15 Object moving from left to right example (case 1)

is given in the cases (1, 2 and 3). Table 7.4 shows the way of calculating the speed using Eq. (7.19).

Case 1: The object is moving from left to right side at the tail end is shown in Fig. 7.15.
    At time $T_1 = 10:59:32$ h, Distance $= 13$ m and Ultrasonic Sensor $= $ US004.
    At time $T_2 = 11:00:43$ h, Distance $= 10$ m and Ultrasonic Sensor $= $ US005.
    Result: VIP will be moved toward left direction
        Actuator left will be activated
        Voice command: MOVE LEFT

Case 2: The object is moving from right to left side at the tail end is shown in Fig. 7.16.
    At time $T_1 = 11:43:34$ h, Distance $= 16$ m and Ultrasonic Sensor $= $ US006.
    At time $T_2 = 11:44:20$ h, Distance $= 14$ m and Ultrasonic Sensor $= $ US005.
    Result: VIP will be moved toward right direction
        Actuator right will be activated
        Voice command: MOVE RIGHT

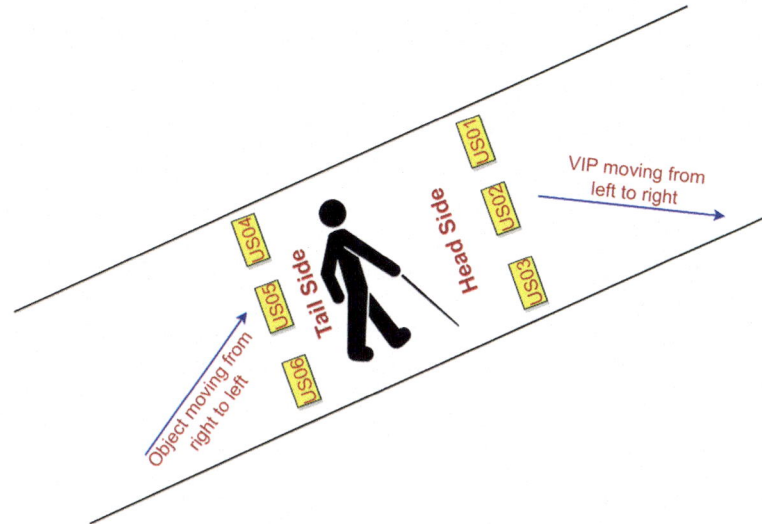

Fig. 7.16 Object moving from right to left example (case 2)

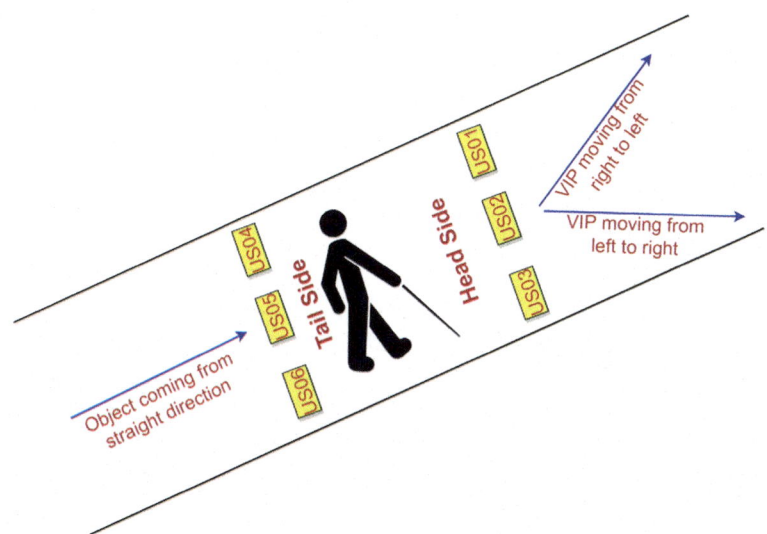

Fig. 7.17 Object moving in straight direction example (case 3)

Case 3: The object is moving in straight direction at the tail end is shown in Fig. 7.17.

At time $T_1 = 08{:}42{:}32$ h, Distance $= 17$ m and Ultrasonic Sensor $=$ US005.

At time $T_2 = 08{:}43{:}59$ h, Distance $= 16$ m and Ultrasonic Sensor $=$ US005.

Result: VIP will be moved toward right or left direction
        Actuator right or left will be activated
        Voice command: MOVE RIGHT or MOVE LEFT

7.6 Conclusion

It is very difficult for the visually disabled to pay their payments for their domestic needs. They cannot travel by bus or any other transport to make their payments. They may face a lot of challenges when they move in the society. The challenges may be in the form of social, technological and environmental. When they move indoor or outdoor, the obstacle creates a major problem during their navigation. The navigation must be supported for their reach toward their destination.

All the subsystem HOD, TOD, PLS, ANS and IMS of this architecture combined together to provide a single integrated solution, that fulfills all the requirements and needs of a VIP to continue their daily activities in a normal way. We included a Selenium architecture, which helps the VIPs to easily communicate with the web server. Through this architecture, they can login into the web server; make payments to meet their domestic and non-domestic needs. We also included a prominent way of detecting the obstacles through three different methods. The speed of the movable obstacles is identified to avoid the collision. By this, we have made them to move in a convenient manner in the society.

7.7 Future Enhancement

In future, the Selenium architecture can be extended to support Google search for sentiment mining (Sivakumar & Rajalakshmi, 2017) based on the VIPs product preference (Rajalakshmi & Agrawal, 2017). In this chapter, only the car object is considered for object classification. The objects like motorcycle, lorry, bus, etc. can also be analyzed in future with improved deep learning models. The VIPs are suffering in taking proper medication given by the doctor. An improved medication box can be introduced, that enables the doctor and caregivers to remotely monitor their activities from their convenient place.

References

AlAbri, H. A., AlWesti, A. M., AlMaawali, M. A., & AlShidhani, A. A. (2014). NavEye: Smart guide for blind students. In *Systems and Information Engineering Design Symposium (SIEDS-IEEE)*, (pp. 141–146). https://doi.org/10.1109/SIEDS.2014.6829872

Baig, M. M., & Gholamhosseini, H. (2013). Smart health monitoring systems: An overview of design and modeling. *Journal of Medical Systems, 37*, 9898. https://doi.org/10.1007/s10916-012-9898-z.

Carlson, R., & Granström, B. (1986). A search for durational rules in a real-speech data base. *Phonetica, 43*, 140–154. https://doi.org/10.1159/000261766.

Chaudary, B., Paajala, I., Keino, E., & Pulli, P. (2016). Tele-guidance based navigation system for the visually impaired and blind persons. In K. Giokas, L. Bokor, & F. Hopfgart-ner (Eds.), *eHealth 360°* (Lecture Notes of the Institute for Computer Sciences, Social Informatics and Telecommunications Engineering) (Vol. 181, pp. 9–16). Cham: Springer. https://doi.org/10.1007/978-3-319-49655-9_2.

Chen, A. Q., & Goh, W. (2015). Two factor authentication made easy. In *International Conference on Web Engineering* (pp. 449–458). New York: Springer. https://doi.org/10.1007/978-3-319-19890-3_29.

Chung, I. Y., Kim, S., & Rhee, K. H. (2014). The smart cane utilizing a smart phone for the visually impaired person. In *3rd Global Conference on Consumer Electronics (GCCE-IEEE)* (pp. 106–107). https://doi.org/10.1109/GCCE.2014.7031333

Eldefrawy, M. H., Alghathbar, K., & Khan, M. K. (2011). OTP-based two-factor authentication using mobile phones. In *Eighth International Conference on Information Technology: New Generations (IEEE)*, (pp. 327–331). https://doi.org/10.1109/ITNG. 2011.64

Elson, J., Douceur, J. R., Howell, J., & Saul, J. (2007). Asirra: A CAPTCHA that exploits interest-aligned manual image categorization. In *Proceedings of 14th ACM Conference on Computer and Communications Security (CCS)*. New York, NY: Association for Computing Machinery, Inc. https://doi.org/10.1145/1315245.1315291.

Fukushima, K. (1980). Neocognitron: A self-organizing neural network model for a mechanism of pattern recognition unaffected by shift in position. *Biological Cybernetics, 36*(4), 93–202. https://doi.org/10.1007/BF00344251.

Gao, M., Hu, X., Cao, B., & Li, D. (2014). Fingerprint sensors in mobile devices. In *9th IEEE Conference on Industrial Electronics and Applications (IEEE)* (pp. 1437–1440). https://doi.org/10.1109/ICIEA.2014.6931 394

Gazdar, G., & Mellish, C. S. (1990). *Natural language processing in Lisp: An introduction to computational linguistics* (Computational Linguistics) (Vol. 16(2)). Boston, MA: Addison-Wesley Longman Publishing Co.

Ghidini, E., Almeida, W. D. L., Manssour, I. H., & Silveira, M. S. (2016). Developing apps for visually impaired people: Lessons learned from practice. In *49th Hawaii International Conference on System Sciences (IEEE)* (pp. 5691–5700). https://doi.org/10.1109/HICSS.2016.704

Huang, X. D., Acero, A., & Hon, H. (2001). *Spoken language processing—A guide to theory, algorithms, and system development*. Upper Saddle River, NJ: Prentice Hall.

Jackson, C. L., Konopka, J. B., & Hartwell, L. H. (1991). *S. cerevisiae* alpha pheromone receptors activate a novel signal transduction pathway for mating partner discrimination. *Cell, 67*(2), 389–402. https://doi.org/10.1016/0092-8674(91)90190-A.

Karthikeyan, C., & Ramadoss, B. (2014). Non linear fusion technique based on dual tree complex wavelet transform. *International Journal of Applied Engineering Research, 9*(22), 13375–13385. https://www.ripublication.com/Volume/ijaerv9n22.htm.

Karthikeyan, C., & Ramadoss, B. (2015). Fusion of medical images using mutual information and intensity based image registration schemes. *ARPN Journal of Engineering and Applied Sciences, 10*(8), 3561–3565. http://www.arpnjournals.com/jeas/research_papers/rp_2015/jeas_0515_1962.pdf.

Karthikeyan, C., & Ramadoss, B. (2016). Comparative analysis of similarity measure performance for multimodality image fusion using DTCWT and SOFM with various medical image fusion techniques. *Indian Journal of Science and Technology, 9*(22). https://doi.org/10.17485/ijst/2016/v9i22/95298.

Karthikeyan, C., Ramadoss, B., & Baskar, S. (2011). Segmentation algorithm for CT images using morphological operation and artificial neural network. *International Journal of Computer Theory and Engineering, 3*(4), 561–564. https://doi.org/10.7763/IJCTE.2011.V3.370.

Kasper, K., & Reininger, H. (1999). Evaluation of pemo in robust speech recognition. *The Journal of the Acoustical Society of America, 104*(2), 1175. https://doi.org/10.1121/1.425502.

Kato, M., & Hirata, K. (2017). Dynamic characteristics of linear resonant actuator using electrical resonance. In *Conference on Electromagnetic Field Computation (CEFC-IEEE)* (p. 1). https://doi.org/10.1109/CEFC.2016.7815963

Kingma, D. P., & Ba, J. L. (2015). Adam: A method for stochastic optimization. In *International Conference on Learning Representations* (pp. 1–13). https://arxiv.org/abs/1412.6980

Krause, J., Stark, M., Deng, J., & Fei-Fei, L. (2013). 3D object representations for fine-grained categorization. In *4th IEEE Workshop on 3D Representation and Recognition, at ICCV 2013* (3dRR-13), Sydney, Australia. https://doi.org/10.1109/ICCVW.2013.77

Lee, J.-H., Kim, K., Lee, S.-C., & Shin, B.-S. (2013). Smart backpack for visually impaired person. In *International Conference on ICT for Smart Society (IEEE)* (pp. 1–4). https://doi.org/10.1109/ICTSS.2013.6588057

Li, Z., Pundlik, S., & Luo, G. (2013). Stabilization of magnified videos on a mobile device for visually impaired. In *IEEE Conference on Computer Vision and Pattern Recognition Workshops.* https://doi.org/10.1109/CVPRW.2013.15

Machida, E., Cao, M., Murao, T., & Hashimoto, H. (2012). Human motion tracking of mobile robot with Kinect 3D sensor. In *Proceedings of the SICE Annual Conference (IEEE)* (pp. 2207–2211). https://ieeexplore.ieee.org/document/6318381

McTear, M. F. (2004). Components of a spoken dialogue system—Speech input and output. In *Spoken dialogue technology* (pp. 79–105). London: Springer. https://doi.org/10.1007/978-0-85729-414-2_5.

Prakash, K. B., & Dorai Rangaswamy, M. A. (2016a). Content extraction of biological datasets using soft computing techniques. *Journal of Medical Imaging and Health Informatics, 6*, 932–936. http://www.aspbs.com/jmihi/contents_jmihi2016.htm.

Prakash, K. B., & Dorai Rangaswamy, M. A. (2016b). Content extraction studies using neural network and attribute generation. *Indian Journal of Science and Technology, 9*(22), 1–10. https://doi.org/10.17485/ijst/2016/v9i22/95165.

Prakash, K. B., & RajaRaman, A. (2016). Mining of bilingual Indian Web documents. *Procedia Computer Science, 89*, 514–520. https://doi.org/10.1016/j.procs.2016.06.103.

Prudtipongpun, V., Buakeaw, W., Rattanapongsen, T., & Sivaraksa, M. (2015). Indoor navigation system for vision-impaired individual: An application on android devices. In *International Conference on Signal-Image Technology & Internet-Based Systems (SITIS-IEEE)* (pp. 633–638). https://doi.org/10.1109/SITIS.2015.66

Rajalakshmi, R., & Agrawal, R. (2017). Borrowing likeliness ranking based on relevance factor. In *Fourth ACM IKDD Conference on Data Science (ACM)*, (pp. 1–2). https://doi.org/10.1145/3041823.3067694

Rajalakshmi, R., & Aravindan, C. (2011). Naive Bayes approach for website classification. In *International Conference on Advances in Information Technology and Mobile Communication* (pp. 323–326). New York: Springer. https://doi.org/10.1007/978-3-642-20573-6_55.

Rajalakshmi, R., & Aravindan, C. (2013). Web page classification using n-gram based URL features. In *Fifth International Conference on Advanced Computing (ICoAC-IEEE)* (pp. 15–21). https://doi.org/10.1109/ICoAC.2013.6921920

Ramani, S. V., & Tank, Y. N. (2014). Indoor navigation on Google Maps and indoor localization using RSS Fingerprinting. *International Journal of Engineering Trends and Technology, 11*(4), 171–173. https://doi.org/10.14445/22315381/IJETT-V11P234.

Ramya, P., Sindhura, V., & Vidya Sagar, P. (2017). Testing using selenium web driver. In *Second International Conference on Electrical, Computer and Communication Technologies (ICECCT-IEEE)* (pp. 1–7). https://doi.org/10.1109/ICECCT.2017.8117878

Rodríguez, J., Goñi, A., & Illarramendi, A. (2003). Capturing, analysing, and managing ECG sensor data in handheld devices. In *OTM Confederated International Conferences On the Move to Meaningful Internet Systems* (pp. 1133–1150). Cham: Springer. https://doi.org/10.1007/978-3-540-39964-3_73.

Sivakumar, S., Arun, P., Lokeshvarma, R., & Krishnakumar, P. (2015). Android based traffic updates. *International Journal of Scientific Research in Science, 1*(1), 161–164.

Sivakumar, S., Brindha, S., Deepalakshmi, D., Dhivya, T., Arul, U., & Nattar Kannan, K. (2017). ISCAP: Intelligent and smart cryptosystem in android phone. In *International Conference on Power and Embedded Drive Control (ICPEDC-IEEE)*, (pp. 453–458). https://doi.org/10.1109/ICPEDC.2017. 8081132

Sivakumar, S., Jennifer, J., Marrison, M. N., Seetha, J., & Sathish Saravanan, P. (2017). DMMRA: Dynamic medical machine for rural areas. In *International Conference On Power And Embedded Drive Control (ICPEDC-IEEE)* (pp. 467–471). https://doi.org/10.1109/ICPEDC.2017.80811 35

Sivakumar, S., Kamatchi, K., Sangeetha, R., Subha, V., & Ramachandran, R. (2017). D2CMUS: Detritus to Cinder conversion and managing through ultrasonic sensor. In *Third International Conference on Science Technology Engineering & Management (ICONSTEM-IEEE)* (pp. 38–43). https://doi.org/10.1109/ICONSTEM.2017.8261254

Sivakumar, S., Kasthuri, R., Nivetha, B., Shabana, S., & Veluchamy, M. (2017). Smart device for visually impaired people. In *Third International Conference on Science Technology Engineering & Management (ICONSTEM-IEEE)* (pp. 54–59). https://doi.org/10.1109/ICONSTEM.2017.8261257

Sivakumar, S., & Rajalakshmi, R. (2017). Comparative evaluation of various feature weighting methods on movie reviews. In *International Conference on Computational Intelligence in Data Mining*. New York, NY: Springer. https://doi.org/10.1007/978-981-10-8055-5_64.

Sivakumar, S., Saranu, P. N., Abirami, G., RameshKumar, M., Arul, U., & Seetha, J. (2018). Theft detection system using PIR sensor. In *4th International Conference on Electrical Energy Systems (IEEE)*, (pp. 321–324). https://doi.org/10.1109/ICEES.2018.8443215

Sivakumar, S., Thirumalai Raj, R., & Sanjay, S. (2016). Digital license mv. In *International Conference on Wireless Communications, Signal Processing and Networking (WiSPNET-IEEE)* (pp. 1277–1280). https://doi.org/10.1109/WiSPNET.2016.7566342

Tahir, A. S. (2015). Design and implementation of RSA algorithm using FPGA. *International Journal of Computers & Technology, 14*(12), 6361–6367. https://doi.org/10.24297/ijct.v14i12.1737.

Van Den Bosch, A., & Daelemans, W. (1993). Data-oriented methods for grapheme-to-phoneme conversion. In *ACL Anthology-A Digital Archive of Research Papers in Computational Linguistics* (pp. 1–9). https://doi.org/10.3115/976744.976751

Van Noord, G., Bouma, G., Koeling, R., & Nederhof, M. J. (1999). Robust grammatical analysis for spoken dialogue systems. *Natural Language Engineering, 5*(1), 45–93. https://doi.org/10.1017/S1351324999002156.

Varadan, V. K., & Varadan, V. V. (2000). Wireless MEMS-IDT based accelerometer and gyroscope in a single chip. *Smart Materials Bulletin, 2000*(12), 9–13. https://doi.org/10.1117/12.436591.

Zang, F., & Zhang, J.-S. (2011). Softmax discriminant classifier. In *Third International Conference on Multimedia Information Networking and Security (IEEE)* (pp. 16–19). https://doi.org/10.1109/MINES.2011.123

Zhou, D., Yang, Y., & Yan, H. (2016). A smart "virtual eye" mobile system for the visually impaired. *IEEE Potentials, 35*, 13–20. https://doi.org/10.1109/MPOT.2015.2501406.

Chapter 8
Intelligent Vision Impaired Indoor Navigation Using Visible Light Communication

Jayakody Arachchilage Don Chaminda Anuradha Jayakody, Iain Murray, Johannes Hermann, Shashika Lokuliyana, and Vandhana Dunuwila

8.1 Introduction

Recent statistics of the World Health Organization (WHO) indicate that over 253 million of the world's population to be visually impaired (World Health Organization, 2017). These vision impaired individuals may come across several challenges in their day-to-day life when self-navigating in unknown environments. For instance, traveling or simply walking down a crowded street could become confounding for those with vision impairment. Furthermore, they may face difficulties in determining the direction of travel without guidance. As a result, vision impaired individuals are often accompanied by a volunteer helper or a caretaker to help them navigate in unknown environments.

The use of technology in facilitating vision impaired navigation has increased over the years with the increasing number of research work. Published literature shows that many researchers have engaged in research work in developing various aids for improving the quality of life for individuals with vision impairment. However, indoor positioning mechanisms require to be sensitive and precise to ensure a high level of positional accuracy.

J. A. D. C. A. Jayakody (✉) · I. Murray · J. Hermann
Department of Electrical and Computer Engineering, Curtin University of Technology, Bentley, WA, Australia
e-mail: j.c.jayakody@postgrad.curtin.edu.au; i.murray@curtin.edu.au; hannes.herrmann@curtin.edu.au

S. Lokuliyana · V. Dunuwila
Department of Information Systems Engineering, Sri Lanka Institute of Information Technology, Malabe, Sri Lanka
e-mail: shashika.l@sliit.lk; vandhana.dunuwila@my.sliit.lk

© Springer Nature Switzerland AG 2020
S. Paiva (ed.), *Technological Trends in Improved Mobility of the Visually Impaired*,
EAI/Springer Innovations in Communication and Computing,
https://doi.org/10.1007/978-3-030-16450-8_8

The Nottingham Obstacle Detector (NOD) (Sakhardande, Pattanayak, & Bhowmi, 2012) is a hand-held sonar device that provides an auditory feedback that indicating eight discrete levels of distance by eight different musical tones. Borenstein and Ulrich built the "GuideCane" (Borenstein & Ulrich, 1997), a mobile obstacle avoidance device that consists of a long handle and a sensor unit mounted on a steerable two-wheel axle. The sensor unit consists of ultrasonic sensors that detect obstacles and help the user to steer the device around them.

A Finnish company, MIPSoft, developed a mobile application for individuals with visual impairment. This application, 'BlindSquare' is the World's Most Popular accessible GPS-app designed for vision impaired individuals (Blindsquare, n.d.). 'BlindSquare' is capable of describing the environment by announcing points of interest and street intersections as the user travels. Vision impaired outdoor navigation could be dealt successfully with the use of GPS. However, GPS receivers cannot be used for indoor navigation as the satellite signals are incapable of penetrating through construction materials (Khudhair, Jabbar, Sulttan, & Wang, 2016).

However, there are several other navigation technologies that could be used to facilitate vision impaired individuals with their indoor navigation. Most popular indoor navigation techniques include RFID, geomagnetism, wireless LAN, IMU (Inertial Measurement Unit), and VLC (Visible Light Communication). The wireless LAN access point method has encountered issues with fluctuating positional accuracy due to reflected signals from the wireless LAN, obstacles, or the surrounding environment (Bai et al., 2014). However, Radio-frequency identification (RFID)-based navigation systems pose no system interference and is resistant to collisions. Moreover, they are capable of identifying the direction accurately and require light maintenance. However, RFID-based navigation systems are susceptible to reader and tag collisions while also consuming much time in deploying the RFID tags (Dharani, Lipson, & Thomas, 2012).

Similarly, inertial navigation is a self-contained navigation technique in which measurements provided by accelerometers and gyroscopes are used to track the position and orientation of an object with a known starting point, orientation, and velocity. However, a paper on "Inertial Sensor Fusion" (Hol, 2011) states that the positioning error of the accelerometer is too high which requires the inclusion of additional positioning sensors for accuracy. Despite its high positioning error, IMU-based navigation systems are comparatively cheaper. As indoor positioning mechanisms require to be sensitive and precise, the authors propose an intelligent indoor navigation system that utilizes Visible Light Communication (VLC), geomagnetism, best path detection algorithms, and obstacle detection to support vision impaired individuals with their indoor navigation.

Visible light communication commonly known as VLC is a communication mechanism that uses LIFI (Light-Fidelity) technology for transferring information between peers (Khan, 2017). VLC enables transmission of data using visible light by encoding data through LED lamps. LEDs are more energy efficient and could be easily illuminated by switching on and off at a higher frequency. Compared to fluorescent light, LED lamps have a long lifespan, low power consumption, and are mechanically robust. Moreover, LEDs are expected to be the next generation of lamps that would be widely installed to replace fluorescent light. Thus, many researchers have studied and published literature on VLC-based indoor navigation systems.

In 2013, a group of Chinese researchers proposed a VLC-based indoor positioning system using dual-tone multi-frequency (DTMF) technique (Luo et al., 2013). This study was based on the different modulation techniques that could be accommodated in visible light communication. The main outcome of this research is that the developed algorithm does not need to synchronize to separate signals from different time slots as it analyses both the frequency domain and the time domain of the received signal to identify the position of the receiver device. This study used image processing to read the data transmitted from the LED lights while the DTMF enabled to distinguish the signals and eliminate inter-LED interference. However, the use of image processing requires a complex algorithm to distinguish the signals while also consuming a high power which is costly.

Similarly, Nakajima and Haruyam (2013) proposed an indoor navigation system that utilized visible light communication technology, which employed LED lights and a geomagnetic correction method, aimed at supporting visually impaired people who travel indoors. Their system composed of LED lights, a smartphone with integrated receiver and headphones. Positional information was obtained and calculated using the route retrieval mechanism together with a positional information base. The LED light sends an ID using visible light communication which is acknowledged by the receiver using Bluetooth technology. The smartphone receives the positional information from the positional information base through Wi-Fi, and the positional information and the guidance content are combined into audio files using a speech synthesizer system and are sent to the user's headphones.

However, the work proposed in this chapter utilizes visible light communication technology, geomagnetism, best path algorithm and database optimization to produce a system that is capable of providing accurate and secure indoor navigation assistance to vision impaired individuals. The integration of several techniques such as geomagnetism, best path algorithm and database optimization differentiate the work carried out by the authors from other researchers.

Benefits of using VLC for the proposed research work include the ability to incorporate communication functionality to the existing lighting equipment, the long operational life and low power consumption of LED lamps, the absence of electromagnetic interference and secure transmission due to limited communication range.

However, knowing the accurate position alone is not sufficient, a navigator should also be aware on the direction of travel. The uniqueness of the magnetic field variations in indoor environments could be used to identify the current position, and possibly the orientation as the three-dimensional magnetic field varies significantly with the position. Through the use of relatively inexpensive three-axis magnetic field sensors, it is possible to estimate the user location in an indoor environment.

Benefits of using geomagnetism for the proposed research work include accurate orientation estimation, direction identification and the use of traveling path correction mechanism to keep the user on the best path and correct direction.

Traditional wireless communication utilizes radio frequencies to transmit and receive data whereas VLC uses the visibility spectrum which offers a great advantage over radio frequency communication due to the free use of visible light. LEDs illuminate by varying its intensity at a faster rate which cannot be identified by the human eye. This is another advantage of LED for visible light communication. Besides, LED bulbs can be controlled by altering the supply voltage at the same power.

In Visible Light Communication, the light source which is used for illumination is also modulated to transmit data to a receiver. This mechanism could be used to provide navigation assistance to users in an indoor environment. In VLC, each LED node is identified by a unique ID number for which navigation is achieved by mapping each ID of the node available in the path to the destination. When transmitting data over a LED light, each LED light should flicker at different rates to provide "1" and "0" (ON and OFF) with respect to the identification number of the LED light. The flickering should happen at a faster rate so that human eye will not be able to detect the change in illumination.

Moreover, there are several modulation techniques available to transmit data using LED nodes. However, VLC cannot accommodate pulse amplitude modulation because of the flicker and dimming of lights (Jha, Kumar, & Mishra, 2017) as data could only be transmitted by changing the intensity of the light wave. Intensity Modulation (IM), Direct Detection Modulation (DD), ON/OFF Keying (OOK), Pulse Width Modulation (PWM), Orthogonal Frequency Division Multiplexing (OFDM), Color Shift Keying (CSK), and Pulse Position Modulation (PPM) are several modulation techniques used in VLC communication.

Since the work proposed in this chapter uses only an ID to transmit data to the receiver, the PWM technique would be the most simple and effective technique to be used. In PWM, the width of the pulses is adjusted according to the encoded ID and the LED light source will be dimmed/flickered based on the ID value which would then carry the modulated data to the receiver.

8.2   System Overview

8.2.1   System Architecture and Framework

Figure 8.1 illustrates the system architecture of the proposed work while Table 8.1 describes the elements of the system architecture.

Figure 8.2 illustrates the framework of the system which consists of four layers namely: the initial layer, interface layer, functional layer, and the backend layer.

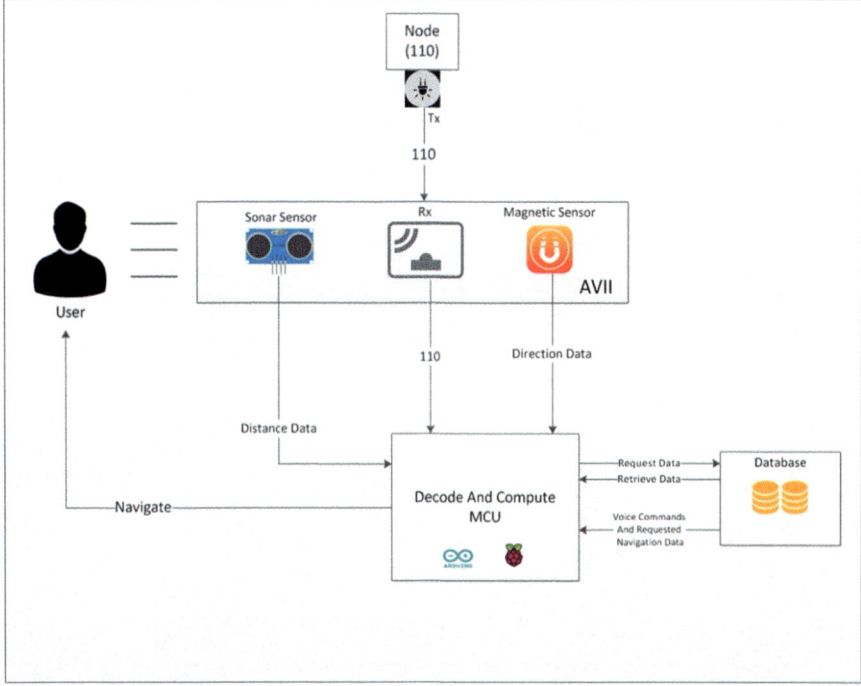

Fig. 8.1 System architecture

Table 8.1 Elements of system architecture

Component	Description
Node (Tx)	The transmitter sends converted digital signals through visible light
Receiver (Rx)	Detects the digital signal and transfer it to the main program which is running in the MCU
MCU	Process the received data and pass it to the backend database
Database	Retrieve only the required data from the DB
Sonar Sensor	Provide obstacle detection
Magnetic Sensor	Provide accurate navigation direction to turn

The initial layer consists of the destination input and the voice output while the interface layer consists of all the sensor functions and user alerting functions. All of the processing takes place in the functional layer while the backend layer consists of the database schema. Figure 8.3 illustrates the workflow of the system.

The proposed navigation system is responsible for guiding the user throughout his/her navigation by determining the optimal route (best path) to reach a specific

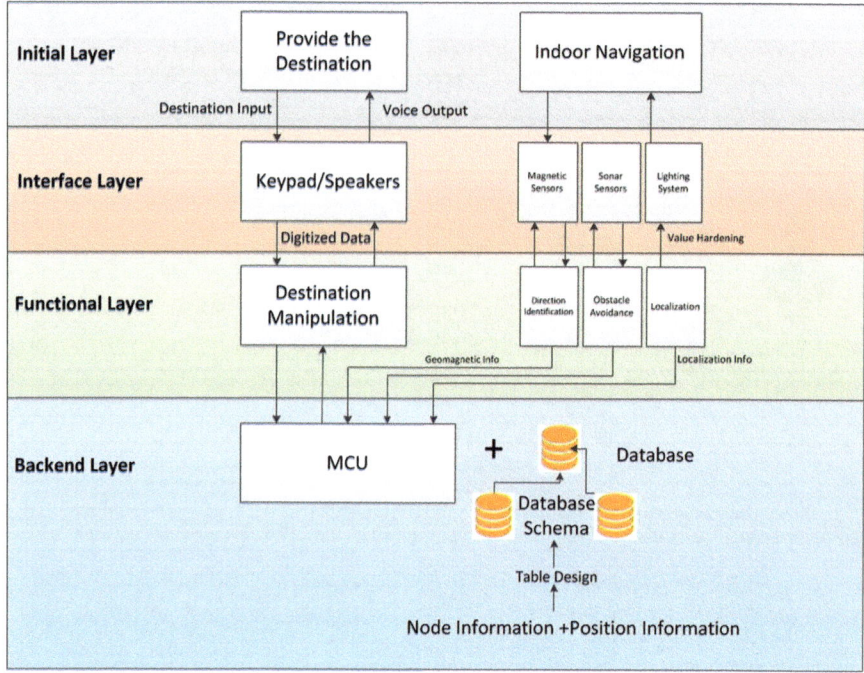

Fig. 8.2 Framework of the system

destination. An algorithm is used to determine the optimal route based on the destination given by the vision impaired individual. VLC is embedded into the indoor lighting system via a Raspberry Pi based embedded device which analyzes the current situation and delivers useful navigation information to the user. The use of a raspberry pi computing module benefits in manipulating the received data as only one serial port can open at a time to receive data from the transmitter which eliminates the receipt of unnecessary data. The system identifies the user's current position by acquiring the node ID (LED ID) transmitted by the LED nodes. The optimal path is then calculated by executing routing algorithms on the data provided by the user and the data stored in the database.

With the best path identified, the system uses voice instructions to guide the user to his/her desired destination. These voice instructions are delivered to the user via an application available in their mobile phones. While in the process of guiding the user, the user's traveling direction is continuously analyzed with the data from the geomagnetic sensor to ensure that the user is travelling in the right direction. If the vision impaired individual is traveling in the wrong direction, the system alerts and guides the user to the correct direction.

A continuous beep sound is generated to inform the user about the distance to the obstacles ahead. A high-frequency beep sound would indicate that an obstacle is very near. As LED lighting is often installed in pathway ceilings, accurate positional

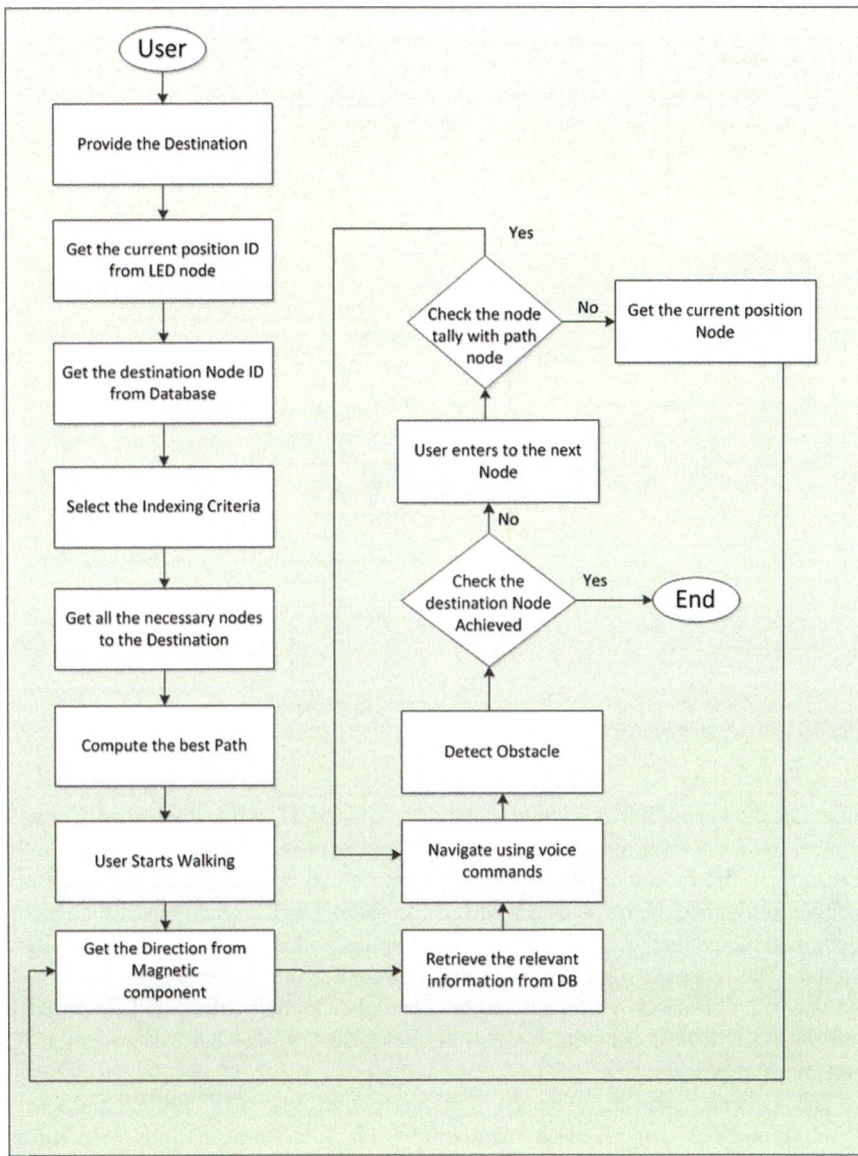

Fig. 8.3 System workflow

information can be obtained naturally above the user's head. The user's direction of travel is obtained by calculating the orientation of the embedded geomagnetic sensor.

In the proposed system design, the LED driver, Controller unit, and LED light will be used as a transmitter. The controller unit will provide a mechanism to

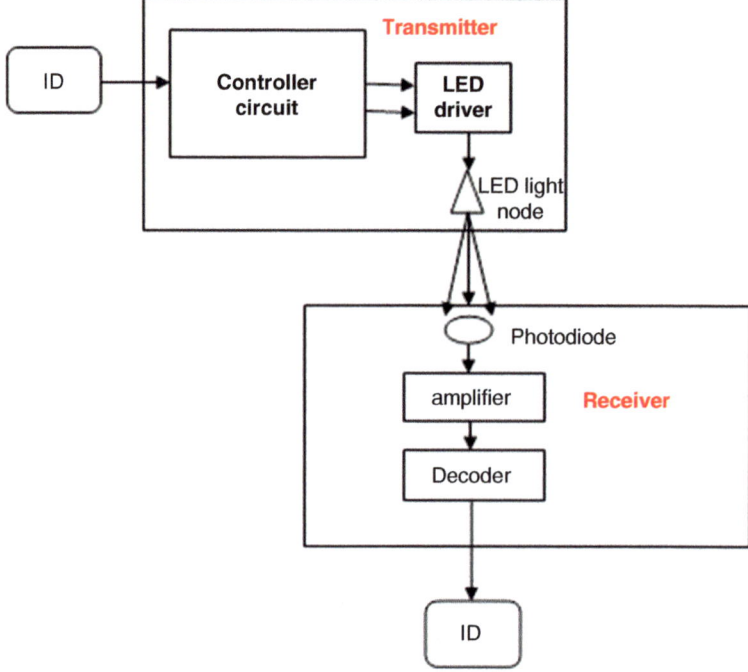

Fig. 8.4 ID transmission process

modulate data using PWM with logical binary "1" and "0" while the LED driver will
control the LED with high switching frequency and the LED node will constantly
transmit the ID by flickering with high frequency so that the human eye will not
be able to identify the changes. However, the sensors at the receiver will be able to
recognize the pattern. At the receiver, photodiodes will be used to identify the light
signals. The received signal will be amplified and errors will be removed through
the use of an error correction algorithm. Thereafter, output values will be decoded
and the ID will be fed to the system for navigation. Figure 8.4 illustrates the ID
transmission process.

The system hardware consists of a microcontroller (MSP430G25530) with
a 16 MHz clock, 16 kB flash memory, 512 B RAM and 20 pins in addition
to two 16 bit timers, one I2C, two Serial Peripheral Interfaces, one Universal
Asynchronous Receiver/Transmitter (UART), MSP430 Launchpad, CSD18503KCS
MOSFET (Metal-oxide-semiconductor field-effect transistor), LD33CV Dropdown
3.33 V regulator, 1 W high power 4×5 LED Panel, 20 W LED driver circuit and
a 12 V constant current voltage dropdown circuit. The microcontroller is used to
transmit the ID to the LED panel one bit at a time. C language is used to program
the MCU (Microcontroller Unit) and code is fed to the microcontroller using the
Launchpad. This transmission is done using the UART module in the MCU. Serial

communication occurs between transmitter (Tx) and receiver (Rx). Both Tx and Rx are configured to use 1 MGHz clock rate and 38,400 baud rate (signal rate).

Baud rate is the factor that decides the amount of information per signal which is the signal rate (Frenzel, 2012). Baud rate factor should match in both Tx and Rx for the communication to occur. If not, the receiving device cannot read the data it receives and the Rx buffer would be filled with garbage values. The UART module can be configured to transmit data using Tx buffer (e.g. TXBUFF = "A"— to transmit node ID 'A') by adding the necessary values to the UART registers in the MCU. This value is converted to an 8-bit frame and each bit is transmitted using the Tx pin of the transmitter. Tx pin of the MCU is connected to MOSFET circuit for the switching function of the LED panel.

In order to receive the data transmitted over LED panel, LiFi receiver is used with a raspberry pi computing module. The LiFi receiver sends the data received to the serial module of the raspberry pi. The Raspberry pi is also configured with the same baud rate to read the received data. This received ID is fed to the navigation function of the system. The indoor navigation system proposed in this chapter uses node IDs with ASCII alphabet values. (A–Z). Hence, the Rx should be calibrated to receive only these values.

The LiFi receiver has an angle of arrival of 90° which helps the Rx to receive data from many angles. The distance between Rx and Tx is 5 cm for three LEDs. By making a 20 LED array with 1 W high power LEDs, the distance increases up to 1.5 m. Since it is the average height of an indoor building, it can receive data without any distortion. This distance could be further increased by using parallel LED panels without increasing the voltage or power. Receiving garbage values are totally eliminated by adjusting the code inside the raspberry pi computing module. Line by line reading provides better accuracy and performance.

8.2.2   Database Optimization

Database management systems should be capable of retrieving the right data to display the desired output. However, this is difficult to achieve when databases deal with high volumes of data. Thus, employing data optimization can reduce the complexity of the data retrieval process by reducing the resources required for the processing to occur. In some database applications, the database management system itself is loaded with features to make querying easy while some database applications have its own flexible language for mediating between peer schemas extending from known integration formalisms to more complex architecture.

Data optimization can be achieved by data mapping, which is an essential aspect of data integration. This process of data optimization includes data transformation or data mediation between a data source and its destination, and in this case, the data sources could refer to the logical schema and the destination the data view schema. Data mapping as a means of data optimization could translate data between various

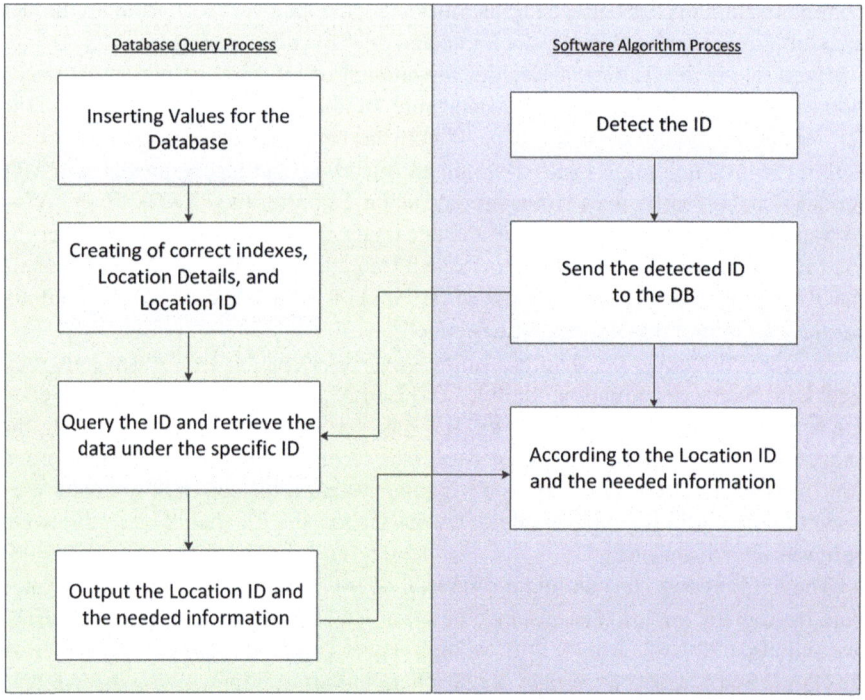

Fig. 8.5 Database function overview

kinds of data types and presentation formats into a unified format used in different reporting tools.

According to the proposed indoor navigation system, there are many nodes in a certain environment. These nodes consist of different ID from one to one, which depends according to the ID given by the controller circuit. Each of these nodes ID should be stored in a database with proper indexing to retrieve the data efficiently. Figure 8.5 illustrates the database function overview.

First the user presses the desired location from the Braille Keypad. Based on the details entered, the program will search the Node details from the table in the Database and retrieve it to the program which runs the shortest path algorithm. Then the shortest path algorithm will output the required nodes. Afterwards the database will retrieve all the information of the nodes given out by the shortest path algorithm required by the user to continue the navigation process. Thus, node by node the algorithm will retrieve data accordingly.

The work proposed in this chapter uses SQLite as its database software. SQLite is an in-process library that implements a self-contained, server less, zero-configuration, transactional SQL database engine whose code is freely available for any commercial or private purpose (SQLite, n.d.). Figure 8.6 illustrates the steps followed in optimizing the SQLite database.

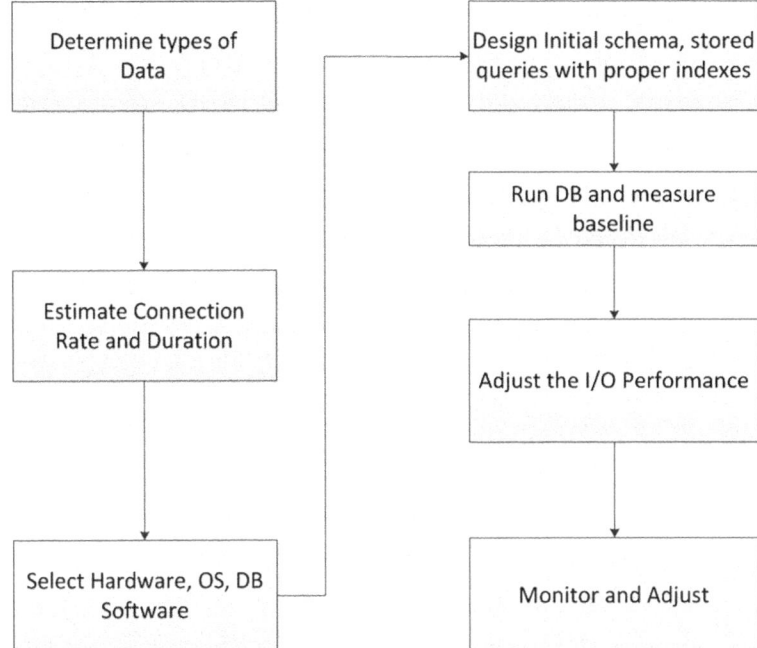

Fig. 8.6 Steps followed in database optimization

- *Determining the Data type* plays a major role in the data retrieval time. In this system, the controller circuit uses binary patterns to process different IDs for the nodes. Using only binary will make the retrieval process much faster than using other data types.
- *Estimating the Connection Rate and Duration* depends on the main system that will be used. It may be an MCU or a mobile phone the connection rate will be varied according to the physical memory of the system that will be used for the processes to be done. Duration depends on the navigation algorithm and the node path. If the required navigation path is long the duration will be high which will require more processing power to complete.
- *Selecting the appropriate hardware, OS, and DB Software* is another challenge in database optimization. The hardware, OS, and the DB software should be carefully decided to achieve maximum efficiency, speed, and reliability.
- *Design Initial Schema, stored queries with correct indexes* is one of the important factors when tuning a database. Many queries rely on sequential (linear) searching. Using default type setting will lead to poor performance when using a database on a set of predefined data. The poorly tuned system can be much slower than a properly tuned one.
- *Run DB and measure baseline* is definitively figuring out, what is normal and abnormal with the database? Without that information, you would be forced to

rely on broad rules that will lead to difficulties in handling the Data inside the database.

- *In Adjusting the I/O performance* Latency, Input/Output Operations per Second (IOPS) and the Sequential Throughput is measured and adjusted. Latency is simply the time that it takes an I/O to complete. This is often called the response time or service time. The measurement starts when the operating system sends a request to the drive (or the disk controller) and ends when the drive finishes processing the request. Reads are complete when the operating system receives the data, while writes are complete when the drive informs the operating system that it has received the data. The Input/Output Operations per Second (IOPS) is directly related to latency. Latency would increase for the increasing number of Ios. Sequential throughput is the rate of data transfer, typically measured in megabytes per second (MB/s) or gigabytes per second (GB/s).

- *Monitor and Adjusting* are the final processes that make the database process fully reliable and error free. Every transaction must be copied and monitored through a log. Future errors could be overcome through regular monitoring. Monitoring and adjusting could be achieved by using a web server connected to the main processing system. Admin can remotely log to the Web server and look into the data movement and can make changes accordingly.

8.2.3   Use of a Best Path Algorithm

The proposed navigation system is responsible for guiding the user by determining an optimal route to reach the desired destination. Each LED node is given a unique ID. The system starts by giving instructions for the user to add a destination (node ID) using the user-friendly braille keypad. According to the destination given by the user from the keypad, an algorithm is used to identify the optimal route.

The system uses a Raspberry Pi microcontroller to process the data collected from the keypad, receiver, and compass module which would then transmit audio signals to the earphone. The LED nodes will continuously transmit the node IDs and receiver will keep track of the user's current position. The system calculates the best path and will guide the user by giving voice commands. Figure 8.7 illustrates how LED nodes transmit IDs.

In order to accomplish all the above-mentioned requirements, the system needs to analyze its environment. It uses three key pieces of information to analyze the current situation and deliver useful navigation information to the user. This key information is the user's current position in the environment, the direction in which the user is moving and the presence of objects in the surrounding area that may be potential obstacles. The navigation mechanism of the proposed research work is illustrated in Fig. 8.8.

With the current position of the user known, it is important to determine the destination that the user wants to reach. The output of this system is an audio instruction that guides the user to their desired destination. The data on the database

Fig. 8.7 LED node transmits ID

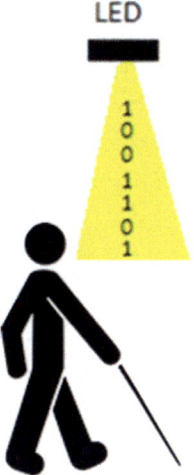

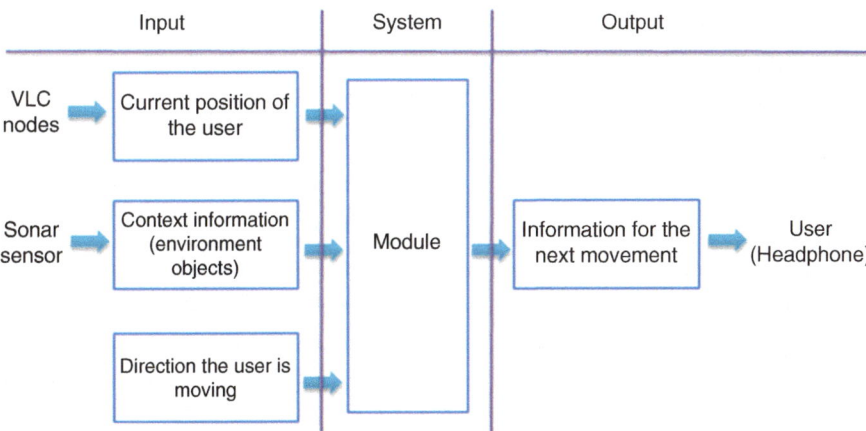

Fig. 8.8 Navigation mechanism

can be a collection of information about nodes that are connected in a tree-like data structure. A node represents a particular position in a building and tells the information about that position. All of these elements will be represented by nodes as shown in the Fig. 8.9 with coordinates and information associated with them. The red color numbers depict the weight (distance) between nodes to explain how the shortest path algorithm works accurately.

The network approach analyzes the indoor environments using topologically based structures that describe the interconnectivity and adjacency between two nodes (Santosa, 2009). The network approach was selected to implement pathfinding for the proposed work due to reasons such as easy implementation and maintenance and low data processing time.

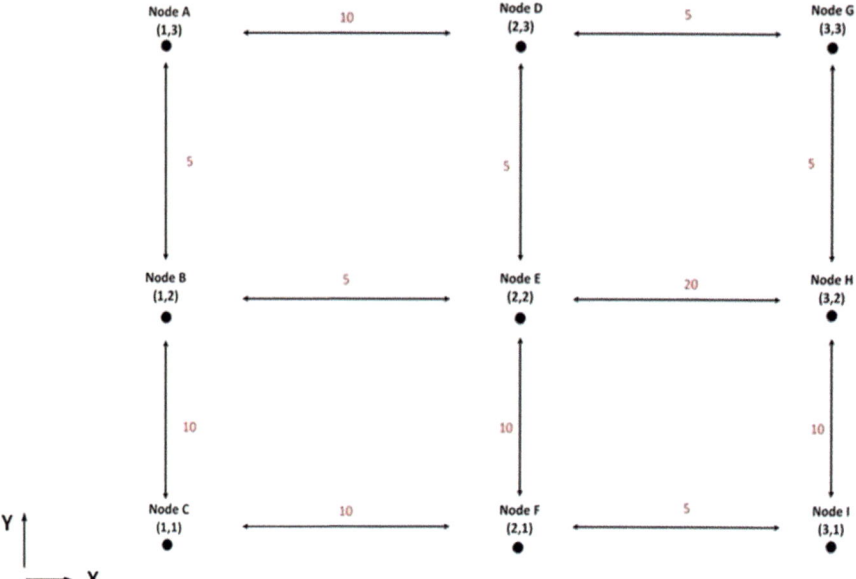

Fig. 8.9 Node map

To select the best path between two nodes, the algorithm must first analyze the assigned cost metrics in each link [path between two nodes] and calculate the cost metrics of all possible paths. From that calculated values, the path with the least value is sorted out as the best path. Figure 8.10 illustrates how each path values are analyzed.

8.2.4   Node Identification and Localization with Direction

A variety of data is required to travel indoors, such as the accurate current position, travel direction, distance to the destination, and information about the obstacles in the surroundings. Geomagnetism is used as the method to survey the travel direction. The travel direction is obtained by calculating the orientation of the embedded geomagnetic sensor as shown in Fig. 8.11. Therefore, compass/magnetic sensor is one of the most important parts of the indoor navigation system.

Geomagnetic field variation in support for indoor positioning and navigation has recently attracted considerable interest as it requires no infrastructure needs. Magnetic field variations could be sensed via magnetometers, also known as compass sensors. The best device to sense the magnetic field variation is a three-axis

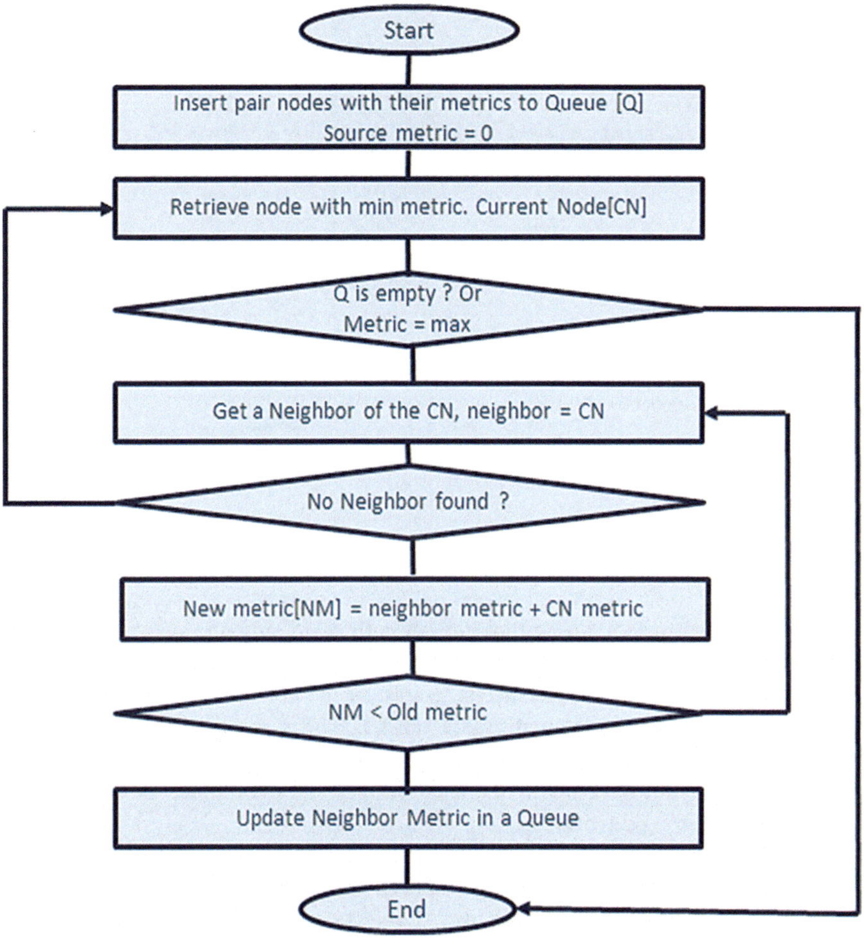

Fig. 8.10 Path value analysis

magnetic field sensor. Even though there are many three-axis magnetic field sensors available in the market, the magnetic sensor for this work should be compatible with Raspberry Pi module and VLC systems. Hence, 3-Axis Digital Compass HMC5883L module is the most appropriate to obtain the geomagnetic field variation in the proposed work.

The system gives voice commands to the user to turn in the correct directions according to the best path. But the system needs to keep track whether the user turns in the right direction. The turning direction is calculated using an algorithm by passing the x and y coordinates of the current and next node according to the best path to the algorithm. Algorithm will return the direction to turn. The value returned from the algorithm is an integer (ID) and direction to turn is predefined for each integer. The voice commands will be given to the user according to the direction (Table 8.2).

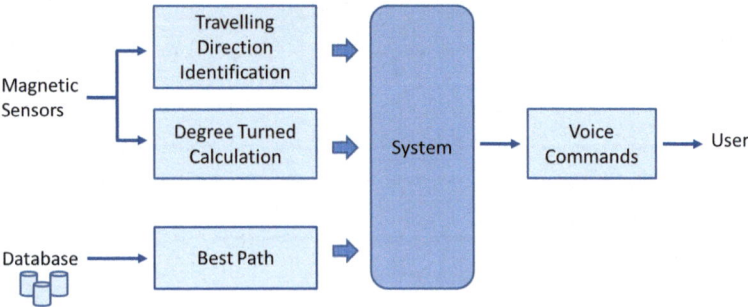

Fig. 8.11 Navigation approach

Table 8.2 Voice commands

Return ID	Direction commands
1	Walk up straight
2	Turn right
3	Turn around
4	Turn left

If the user turned to a wrong direction or path accidently, the system detects the path and alerts the user by giving appropriate warning commands. When there is a bend in the path that the user needs to turn in the correct direction, the system will give voice commands to the user until he/she turns to the right direction by calculating the degree turned. The system will accurately guide the visually impaired individual by correcting the user through voice commands if he/she starts walking in the wrong directions.

The HMC5883L magnetometer plays a major part in guiding the user to the destination. The HMC5883L compass module takes the current position heading/degree and calculates the heading that the user should be after taking the turn. Compass module then continuously checks the heading/degree change, until the user turns to the direction given by the system. When the user reaches the correct position compass module will detect the heading and system will give voice commands to stop turning and to proceed on the path. Heading after tuning is calculated according to the direction that requires to be turned as illustrated in Fig. 8.12.

$$\text{Heading after turning} = \text{Initial Heading} + \text{Degree needed to be turned according to the direction}$$

Vision impaired individuals usually build pictures using his sense of touch and mostly by listening to the sounds that bounce off objects in his/her surroundings. The audio guidance system used in the proposed work will output a voice command with accurate directions to guide the blind individual to the desired destination and warning beep sounds would be emitted to alert the user on obstacles.

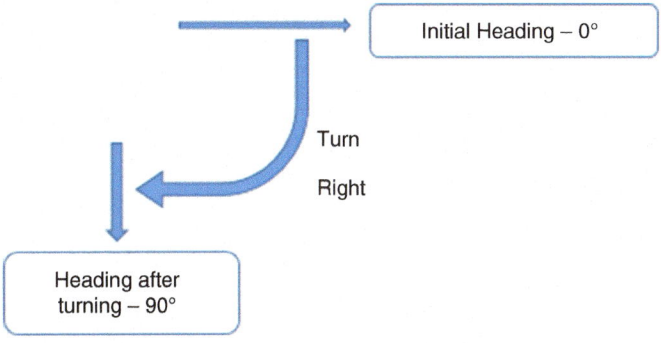

Fig. 8.12 Heading calculation

8.3 Evaluation

8.3.1 Test Case 01: Navigation System Testing

Current position—C
　Destination—A
　VLC receiver identifies the current LED node and then the system calculates the best path by obtaining the current position and destination given by the user.
　Best path—C → B → A
　Navigation to the destination starts.
　Current node—C
　Next node—B
　Walk straight to go to the next node according to the best path.
　Current heading—88.26′
　Heading while walking—88.26′
　Current node—B
　Next node—A
　Turn right to go to the next node according to the best path.
　Current heading—96° 48′
　Degree needed to be turned—90° to the right
　Heading after the right turn—186° 48′
　Stop after turning right (after turning 90°) to continue to the destination.
　Current node after right turn—B
　Destination—A
　Walk straight to go to the destination according to the best path.
　Heading while walking—185° 33′
　User has successfully arrived at the desired destination

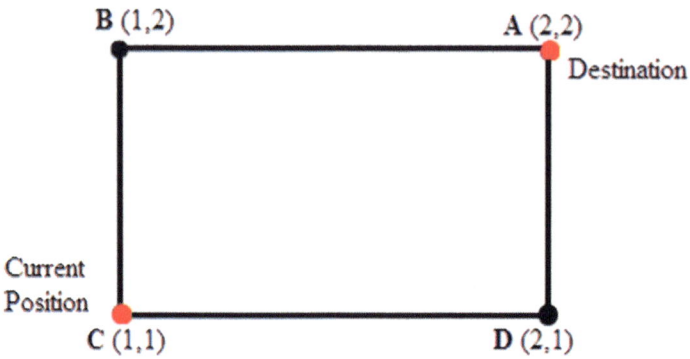

Fig. 8.13 Test map 1

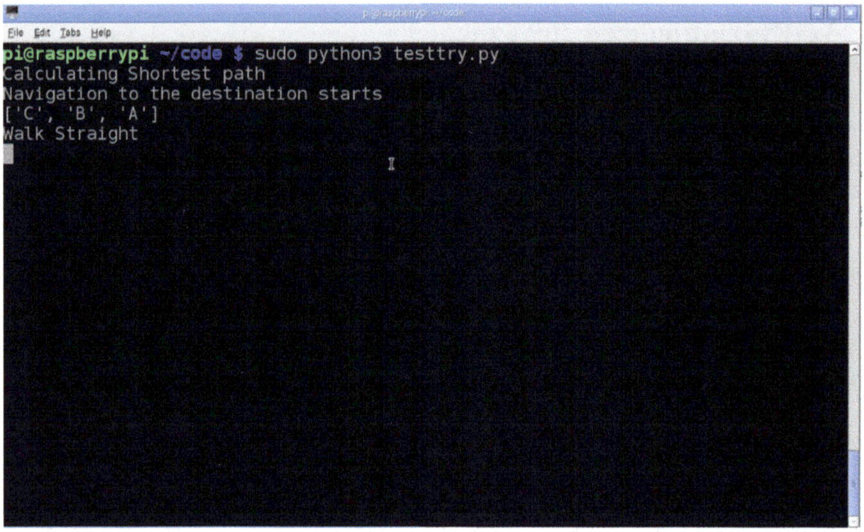

Fig. 8.14 Best path testing

8.3.2 Test Case 02: Navigation System Testing (Test Map 2)

Current position—C

Destination—G

VLC receiver identifies the current LED node and then the system calculates the best path by obtaining the current position and destination given by the user.

Best path—C → B → E → D →G

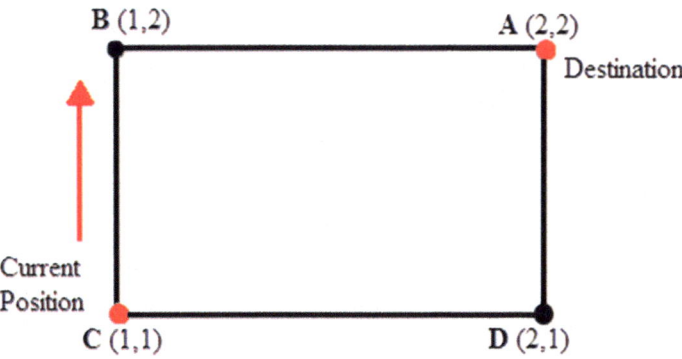

Fig. 8.15 Test map 1 - Walk straight

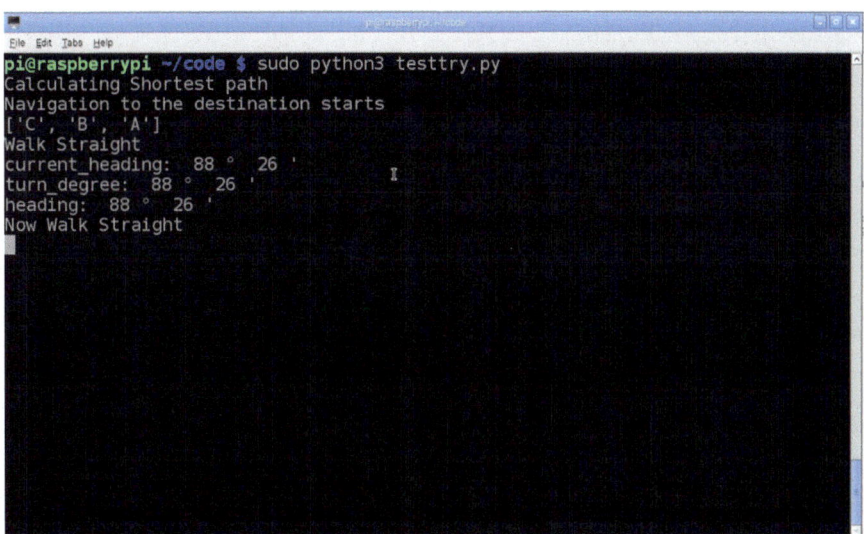

Fig. 8.16 Walk straight testing

8.3.3   Test Case 03: Wrong Direction Navigation Testing (Test Map 2)

Current position—C

    Destination—A

    VLC receiver identifies the current LED node and then the system calculates the best path by obtaining the current position and destination given by the user.

    Best path—C → B → A

    Navigation to the destination starts.

    Current node—C

    Next node—B

B (1,2)
A (2,2)
Current
Position
Destination
C (1,1)
D (2,1)

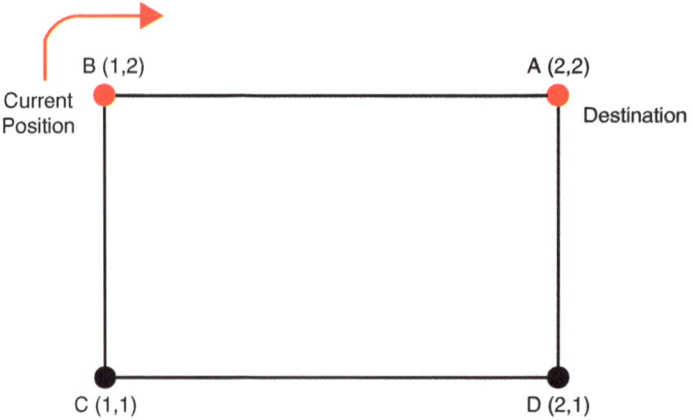

Fig. 8.17 Test map 1 - Right turn

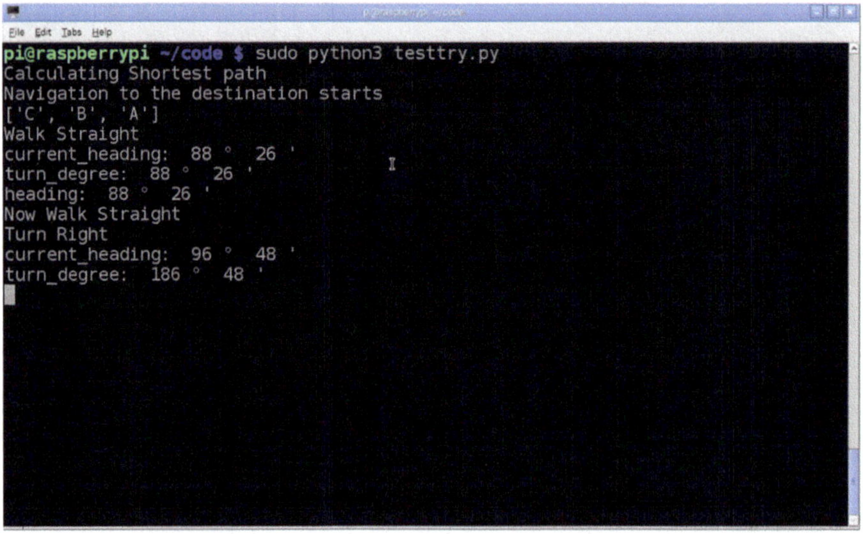

File Edit Tabs Help
pi@raspberrypi ~/code $ sudo python3 testtry.py
Calculating Shortest path
Navigation to the destination starts
['C', 'B', 'A']
Walk Straight
current_heading: 88 ° 26 '
turn_degree: 88 ° 26 '
heading: 88 ° 26 '
Now Walk Straight
Turn Right
current_heading: 96 ° 48 '
turn_degree: 186 ° 48 '

Fig. 8.18 Right turn testing

Walk straight to go to the next node according to the best path.

Current node—B

Next node—A

Walk straight to go to the next node according to the best path.

But the user turns right accidently without following the instructions to the node E.

System inputs the correct destination again to correct the path.

Current node after the wrong turn—E

Destination—A

B (1,2)
A (2,2)
Current Position
Destination
C (1,1)
D (2,1)

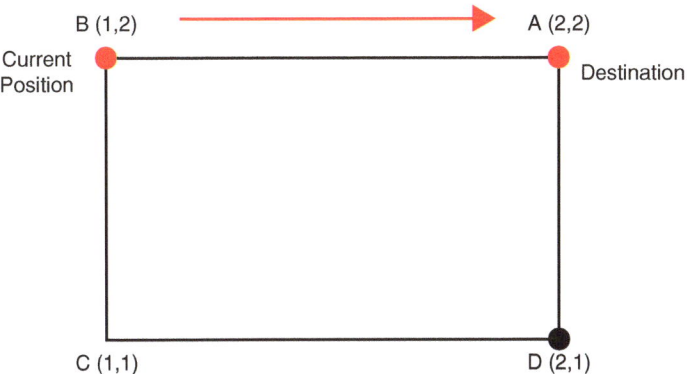

Fig. 8.19 Test map 1 - Walks straight

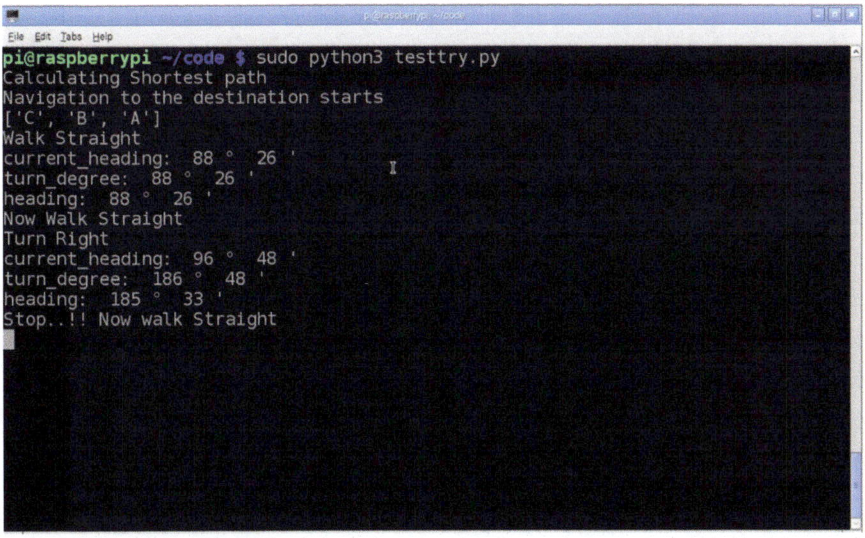

File Edit Tabs Help
pi@raspberrypi ~/code $ sudo python3 testtry.py
Calculating Shortest path
Navigation to the destination starts
['C', 'B', 'A']
Walk Straight
current_heading: 88 ° 26 '
turn_degree: 88 ° 26 '
heading: 88 ° 26 '
Now Walk Straight
Turn Right
current_heading: 96 ° 48 '
turn_degree: 186 ° 48 '
heading: 185 ° 33 '
Stop..!! Now walk Straight

Fig. 8.20 Walk straight testing

The system calculates the best path according to the current position and destination gave by the user.

Best path—E → B → A

Navigation to the destination starts.

Walk straight to the node B go to the destination according to the best path.

Current node—B

Next node—A

Turn right to go to the next node according to the best path.

Since all the three test scenarios have been executed successfully as expected, it can be concluded that the proposed VLC-based indoor navigation system is

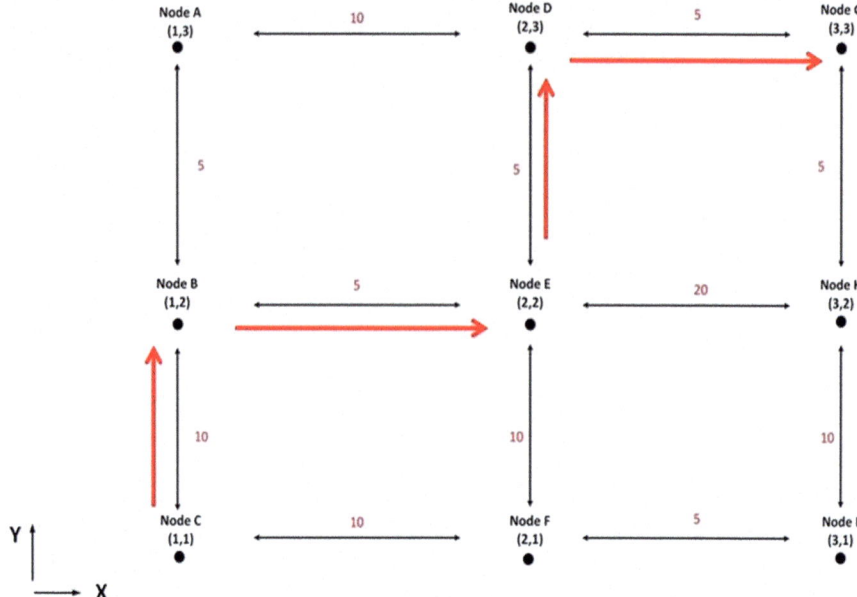

Fig. 8.21 Navigation path - Test map 02

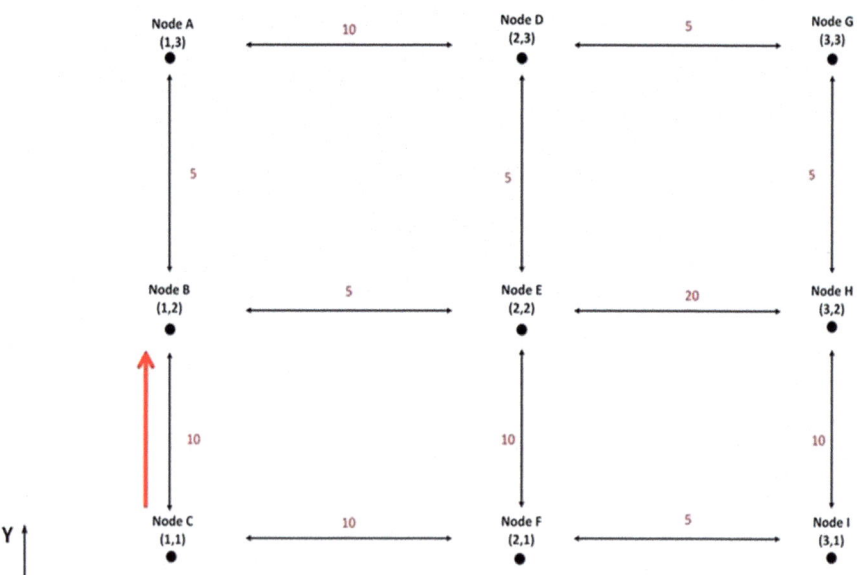

Fig. 8.22 Node map

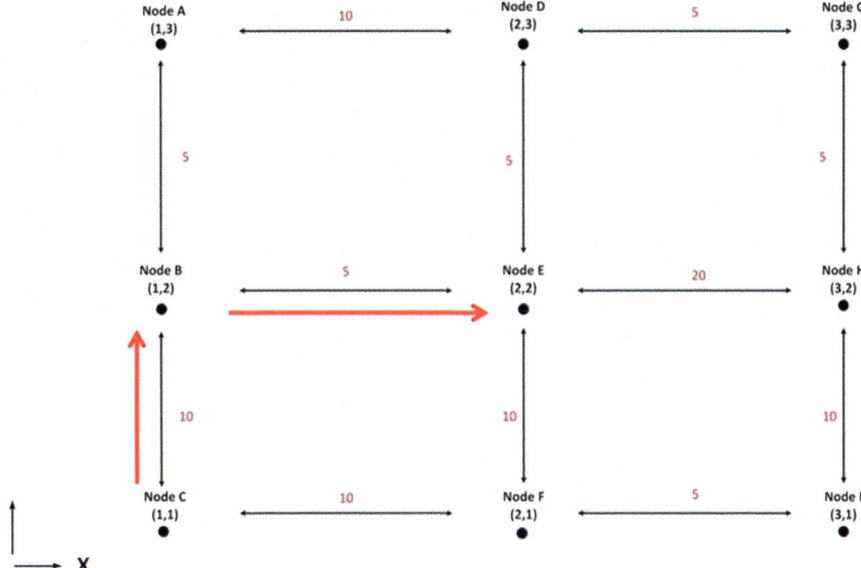

Fig. 8.23   User walks in wrong turn

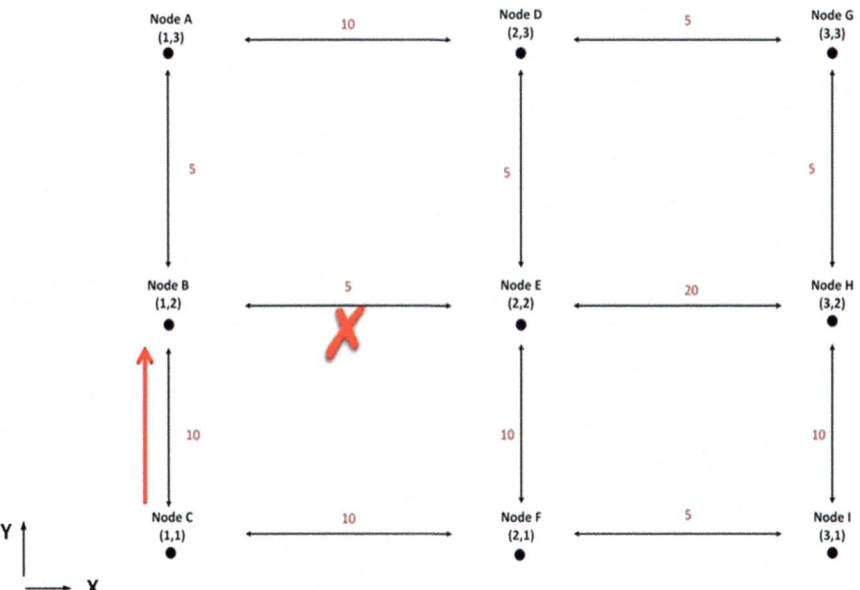

Fig. 8.24   Test map 02 - Wrong path

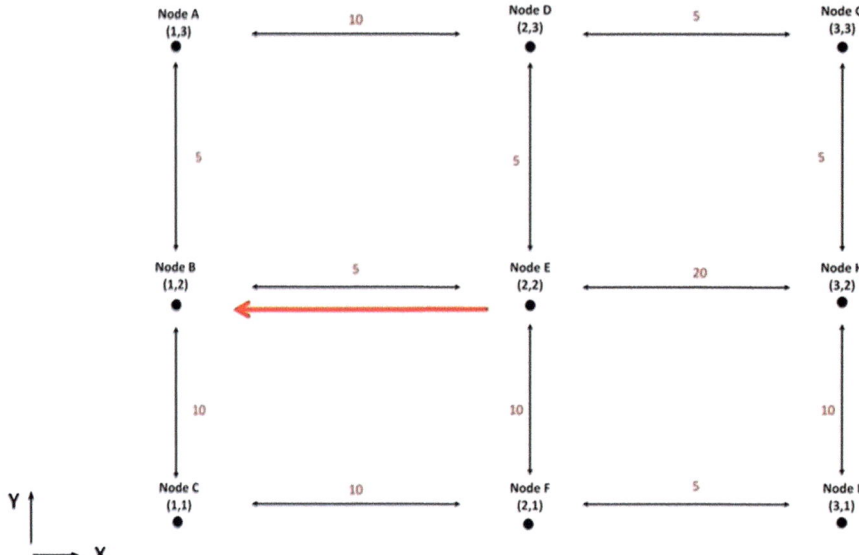

Fig. 8.25 Test map 02 - Correct path

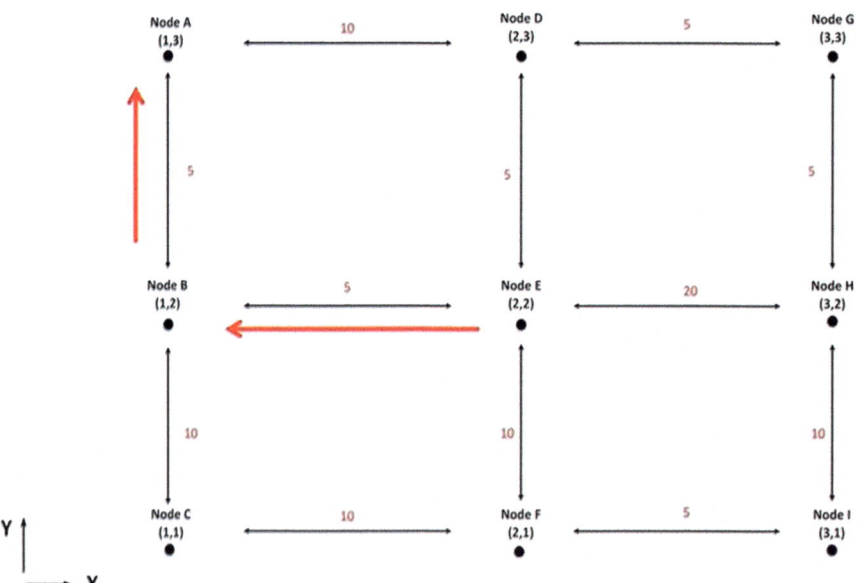

Fig. 8.26 Test map 02 - User walks in wrong turn

reliable to be used by vision impaired individuals in their day-to-day navigation. Furthermore, the system was tested with the aid of eight vision impaired individuals for which they were asked to rate the aspects such as usability, reliability, and satisfaction. The mean scores for usability, reliability, and satisfaction were 72.6%, 78%, and 84% respectively.

8.3.4   Issues in Implementation

The major issues encountered during the actual implementation were the fact that humans do not always walk straight as they tend to hitch while walking which results in the receiver being incapable of retrieving data at times. Additionally, at the receiver, the node ID is received after a difference of 0.5 s.

8.4   Conclusion

The work proposed in this chapter consists of a substitute vision system designed to assist vision impaired individuals using Visible Light Communication and Geomagnetism. It is designed as a product, which provides efficient and accurate guidance for the blind individuals to navigate in an unfamiliar indoor environment without any difficulty. Though many navigation systems to support the visually impaired domain are available, there is no such system that uses both visible light communication and geomagnetism in their work to produce a system that has the capability of providing accurate and secure indoor navigation assistance, which in turn would increase the overall satisfaction of the system users.

The proposed navigation system is responsible for guiding the user throughout map and determining an optimal route to reach the destination. An algorithm is used to determine the optimal route and according to the destination given by the user as a keypad input. The user needs to turn to different directions to reach the desired destination. There will be a large difference in paths if the degree turned is less or more than the desired amount. Therefore, the system checks the angle or the degree turned by the user to give further directions using magnetic sensors. The system guides the user to his/her desired destination through audio instructions via an earphone. A microcontroller is used to process the data collected from the keypad, receiver, and compass module.

Future work could focus on developing and enhancing the system for the use in larger environments. Hence, it could be concluded that the proposed indoor navigation system is capable of eliminating the difficulties prevalent among vision impaired individuals thus providing them with navigation assistance in their day-to-day activities.

References

Bai, Y. B., Wu, S., Retscher, G., Kealy, A., Holden, L., Tomko, M., et al. (2014). A new method for improving Wi-Fi-based indoor positioning accuracy. *Journal of Location Based Services, 8*(3), 135–147.

Blindsquare. (n.d.). *Blindsquare.* (Blindsquare) Retrieved June 21, 2018, from http://www.blindsquare.com/

Borenstein, J., & Ulrich, I. (1997). The GuideCane—A computerized travel aid for the active guidance of blind pedestrians. In *Proceedings of the IEEE International Conference on Robotics and Automation*, Albuquerque.

Dharani, P., Lipson, B., & Thomas, D. (2012). *RFID navigation system for the visually impaired.* Worcester, England: Polytechnic Institute.

Frenzel, L. (2012, April 27). *What's the difference between bit rate and baud rate?* (Electronic Design) Retrieved June 21, 2018, from http://www.electronicdesign.com/communications/what-s-difference-between-bit-rate-and-baud-rate

Hol, J. (2011). *Sensor fusion and calibration of inertial sensors, vision, ultra-wideband and GPS.* Linköping, Sweden: LiU-Tryck.

Jha, P. K., Kumar, D. S., & Mishra, N. (2017). Challenges and potentials for visible light communications: State of the art. In *American Institute of Physics Conference*.

Khan, L. U. (2017). Visible light communication: Applications, architecture, standardization and research challenges. *Digital Communications and Networks, 3*(2), 78–88.

Khudhair, A. A., Jabbar, Q. S., Sulttan, Q. M., & Wang, D. (2016). Wireless indoor localization systems and techniques: Survey & comparative study. *Indonesian Journal of Electrical Engineering and Computer Science, 3*(2), 392–409.

Luo, P., Zhang, M., Zhang, X., Cai, G., Han, D., & Li, Q. (2013). An indoor visible light communication positioning system using dual-tone multi-frequency technique. *2013 2nd International Workshop on Optical Wireless Communications (IWOW)*, Newcastle upon Tyne.

Nakajima, M., & Haruyam, S. (2013). New indoor navigation system for visually impaired people using visible light communication. *EURASIP Journal on Wireless Communications and Networking, 2013*, 37.

Sakhardande, J., Pattanayak, P., & Bhowmi, M. (2012). Smart cane assisted mobility for the visually impaired. *International Journal of Electrical and Computer Engineering, 6*(10), 1262–1265.

Santosa, S. (2009). *Indoor Centrality.* Master thesis, Melbourne.

SQLite. (n.d.). *About SQLite.* (SQLite) Retrieved June 21, 2018, from https://www.sqlite.org/about.html

World Health Organization. (2017, October 11). *Blindness and Visual impairment key facts.* Retrieved June 19, 2018, from http://www.who.int/news-room/fact-sheets/detail/blindness-and-visual-impairment

Chapter 9
AmIE: An Ambient Intelligent Environment for Blind and Visually Impaired People

Marwa Kandil, Fatemah AlAttar, Reem Al-Baghdadi, and Issam Damaj

9.1 Introduction

With the rise of new technologies affecting every aspect of our lives (Abdullah, Enazi, & Damaj, 2016; Al-Chalabi, Shahzad, Essa, & Damaj, 2015; Al-Fadhli, Ashkanani, Yousef, Damaj, & El-Shafei, 2014; El-Shafei, Al Shalati, Rehayel, & Damaj, 2014; Raad, Makdessi, Mohamad, & Damaj, 2018), it is imperative that we use these new and innovative technological advances to help improve the lives of those with disabilities; this is what AmIE aims to do. The main goal of this project is to develop a strong relationship between a context-aware system and a wearable device that will improve the assisted living of blind and visually impaired (BVI) people in unfamiliar indoor environments.

Ambient intelligence and context-aware systems are rapidly maturing to transform daily life by making the environment and surroundings more interactive. With the growth of this discipline, it is the perfect time to advance the field of disability services (Zhu & Sheng, 2011). Context awareness enables the system to take action automatically and reduces the burden of excessive user involvement and provides intelligent assistance which is an extremely important feature in a system to aid blind people. In a context-aware environment, there should be three levels of data collection from the environment. The first level is called the perception level which includes sensors and other hardware that need to collect the data from the

M. Kandil (✉) · F. AlAttar · R. Al-Baghdadi
Electrical and Computer Engineering Department, American University of Kuwait, Kuwait City, Kuwait
e-mail: s00030752@auk.edu.kw; s00027443@auk.edu.kw; s00029415@auk.edu.kw

I. Damaj
Electrical and Computer Engineering Department, Rafik Hariri University, Mechref, Lebanon
e-mail: damajiw@rhu.edu.lb

© Springer Nature Switzerland AG 2020   207
S. Paiva (ed.), *Technological Trends in Improved Mobility of the Visually Impaired*,
EAI/Springer Innovations in Communication and Computing,
https://doi.org/10.1007/978-3-030-16450-8_9

environment. The next layer is the network level which deals with communication and finally there is the application layer which consists of four parts. This layer should collect all the data gathered and then start preprocessing it. This means filtering and classifying all the data while removing the unnecessary noise and integrating it from all the sensors together. Afterwards, context detection is needed using the classified data from different sensors, which will help to infer important information from the environment that the user should be informed about.

Although there are many projects focused on the field of blind navigation, they mainly focus on outdoor navigation while AmIE is a system meant for in-door navigation and many of these projects are not hands-free which can greatly limit the user (Wafa & Elleithy, 2017). Context awareness is a valuable feature to such a project; however, it has not been exploited as much as possible so far, and the current existing projects focus only on having a device with the user instead of having both an ambient intelligence environment and a smart device connected.

According to the World Health Organization (WHO) there are about 253 million people with vision impairment and 36 million who are blind (World Health Organization, 2018). This makes up a considerable amount of the population and so identifying the problems they face and proposing possible solutions is critical. Such problems include the facts that it is very difficult for BVI people to be completely independent when they are by themselves in an unfamiliar environment and they usually need a guide dog or another person assisting them in order for them to reach their destinations and complete their tasks. Implementing AmIE, solves this problem as BVI people will have much more independence and be able to manage unfamiliar environments without assistance from others. Introducing an ambient intelligent and context-aware system to indoor environments will significantly enhance the living standard of BVI people. AmIE will benefit BVI people of all ages, whether they have only some vision impairment or are fully blind and can be used in a wide range of countries as it is a multilingual system. Altogether, the AmIE will help increase the chances if BVI people becoming more integrated into society and it will increase the number of their opportunities and make many more areas available to them that may have been hard to access before.

This chapter is organized such that the Sect. 2 presents related work. Section 3 presents the motivation behind the system. In addition, Section 4 presents AmIE system development, while Sect. 5 represents the main implementation steps. Section 6 thoroughly analyzes and evaluates the proposed model and Sect. 7 concludes the chapter and sets the grounds for future work.

9.2 Literature Review

Technological research has led, thus far, to the creation of Assisted-living technology along with IoT systems to aid the blind and visually impaired (BVI). As a result of this research, system proposals vary between mobile cloud-based systems, smart cane-based system, and Ambient intelligent and context-aware systems (Domingo, 2012). The majority of the systems approaches include indoor navigation, out-door navigation, object recognition, and avoidance, to name a few. The focus of this section is to provide background information on IDM techniques to create and represent the system and to compare the surveyed systems with AmIE functionalities. The papers are categorized according to two main functions: Indoor positioning and navigation, and context-aware and Ambient Intelligence systems.

9.2.1 Indoor Positioning and Navigation

One of the hardest tasks for a BVI person is finding their way through a building. Most research papers discussed in this section used obstacle avoidance as a way for navigation. Some systems depended on GPS to locate the user and then navigate them through a chosen path.

Angin and Bhargava (2011) propose Mobile-Cloud Computing approach for context-aware navigation of the BVI through unfamiliar places. One of the main system components used is the hand-held device that can receive commands on the required destination from the user. For positioning they used Skyhook Wireless positioning module that collects raw data from Wi-Fi access points distributed through the building, GPS satellites and cell towers with advanced hybrid positioning algorithms in addition to the integrated campus of the Mobile phone. The system was designed for indoors and outdoors.

CASBlip (CMOS sensor-based acoustic object detection and navigation system for blind people) (Dunai, Garcia, Lengua, & Peris-Fajarnés, 2012) allows navigation through converting objects detected in the surrounding indoor environment into sound signals by Ultrasonic sensors, using a Field Programmable Logic Array (FPGA) and an acoustic module. An FPGA is used to control the collision with approaching objects by calculating the distance, processing the data, and displays the directions through a headset. The acoustic module was used to allow the user to choose a path after detecting the obstacle. One of the issues with this system is that it works for short-range obstacles only and this might not be very safe for blind people.

Another similar system that uses images is the Navigation assistance for visually impaired using RGB-D sensor with range expansion (Aladren, Lopez-Nicolas, Puig, & Guerrero, 2016). The device will be worn on the user's neck and it takes images of the surroundings and then analyzes it. After that it identifies the obstacles that face the user. RGB detector and two IR sensors were used to collect information from the surroundings. A 3D point was used to extract the main features and filter all points that are representing each cube of taken images to one image. This step is repeated until the system can classify these images. Then they used Hough Line Transform and Canny edge detector to generate board line between obstacles and floors. The system shows good performance in identifying a floor from obstacles in very small areas. However, once area is increased it becomes difficult to detect further obstacles. In addition, the system faces many issues when it is used in a place with windows in the morning as the sunlight interferes with the infrared waves.

Silicone Eyes (SiliEyes) (Prudhvi & Bagani, 2013) uses GPS and GSM coordinators that are integrated in a wearable silicone glove to help position and navigate the user inside a building and provide wide range of information from getting their current location, the current time and the color of the object in front of them. Navigation and data are displayed as audio. A set of sensors are used to give details about the environment, these include a 24-bit color sensor, light sensor, temperature sensor, and a SONAR to detect the obstacles. The system also supports a touch keypad using Brielle technique to enter the desired location. In case of emergency the current location of the user will be sent to someone whose phone number is stored in the system. The emergency message sends the current location of the user by using the GPS.

Using BAN (body area network) is another approach to navigate BVIP which was developed in the article Blind Guide: an ultrasound sensor-based body area network for guiding blind people (Pereira et al., 2015). In this article, the authors propose the use of an ultrasound-based body area network for obstacle detection and warning as a complementary and effective solution for aiding blind people navigate from place to place. The Body area network is embedded in the clothing fabric, freeing blind people to continue using the white cane or Seeing Eye dog. The jacket is used to detect the head and chest level obstacles. They used two Mica2 motes placed at each shoulder, to connect these motes to the ultrasonic sensors and prototype board Mica2 mote was used. They were programmed using MantisOS and C programming language. Elastic bands were used to detect the foot level obstacles. Each elastic band embeds a Mica2Dot sensor node and each sensor node has one ultrasound sensor connected through the MDA500CA data acquisition board. Just like the previous discussed systems, this system navigates the user by obstacle avoidance, and it does not offer a positioning function that would help the user in case of emergency. A buzzer was used to inform the user about the approaching obstacle, a different tone was displayed for each obstacle type. This might be an issue as information delivered is limited and it might be confusing if the users were not trained with it.

9.2.2   Context-Aware and Ambient Intelligent Environments

The ability of an environment to react according to our actions is known as context-aware environment. This concept provides us with many possibilities to develop assistive technologies that can help BVI to have a better lifestyle. Some of the research papers discussed in this section used Ambient Intelligent for health care in general, some papers also explain how to develop better context-aware environment.

RUDO System (Hudec & Smutny, 2017) is a home ambient environment that comprises several modules that mainly support recognition of approaching people, alerting to other household members' movement in the flat, work on a computer, supervision of (sighted) children, cooperation of a sighted and a blind person (e.g., when studying), control of heating and zonal regulation by a blind person. The interface for blind people aids with work on a computer, including writing in Braille on a regular keyboard and specialized work in informatics and electronics (e.g., programming). RUDO system is a network-oriented product that runs within a local computer network and is implemented on OS Linux Debian. Over four versions of the system where implemented, the fourth version includes a "mini server" that communicates with various modules in the home of the blind individual via LAN. It also implements several external microphones and speakers for the sake of child supervision by the blind parent. The problem context of this system considers only the fully blind people and not the visually impaired limiting its usage. The system was designed to provide a smart environment inside the homes of the Blind people, however it is not designed to facilitate their interaction in unfamiliar environments.

ISAB (Integrated Indoor Navigation System for the Blind) (Abu Doush, Alshatnawi, Al-Tamimi, Alhasan, & Hamasha, 2016) helps blind users accomplish two main tasks: perform indoor navigation to a certain office or room and fetch a specific item located on a shelf with a high level of accuracy using context data collected from sensors placed all over the building. The system uses multiple indoor localization technologies such as Wi-Fi, Bluetooth and RFID. The Wi-Fi is used to locate the user inside the building, floor plans of the building are sent to the user and it is represented as a graph of connected nodes. The path planning algorithm Dijkstra was used to determine the location of the desired room. Bluetooth is used to locate desired shelf by the self-readers Bluetooth modules placed at the end of each shelf. The user's phone is only paired with the desired shelf. Finally, RFID are used to identify the desired object as the user would use the shelf-Reader device to identify the object they want using the RFID code. This system is considered a context-aware system as it provides the user with context-related data, in this case it provides the user with directions to reach a specific object.

The systems discussed in this section were developed to navigate and assist BVI people. The papers that examined positioning and navigation used many different methods such as obstacle avoidance using ultrasonic sensor, image processing for obstacle recognition, BAN for navigation, and GPS for positioning. A few papers considered providing environment-related information to the user such as details of the approaching obstacles, current time and location as well as features that considers the safety of the user. Some papers discussed used context awareness and ambient intelligence to facilitate lives for BVI such as RUDO (Hudec & Smutny, 2017) where a smart house environment was designed specifically to accommodate blind working parents. Other papers such as ISAB (Abu Doush et al., 2016) used context-related data to help navigate and assist the BVI to their desired location. Speech recognition in Arabic was part of the reviewed literature as it is considered one of the main functionalities of AmIE. Using Android platform and google speech cloud is considered as one of the best available open sources for speech recognition in Arabic and other languages.

9.2.3 Background

To integrate BVI people in their environment, an IoT system is developed to facilitate their interactions with the surrounding. To represent our IoT system, the IoT Development Model (IDM) of Damaj and Kasbah (2019) is used to design, represent, and analyze the system through set of Concept Refinement Pyramid (CRP), Decision Trees (DTs), Architecture and Organization Diagram (AOD), Communication Interfaces (CIs), Use Case Diagrams (UCDs), Realistic Constraint List (RCL), Menu of Analysis Metrics (MAMs), and Evaluation Indicators Graph (EIG). The diagrams discussed in this section are used in the development and evaluation of the AmIE system.

CRP is a pyramid that summarizes the system's functions and technologies. The CRP consists of three levels where each level is described with concise and short statements. The highest level of the CRP is title that defines the concept. The other levels aim to briefly describe the system's concept, design, and implementation main parts while maintaining professional ethics and socioeconomic factors.

DTs, UCDs, and AODs represent the functional requirements of the system. The DTs are multi-leaf-node trees that demonstrate alternate designs or implementation option at the technology level. One of the nodes in a DT is selected as the designer's implementation option. The UCDs are adopted from the UML to interpret the system interactions between the actors and the system functionalities, such as managing, using, extending, and including. They also represent the system events flow. In addition, the AOD illustrates the architecture and organizational structure of the system. Moreover, it shows the communication of the different technologies, subsystems, and platforms used within the system.

RCL, MAMs, and EIG express the non-functional requirements of the system. Realistic constraints can be tight; they are, usually, critical requirements during system development. The clear identification of the system constraints; using the RCL; helps in predicting possible limitations to the system. There are two types of Menu of Analysis Metrics (MAMs), the general metrics and the application-specific metrics. General metrics are typical to all systems, however the application-specific are more focused on the metrics for AmIE itself. MAMs aids the evaluation of the robustness, thoroughness, and adequacy of AmIE and its chosen metrics.

9.3 Motivation and Objectives

The motivation behind this chapter exists as it explores the future of mobility and different methods of indoor positioning and navigation which is still a growing field compared to outdoor navigation. It also addresses the pressing issue that BVI people face when trying to navigate in an unfamiliar indoor environment. They may have trouble finding their way in new areas as they are not as aware of their surroundings and may need to rely on other people for assistance or they would need to use canes or service dogs to help them get around, which both have many limitations such as the user not having the freedom to use both hands in case they need them as they will be holding the cane or the dog's leash. The walking canes they use also cannot give them a full idea of their surrounding areas and cannot help them locate a specific destination, and in the case of the service dogs, it is likely that they will not be allowed in certain areas.

Blind and visually impaired people no longer have to be isolated from the society. AmIE system helps BVI users to navigate through indoor environment with minimum assistance required from others. In addition to indoor navigation, a context-aware environment is proposed to provide the BVI user a comfortable assisted and secure/safe living. Moreover, the speech recognition feature supports both English and Arabic languages so that it fits the preferences of both Arab and non-Arab users. Altogether, AmIE will help increase the chances if BVI people getting jobs and allow them to be more integrated into the society.

AmIE provides an interactive ambient intelligent and context-aware environment for BVI people through multiple sensor nodes located around the building and a voice-controlled application. The following are the objectives for AmIE:

- Provide the user with details about their current location.
- Automated indoor navigation of the user.
- Voice controlled system using Arabic language.
- Direct the user to the nearest exit in case of emergency.
- Allow the user to place calls when necessary.
- Informs the user if there is emergency in the building.
- Informing the user about the weather conditions as they approach the exit.
- Inform the user about the room temperature when requested.
- Inform the user if there are people in the room they entered.

9.4   Amie System Development

This section focuses on representing the CRP diagram, explaining the different design alternatives and choices that were considered for AmIE, and an in-depth study of each design alternative is done to choose the most suitable one to implement. The advantages and disadvantages of the different hardware components of each design are explained to verify the appropriate choice based on the project requirements. After discussing each of the designs alternatives and deciding on the best one, an AOD is created to explain the system clearly. A UCD is provided to further clarify the chosen design. In addition, this section includes RCL and MAMs to articulate the non-functional requirements of AmIE. In addition, it includes information on the prototype developed and its budget.

AmIE is designed to provide an ambient intelligent environment that helps BVI people to navigate in unfamiliar indoor environments. AmIE also implements a context-aware environment that informs the BVI user on relevant information for the surrounding such as current room temperature, people availability in the room, emergency evacuation alert and displays their current location. Moreover, there are extra features that help integrating the BVI user more into the environment such as the phone call feature and the outside weather alert. The main form of interaction between the user and the system will be done through a user application that is connected to the system's control unit through the internet. Multiple sensor nodes will be distributed around the building to communicate environment-related information such as the location of the user, room temperature, and people availability in the room. These sensor nodes consist of microcontrollers, temperature sensors, proximity sensors, and wireless transceivers. A fast and multi-threaded control unit is needed such as the Raspberry pi alongside wireless transceivers to communicate with the sensor nodes. Furthermore, all the collected data will be uploaded to a webserver database to be used later. AmIE's CRP diagram in Fig. 9.1 shows the main concept of the system, the functionalities, and the technologies used.

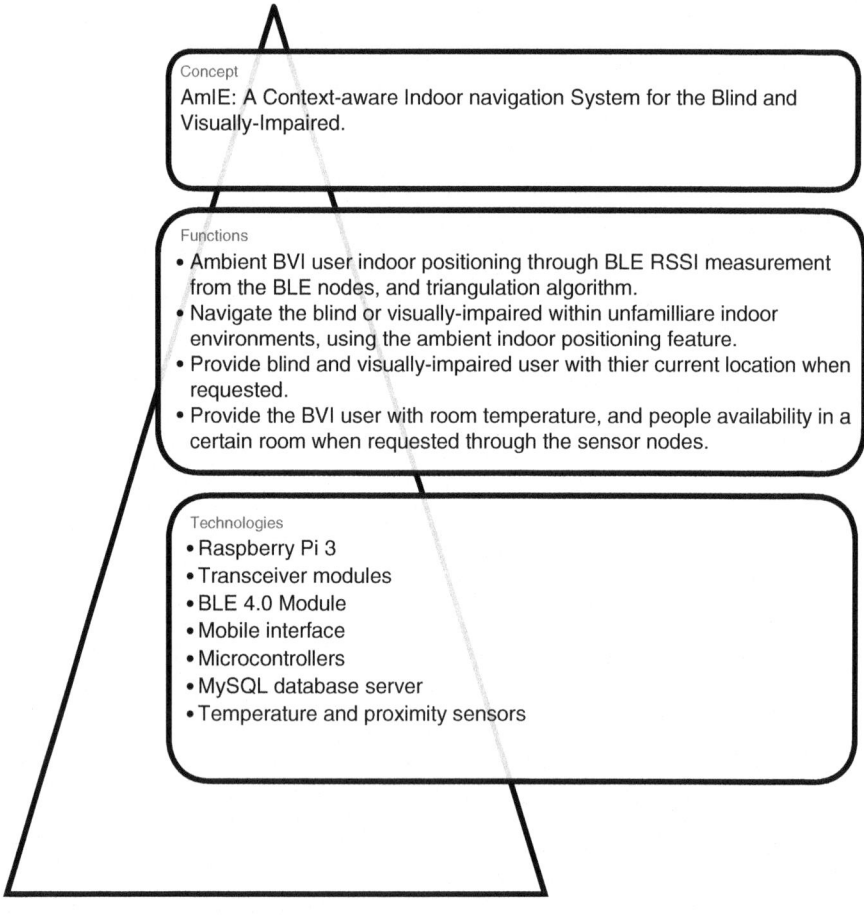

Fig. 9.1 Concept Refinement Pyramid (CRP) of AmIE

The proposed design for AmIE system consists of three main parts: the wearable device, sensor nodes, and a control unit. Different components were compared using the DT diagrams and the design chosen is the most suitable in terms of accessibility, cost efficiency, and quality. The wearable device is chosen to be the SONY SRW50 Android watch. The advantage of this specific watch is that it has Android Wear operating system which makes it programmable and it has open source developer option. Another advantage is that the watch supports google cloud, which allows access to its features such as google speech which has libraries that supports voice recognition in both English and Arabic languages.

The second part of the system contains the sensor nodes. A single node is composed using a sensor module, a microcontroller, and wireless communication module. There are two types of sensors used for the nodes: temperature sensor and motion sensor. The microcontroller used for the node is Arduino Nano microcontroller because it has a cheap and open source platform. As for the wireless communication, nodes communicate with the Raspberry Pi via Wi-Fi as it covers wide range with fast data rates.

The DT diagram shown in Fig. 9.2 is used to decide on the type of system-control unit to use. Raspberry Pi model 3 is the most suitable control unit for AmIE system because it has a fast processor and it already has embedded Wi-Fi standard. It also

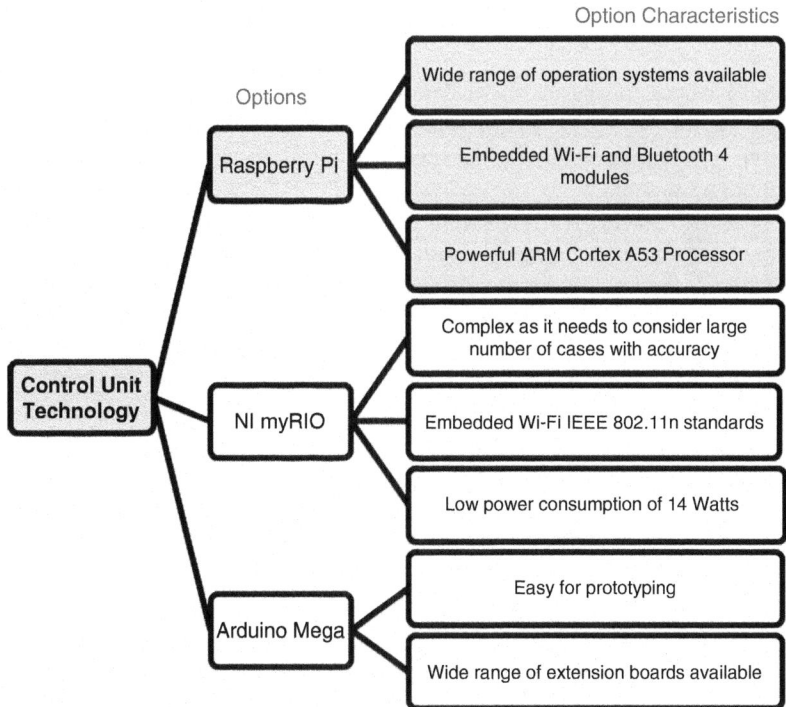

Fig. 9.2 AmIE Control Unit DT. The decision branch is highlighted

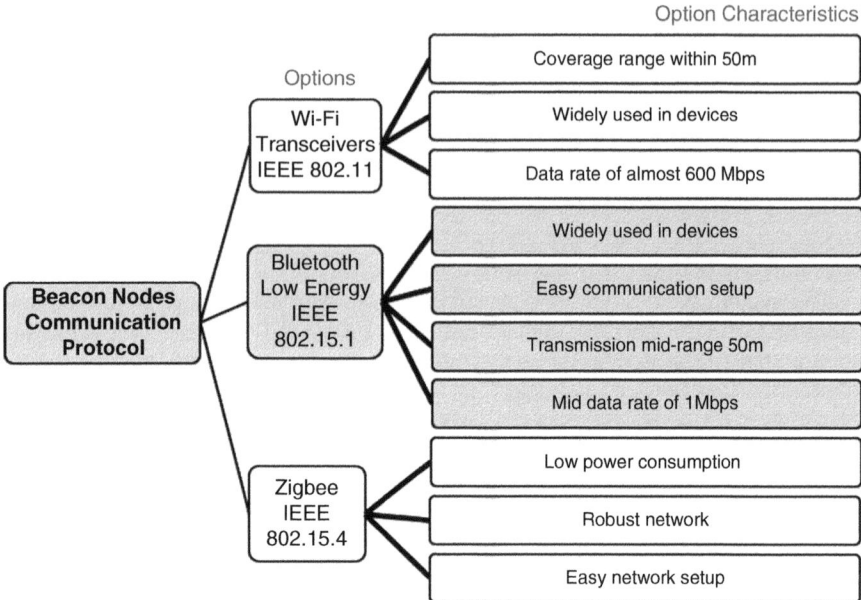

Fig. 9.3 AmIE Beacons Wireless Communication Protocol DT. The decision branch is high-lighted

has multiple operating systems where programs can be written in different languages and use multithreading to execute tasks concurrently for optimum performance. In addition, it communicates with the mobile application through the internet using socket programming.

As for the ambient intelligent features, these features are activated according to the user's request. The features include locating the user, navigating the user, and send emergence alerts to the user. The location of the user can be identified using the Received Signal Strength Indicator (RSSI) from wireless devices around the building (Wang, Yang, Zhao, Liu, & Cuthbert, 2013). Therefore, the DT diagram in Fig. 9.3 shows all three possible communication platforms: Wi-Fi, Bluetooth Low Energy (BLE), and Zigbee. The chosen protocol is the BLE of standard IEEE 802.15.1 because they are constantly sending signals with the lowest energy possible. In addition, BLE modules can communicate easily with current mobile devices as most have Bluetooth embed inside of it. Moreover, the signal produced from the BLE modules can approximate distance as the further the user is from the device the weaker the signal is and the smaller the RSSI value gets.

Location nodes must be placed in a way such that the maximum possible area is covered and provide a range for the RSSI readings below −90 dB as otherwise the readings are considered meaningless (Wang et al., 2013). Two possible placement strategies are represented in Fig. 9.4. The Point of Interest (POI) strategy depends on placing nodes at specific checkpoints such as room entrances, stairs, and elevators.

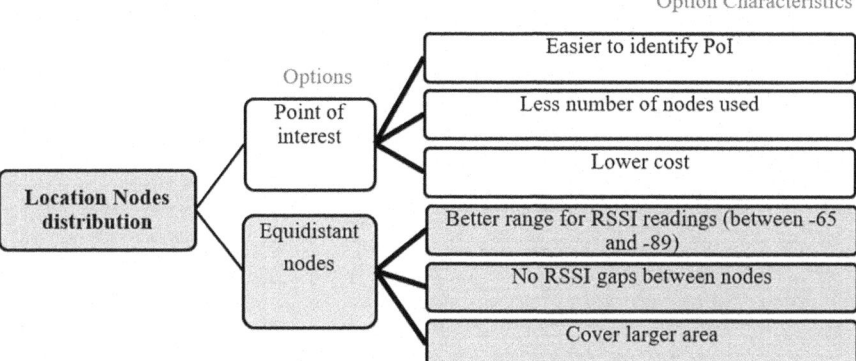

Fig. 9.4 AmIE Location Nodes distribution DT. The decision branch is highlighted

This strategy might be cost efficient, however in some locations there might be gaps between the nodes that cannot be covered. The system will not be able to identify the location of the user in these gaps. On the other hand, the equidistant approach ensures that there are no gaps between the nodes. In addition, some the RSSI readings are guaranteed to be below -90 dB which means that the location of the user relevant to the nodes can be identified. Since AmIE provides the users with their current location and navigation the Equidistant approach is more suitable.

The use-case diagram (UCD) for the AmIE system is shown in Fig. 9.5. It displays all the possible functions that the user can access and the possible exceptions that could occur from each function if there is an error or inaccurate information and such. Through voice commands the user can navigate through the building, provided that they have an accurate location and the destination they wish to reach exists. The BVI user can also make an emergency request which will be sent to the admin, and they can place calls and request the room temperature and the people availability in a room. As for the ambient intelligence features, these can be activated or deactivated by the user depending on if they want them or not. These include hearing details about the room they are approaching and getting information about the weather as they approach the exit. However, they cannot disable the building emergency feature for safety reasons. It also shows the admin who inherits from the user but can also view the location of the user if there is an accurate location displayed and receive emergency messages that the user sends. They also have access to the whole network unless there is no signal.

The Architecture and Organization Diagram (AOD) in Fig. 9.6 is based on the design decisions of AmIE discussed earlier. The control unit, Raspberry pi, communicates with the user's application through the internet, and with the sensor nodes through Wi-Fi transceivers. The user's application interacts with the user through the watch utilizing voice commands. Moreover, the application is constantly scanning for the nearby BLE devices to locate the user and communicates the user's requests through internet connection with the Raspberry pi.

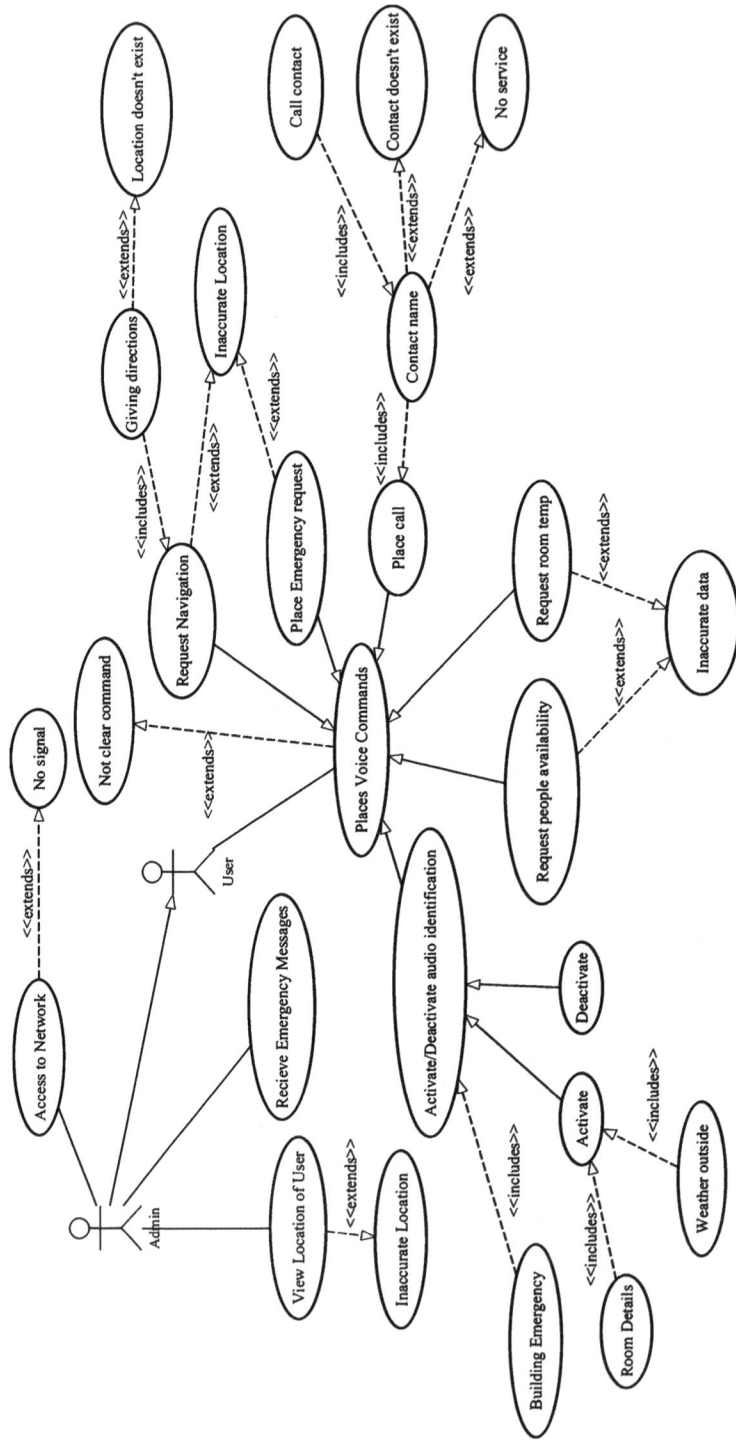

Fig. 9.5 AmIE Full Use Case Diagram (UCD)

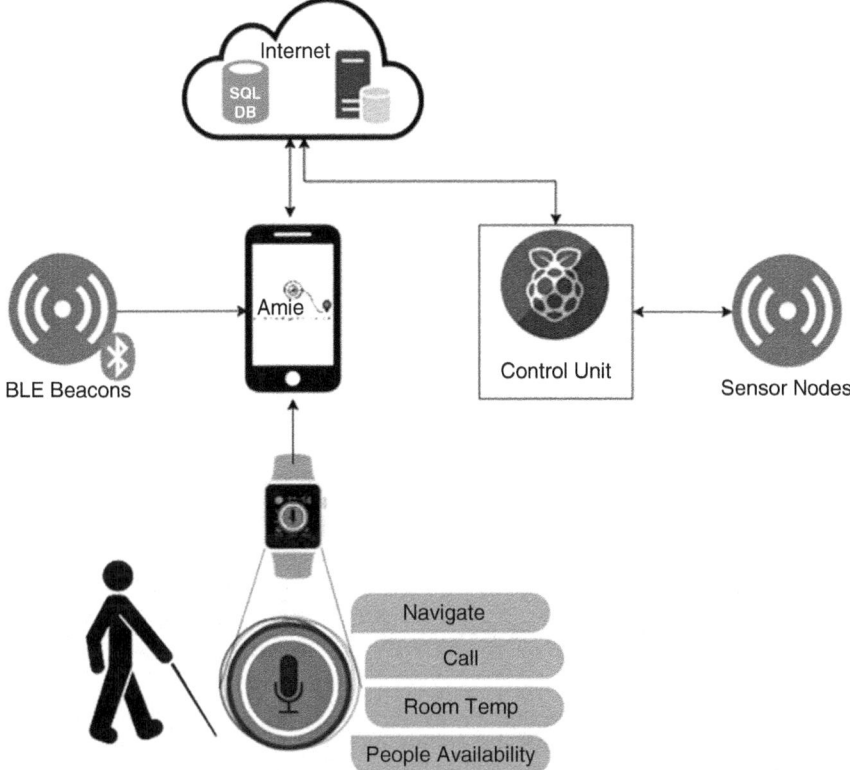

Fig. 9.6 AmIE Architecture and Organization Diagram (AOD)

9.5   Implementation Aspects

The proposed system was implanted and tested. The system implementation is divided into four main parts: the sensor nodes, the location nodes, the control unit, and the mobile application. This section discusses the system features in detail, the main procedures used to implement each system part and integration of the whole system.

9.5.1   Project Features

As discussed earlier there are seven system features which include the navigation request, location request, phone call request, room temperature request, people availability request, emergency request, and weather forecast request. All the system features are activated using voice commands from the user. AmIE implements the system using English and Arabic languages. Specific key words are used to activate each of the requests. The response contains audio messages respectively. The responses consist of either simple directions, the user's location, sensor data, or emergency warning.

The navigation feature is activated by the keyword "Navigate" followed by their requested destination. The user's current location and the requested destination are sent the control unit. The user's direction is determined by tracking the user.

The location request is initiated by the keyword "Location". The application sends the command to the Raspberry Pi along with the RSSI (Received Signal Strength Indication) of the location nodes. The Pi calculates the user's current location using location algorithm developed and represent it using Cartesian coordinates. According to these coordinates the user's location is identified and sent back to the application.

The phone call request is activated using Google API along with access to the user's contact list. This feature is simply initiated by the user when keyword "Call" followed by the desired contact name. The speech recognizer embedded in the smart watch will process the necessary commands and initiates a call via smartphone connection.

The room temperature and the people availability requests are activated when the user uses the keywords "room temperature" or "check for people". The request is sent to the control unit and the control unit retrieves the data from the sensor nodes distributed around the room. Each room consists of one temperature sensor and four motion sensors.

There are two implementations for the emergency request. The first implementation requires the user to utilize the keyword "Help", this will activate the calling feature and it will call a saved number (security number) in case the user needed some immediate help. The second implementation is used when there is emergency in the building. The current location of the user is identified, and the user will be navigated to the nearest exit identified by the system.

The weather forecast notification is available when the user is exiting the building. The user's phone will detect the node that is next to the building door and it will automatically fetch the weather information from the "openweathermap" web API. The desired information is retrieved from the web API which are the temperature and the weather description. That information is then conveyed to the user through text to speech features.

9.5.2 Nodes Implementation

There are two types of nodes in the system, these are the sensor nodes and location nodes. The sensor nodes are responsible for collecting environment-related information such as the room temperature and detect motion in the room. On the other side, the location nodes detect the location of the user through the RSSI of the distributed devices from the user.

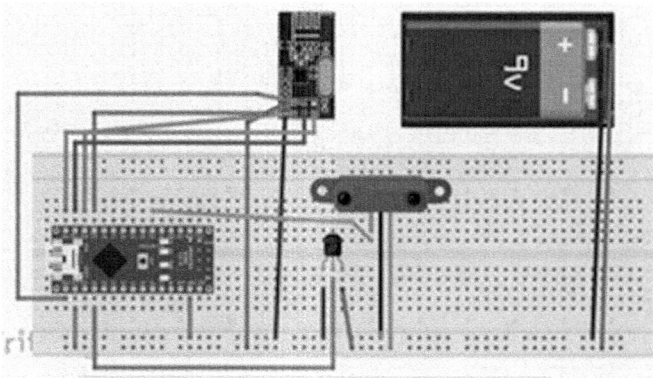

Fig. 9.7 Sensor Node Circuit Schematic

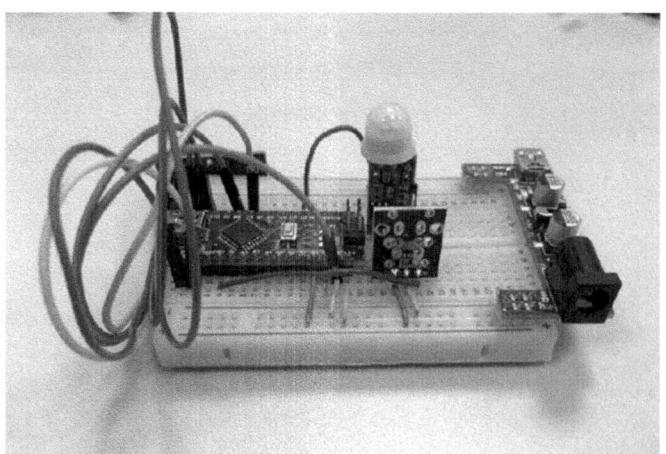

Fig. 9.8 Sensor Node Circuit

According to the design decisions the sensor nodes are implemented using Arduino Nano, analog temperature sensor, motion sensor, and nrf24l transceiver. Each room consists of four sensor nodes placed on the corners of the room. Only one temperature sensor is used per room. The connections of the components are shown in Figs. 9.7, 9.8, and 9.9.

Location Nodes use BLE (Bluetooth Low Energy) as per the design decisions to track the user's location in the building. The module follows the IEEE 802.15.1 standards. Using the signal emitted from each BLE module it is possible to track the location of the user through measuring the RSSI of the Bluetooth signal using the created mobile application. Figure 9.10 shows the location nodes. The testing area is in the American University of Kuwait B building first floor engineering corridor. Since the Equidistant approach is the chosen distribution method six nodes are used to cover the area, a set of three nodes would form a triangle to increase the accuracy

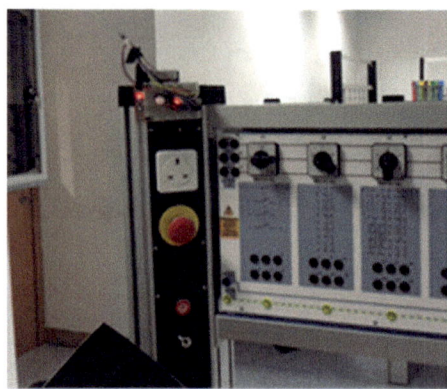
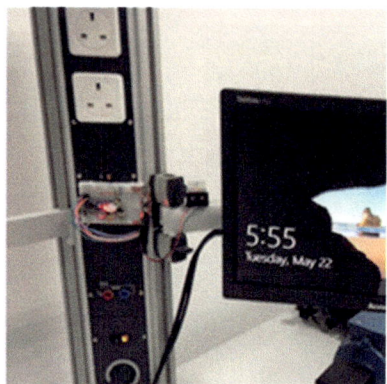

Fig. 9.9 Sensor Node placement

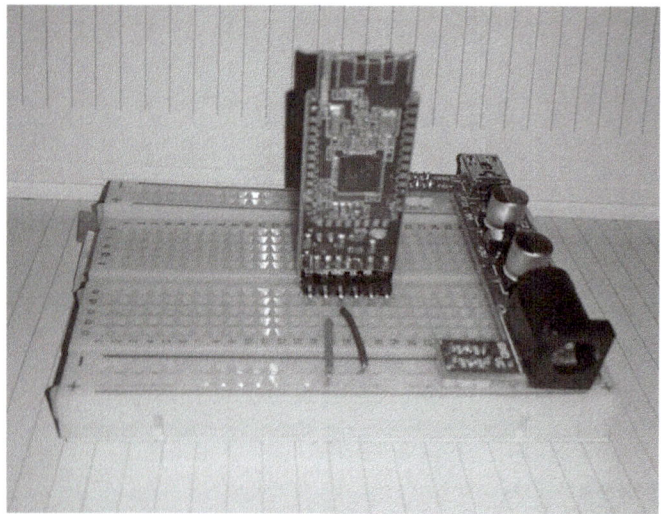

Fig. 9.10 Location Node Circuit Connection

of the results. The nodes were set on Cartesian coordinates where the first node was located at the origin and the axis were aligned according to its position. The nodes were placed at 2.5 units away in terms of the x-axis, and 5 units apart in terms of the y-axis. Figure 9.11 shows the map and the nodes placement:

9.5.3 Distance Measurement and Algorithms

To identify the location the RSSI was measured from each location node to calculate the distance between the user and these nodes and then identify where

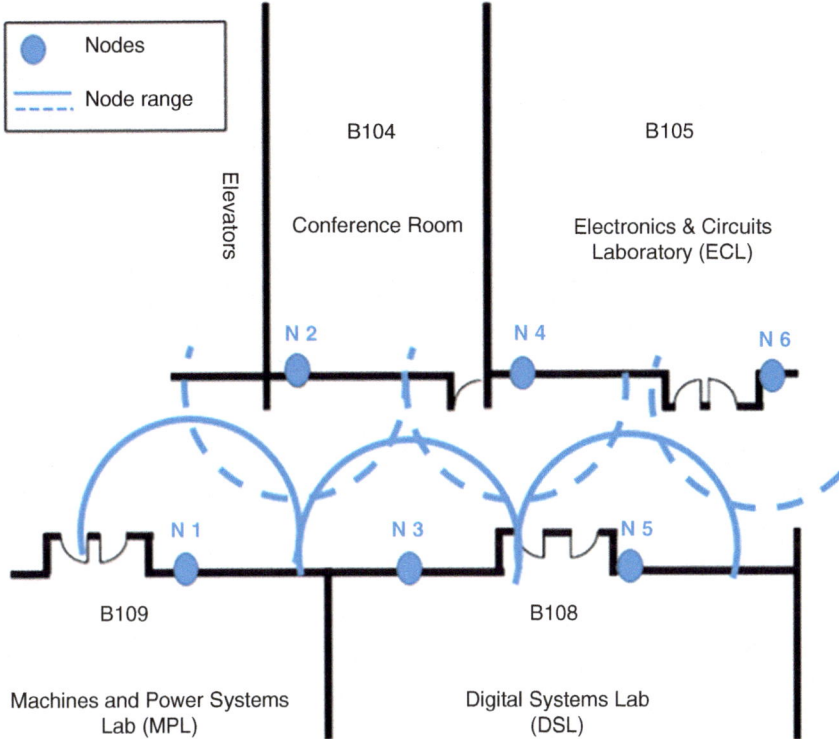

Fig. 9.11 Approximate locations of nodes in a university building of several laboratories and conference room

exactly the user is located. Calculating distance according to the Received Signal Strength (RSS) is a method that is based on the characteristics of radio waves progression with change in distance. The RSS indicates the power level between the transmitter (BLE device) and the receiver (user), it is measured in dB and gets more negative as the user moves further from the nodes. The location of the user can be estimated using positioning through Bluetooth RSSI and triangulation methods. To calculate the distance, an equation is created that represents a function of the RSSI. This equation was created from multiple tests of specific distances with their corresponding RSSIs from the BLE nodes and from multiple directions. The RSSIs were measured from distances of 0.5, 1.0, 1.5, 2.0, 2.5, and 3.0 m. Multiple readings were taken at the same distance to calculate the average and minimize the error. Interpolation of the results was done using MATLAB along with the curve fitting function interp1(..) to find the distance equation. The following equation shows the distance equation.

$$D(x) = \left(-31 \times 10^{-5}\right) x^3 - \left(73 \times 10^{-2}\right) x^2 - 150 \tag{9.1}$$

After calculating the distance from each node, the location algorithm will identify the position of the user in terms of Cartesian coordinates and map it with respect to the nodes. The application will measure all RSSIs from all nodes. Only the closest three nodes to the user are considered in the calculations to have better prediction of the location and eliminate possible errors. The closest three nodes have the lowest RSSI values. The nearest three nodes must be nodes that are close to each other to reduce reading errors. Otherwise the closest two nodes are considered. The distances between the user and these three nodes are calculated using the equation discussed earlier. The assumption that the signals produced from the BLE forms a circular shape for simplicity is used. Therefore, the calculated distances are the radiuses of the circles that represent possible location of the user. The average of the circle intersections is considered the position of the user. Algorithm 9.1 is used to construct circular shapes around each of the nearest nodes assuming that this shape represents the range in which the user exists. The average of the circles intersections is the approximated location of the user. Equation (9.2) shows the average intersections equation. The average point is then represented on a graph representing the closest three nodes, the intersection points and the approximated location of the user relative to the testing area.

Algorithm 9.1 NodesIntersection (nearestRssi[0.. n-1], distances[0.. n-1], centers[(0,0)...]){
// NodesIntersection constructs circles around the nearest nodes and finds the average of the intersection points
//INPUT nearestRssi[] array containing the nearest 3 nodes, distances[] array containing the distances between the user and the nodes, centers[] array containing the location of the nodes
//OUTPUT location point containing the user's coordinates
    Circle circles= [];
    for m=1:nearestRssi.length
        circles[m]= new Circle (centers[m], distances[m]);
    end
    intersections= circleIntersection(circles);
    location = Mean(intersections);
return location;

$$\text{avgPoint} = \frac{\sum_{n=0}^{i} \text{intersections}}{\text{Number of points}} \tag{9.2}$$

Since the user needs simple directions and the testing area is a corridor a set of simple preset directions is used in the navigation algorithm. Initially the current location of the user and the destination are taken from the user's application. The direction of the user is predicted from tracking the user and comparing the X coordinate of the previous location and the current location. There are specific points on the graph that are marked as destination points. There are four directions used, which are Forward, Backward, Right, and Left. The user is asked to move forward or backward every 2.5 units in the graph and depending on the direction of the user. Once the user is in the correct X coordinate range the user is then asked to move either left or right depending on the position of the destination. Once the direction is identified Algorithm 9.2 is executed to develop the directions needed for the user to reach his/her destination point.

Algorithm 9.2 Navigate (currentLocation, distinationPoint, isForward){
// Navigate provide directions to the user to reach their distination
//INPUT currentLocation point, distinationPoint point, isForward boolean
//OUTPUT String of directions
    directions=""
    While (currentLocation.x != destinationPoint.x):
        If (isForward):
            nextLocation= Point (currentLocation.x +2.5, current-Location.y)
      directions = directions + 'Forward'
        else If (!isForward):
            nextLocation= Point (currentLocation.x -2.5, current-Location.y)
            directions = directions + "Backward'
      While (currentLocation.y != destinationPoint.y):
        If (isForward):
            nextLocation= Point (currentLocation.x, currentLoca-tion.y+2.5)
      directions = directions + "Left'
        else If (!isForward):
            nextLocation= Point (currentLocation.x, currentLoca-tion.y-2.5)
            directions = directions + "Right'
return directions;

9.5.4 Control Unit Communication with Sensor Nodes

The nodes communicate using Wi-Fi transceivers NRFL24L01 modules and send to the raspberry pi through the same channel but one after the other to avoid interference and data loss. Figure 9.12 shows the raspberry pi full connections.

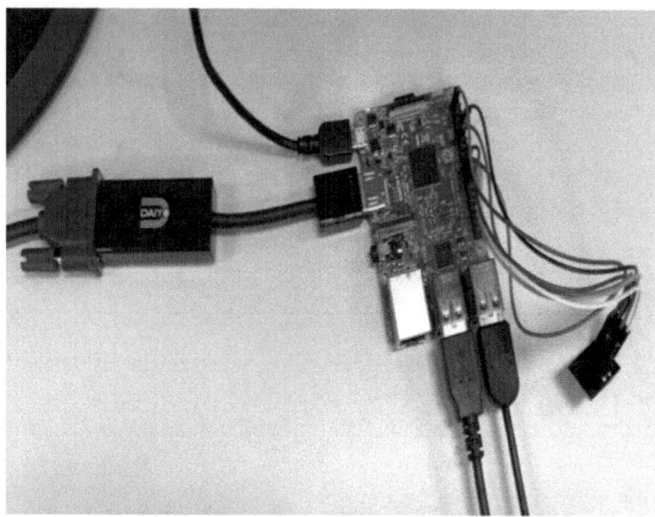

Fig. 9.12 Raspberry pi full connection with NRFL24L01 module

The raspberry pi sends messages to the sensor nodes; however, each sensor node responds only to specific messages. All nodes will receive the message and manage to decode it. Only one sensor node replies if the message fits the commands that the node should reply to. Finally, the Pi receives the data, decode it and send an ACK back to that node. This data gets stored in a database for later use.

9.5.5   Control Unit Communication with Mobile Application

For the pi communication with the mobile phone TCP communication protocol is used and this is achieved through socket programming which involves server-client communication. In this system the mobile device sends either requests or the RSSI readings of the location nodes to the pi. In return, the pi replies according to the request through a new socket. Therefore, the communication is two sided. In case of the pi receiving requests, it acts as the server and the mobile device as the client. However, in case of the pi sending the requests the mobile device acts as the server and the pi as client. The used sockets are then closed and re-opened for new communication. For this communication to be successful both devices must be on the same network and the requests sent in between must be the same to identify the function. The keywords are case sensitive, and they must match in both the application and pi.

9.5.6   Mobile Application Development

Voice recognition is the main input to AmIE. An Android Wear application was created using Android studio 3.0 to receive commands in English and display them on the screen. To implement voice commands, android voice recognizer SDK is used such that if the code received from the user's voice note matches the request code this means that a word was recognized (Android Developers, 2017). For example, when the user wants to identify his/her location the keywords "my location" must be used, and the response is an audio message that specifies his/her location according to the nearest point of interest. The audio message that the user receives as a response to their requests is done by playing pre-recorded messages and instructions both in English and Arabic, rather than using Google Speech response to avoid delay.

For the mobile device to measure the BLE RSSI, a background thread is created to scan for devices and measure the signal strength. The HMsoft BLE nodes appear on the application in order based on the number of nodes that are previously assigned. The measured RSSIs, then, is sent to the Raspberry Pi where it is processed. Figure 9.13 shows the interface of the testing application representing all the RSSI readings of the BLE modules, and Fig. 9.14 shows the user-interface of the application.

Fig. 9.13 The testing application interface

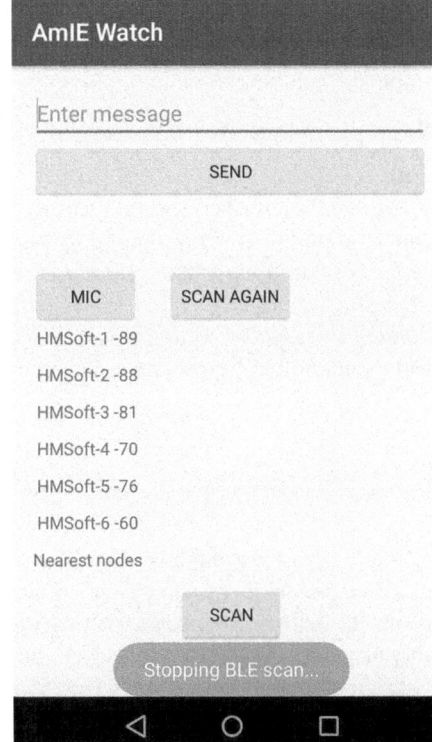

Fig. 9.14 The user-interface
on the watch

9.6 Analysis and Evaluation

The evaluation of the proposed AmIE system considers the aims, implementation, and advantages of the proposed system. In addition, the system effectiveness is evaluated based on small-scale measurements study. Moreover, the system's real-life testing is carried on blind-folded participants and the results are discussed in this section. Finally, the section is concluded by presenting the limitations, challenges, and the identified opportunities for future work.

9.6.1 System Testing and Results

Multiple tests were conducted by blind-folded participants to mimic the situation of the BVI person using the system. Before tests were conducted participants were given the list of commands needed to activate the functionalities of the system shown in Table 9.1. Participants were bilingual therefore they tested the system with both English and Arabic languages. All system functionalities were tested during

Table 9.1 Requests performed by visually impaired people to test AmIE

English request	Arabic request
Navigate...	توجه إلى
My location	مكاني
Get room temperature	درجة الحراره
Check for people	في ناس
Call...	اتصل ب
Request help	المساعده
Get weather	الطقس الان

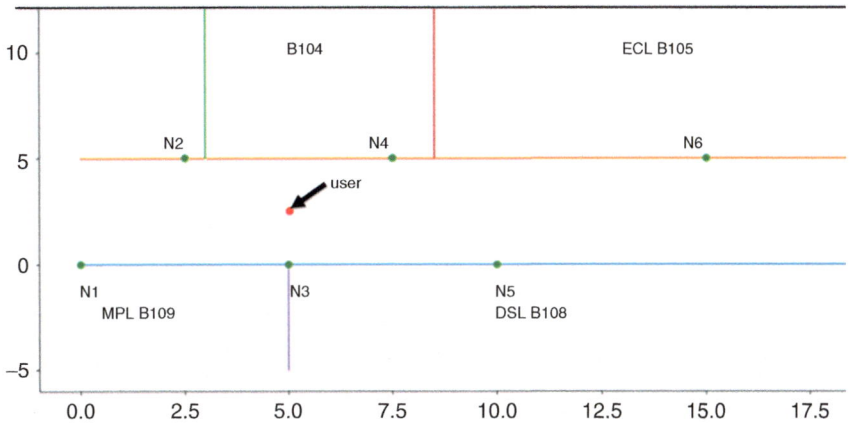

Fig. 9.15 Raspberry Pi screen output of user's location during emergency evacuation

a normal university day and the testing area was in the American University of Kuwait, Liberal Arts Building first floor. Testing of the system showed that it works perfectly and achieves all of the required function. The testing consisted of three parts, which are the location and navigation, sensor node, and the mobile application features.

Participants were asked to move to random locations on the map and request their current location. The result of this test showed that the system managed to identify the closest nodes to the user and display the name of the closest room. In addition, the exact location of the user was displayed on the screen connected to the Raspberry pi as shown in Fig. 9.15. Participants then tested the navigation feature by requesting navigation to one of the saved locations in the system such as Digital Systems Lab and Electric Circuits Lab. The direction of the user was identified from his/her previous changes in locations. The positive change represented facing forward (+ve x axis) and the negative change represented facing backward (−ve x axis). The navigation result was represented as set of directions displayed to the user in audio, an example is shown in Table 9.2. The directions were clear and allowed the user to reach the destination without assistance. The system identified that the user reached the destination by calculating the location and comparing the

Table 9.2 Response to the navigation request

Request	Responses	
	English response	Arabic response
Navigate Digital Lab	Move Forward	تحرك الى الامام
	Move Forward	تحرك الى الامام
	Move Forward	تحرك الى الامام
	Turn Left	تحرك الى اليسار
	You have reached your destination	لقد وصلت الى المكان المطلوب

results with the saved location of that destination. To test the system's emergency evacuation, feature the last node (node 6) was set as the exit node and the emergency evacuation was activated manually for testing. The participants were informed that emergency evacuation will start and were navigated to the exit node regardless of their location.

Participants tested the results of the sensor nodes where they were in the testing room. When room temperature and people availability were requested the system replied quickly with the needed data. However, the people availability function was not accurate in times when there were people in the room but not moving. The participants reported that identifying people availability helped them in understanding the surrounding more and avoid accord situations. In addition, they stated that knowing the room temperature would help in case they wanted to adjust it.

The mobile application features such as calling, outdoor weather, and help request were tested by the participants. The calling option worked as expected when calling numbers that are already in the contact list. The weather option requires the user to activate their location through google services to get the weather of the city that the user. The data that was displayed to the user were the outside weather temperature and the weather description. The help request is placed by the user where the number of the security of the building is called and the location of the user is displayed on the Raspberry pi screen.

9.6.2 System Effectiveness and Evaluation

To analyze and evaluate AmIE's effectiveness the Menu of Analysis Metrics (MAMs) of AmIE shown in Fig. 9.16 shows the non-functional requirement of general IoT system as well as specific requirements regarding AmIE. The system was evaluated based on the user friendliness, system performance, and accuracy of the location.

User friendliness is measured by the ease of use of the system by the user while considering the situation of the BVI person. This includes the simplicity of user interface design and the response to the user's requests. The application is designed

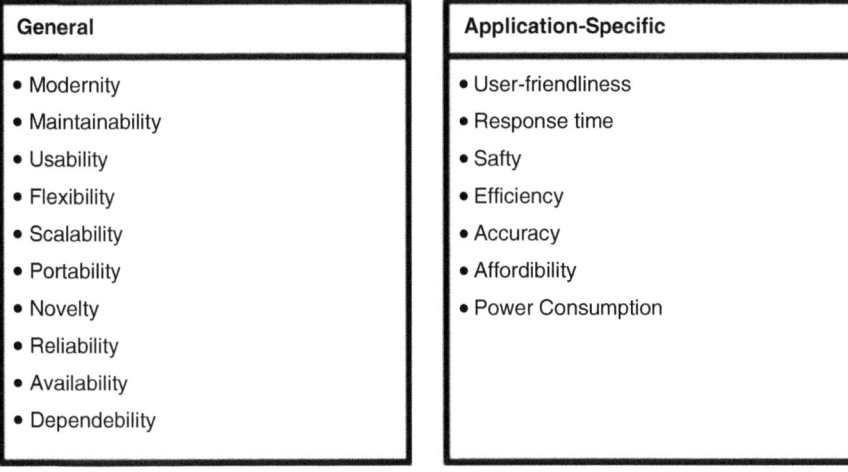

General	Application-Specific
• Modernity	• User-friendliness
• Maintainability	• Response time
• Usability	• Safty
• Flexibility	• Efficiency
• Scalability	• Accuracy
• Portability	• Affordibility
• Novelty	• Power Consumption
• Reliability	
• Availability	
• Dependebility	

Fig. 9.16 Menu of Analysis Metrics (MAM) of AmIE

in a simplified way such that all the user needs is one press on a huge button covering most of the screen to place a request. The responses to the user are in clear simple words in both English and Arabic languages. The responses are recorded to eliminate the delay that happened when Google text-to-speech services were used. Since the responses are recorded, the Arabic responses are in the Kuwaiti accent making it easier for locals of Kuwait to follow it.

Performance is measured by the response time from the user command to the result the system provides. The result should be a correct and delivered to the user in a short amount of time for the system's performance to be suitable. In terms of communication between the pi and the mobile application the performance is quite fast and real-time because it uses wireless communication through the internet. However, some functions such as location and navigation take longer because of the extensive calculations involved. The average response time for the location feature is around 7 s after the request is sent. However, since it is less than 10 s it is still considered as a real-time system. The performance of the mobile application features such as the calling and placing an emergency request, as well as the sensor nodes requests were all fast in response time. However, the weather feature depends on the internet connection; the faster the connection the shorter the response time is.

Accuracy is measured by having more than 30 tests conducted to assess the error percentage of the user's positioning. To measure the accuracy of the positioning algorithm, the error between the user's actual location and measured location is calculated by Eq. 9.3. The average of the errors showed error of $\pm 11.6\%$ in the x axis and $\pm 14.7\%$ in the y axis, which means that the system has accuracy of almost 85% in approximating the location of the user. Despite this, this result can be affected by the nearby Bluetooth devices due to interference. The sensor nodes were quite accurate, but the motion sensors did not detect people who were very far from them. The weather feature collected data from web API therefore the data are accurate and updated regularly. Accuracy of the system's emergency evacuation depends highly on the accuracy of the system's location and navigation algorithms.

$$\text{Error} \% = \frac{\text{Actual position} - \text{Calculated position}}{\text{Actual position}} * 100 \qquad (9.3)$$

In terms of system affordability, AmIE is cheap for the BVI users as all they need are either an android smart watch or phone to download the application, and a headset for clearer responses. In the tested prototype the cost of the system was almost $830, therefore for large buildings to implement AmIE the cost will be high as more nodes are needed.

9.6.3 Closely Related Work

One way to evaluate our system is to compare it with similar systems. In a paper by Cheragh et al. GuideBeacon system is discussed that navigates BVI people indoors using BLE technology (Cheraghi, Namboodiri, & Walker, 2017). The system is designed for a multi-layer indoor area and multiple BLE nodes were distributes in the area to identify the location of the user using the RSSI values received from these nodes. One of the similarities is that both systems rely on speech recognition APIs through Android-based application and audio messages as a way to respond back to the user. In addition, both systems rely on six BLE devices to identify the location of the user through the value of the RSSI measured using the Android application. Despite the similarities, the testing area for AmIE was a hallway, however the testing area for GuidBeacon is a two-layered map. Smaller distance between devices in AmIE might result in higher interference than BLE devices in GuidBeacon thus reduce their effectiveness. Furthermore, the placement of BLE devices in AmIE followed the Equidistant approach, but the GuidBeacon followed the POI approach such that devices are placed on doors, windows, etc. to facilitate identification of the location. In addition, mobile phone compass was used to identify the user direction and they stated that it is sometimes off and needs calibration. However, AmIE keeps track of the user to predict his direction and no calibration is needed. Finally, the calculation of the user's location in GuideBeacon depends on a weighted graph that represents the distances between different BLE devices. AmIE on the other side considers the closest three nodes and constructs circles using the RSSI readings to identify the location of the user by the average intersection point. Both ways work perfectly as indoor positioning algorithms. However, a major difference is that AmIE provides the user with multiple features that increase awareness of BVI people and the surrounding through sensor readings, emergency alerts, and weather functionality.

To assess accuracy of the location algorithm, AmIE is compared with the system proposed by Adam Satan and Zsolt Toth (Satan & Toth, 2018). They present a Bluetooth-based indoor positioning mobile application, specifically designed for offices to notify the users of the nearby offices. The approach is based on RSSI measurement to estimate the user's distance from the Bluetooth beacons. Their application "maps" or associates the beacons to specific rooms, allowing it to specify the closest rooms to the user. User's location is identified using Log-distance Path Loss Model based on the averages of RSSI values. The estimated position is used to acquire the nearest rooms from the database accordingly. The steps of the algorithm are very similar in AmIE. However, AmIE does not take into consideration the height of the Bluetooth beacon as this system does. In addition, AmIE's mathematical model that relates the RSSI values to the user's distance from the nodes is generated through Interpolation using Matlab, whereas this system uses the Log-distance Path Loss Model. Similar to AmIE, the system was tested through a 29 m hallway making the comparison between both system accuracy fair. The system produced an accuracy percentage of 88%. On the other hand, AmIE was capable to locate the user within accuracy percentage of 85%, the difference between both accuracies is small especially that the user's exact location can be estimated correctly. In addition, the extra ambient intelligent and context-aware features allow AmIE to be used by BVI user and help them in interacting with the surrounding. Therefore, AmIE provides a very good and functioning platform for BVI people indoors. This shows that the location algorithm has great potential alongside improving it in the future.

9.6.4   Limitations and Future Work

After various testing and evaluations of the system, some limitations appeared in the process of designing and implementation of the system however they were overcome by applying appropriate solutions. One of the limitations faced was regarding the sensor nodes, as their range was not enough to cover the whole room so more than one sensor node had to be used in a single room to measure the people availability. This is still slightly limited as the range of each sensor node is not very large, but this can be solved by using bigger antennas later. Another limitation is that at times the speech recognition can be inaccurate, and other than that there is sometimes wireless connection attenuation which will cause the whole system to stop working. The wireless network used did not allow static IP addresses, so a dynamic address had to be used although it kept changing. Moreover, the realistic constraints of AmIE are presented in the RCL diagram in Fig. 9.17 which are refinements of the non-functional requirements of the system.

As for future work, AmIE will be tested with real BVI people instead of a blind-folded person by co-operating with Kuwait Association for the Blind for them to provide willing BVI people who would test the system. Since the current testing area was a simple hallway more testing will be conducted in complex areas with

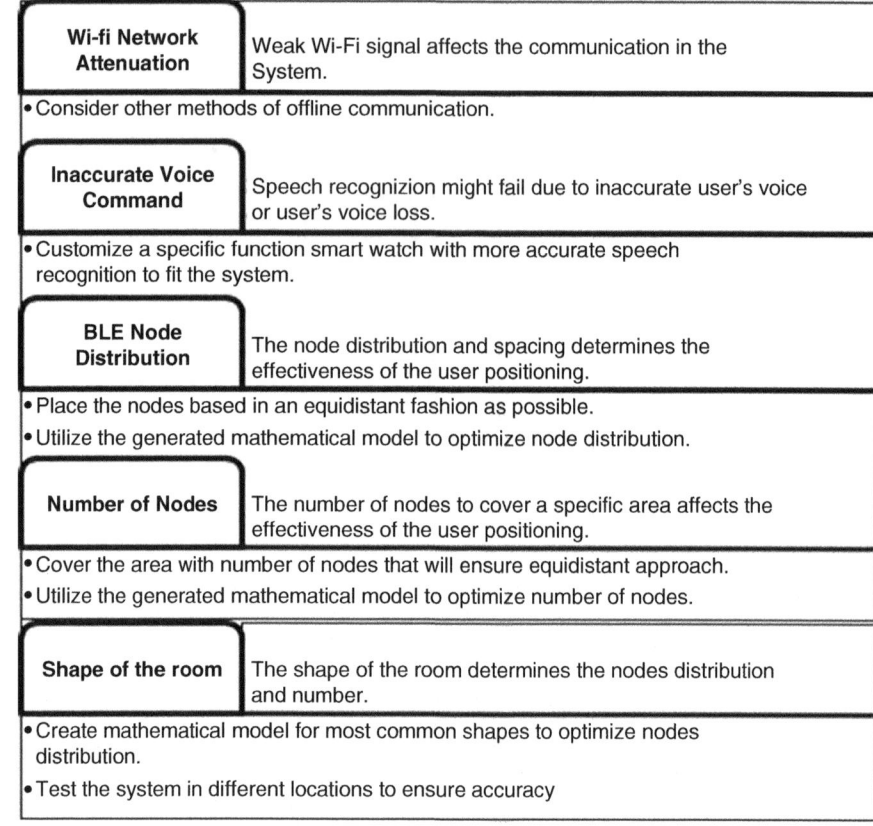

Wi-fi Network Attenuation	Weak Wi-Fi signal affects the communication in the System.
• Consider other methods of offline communication.	
Inaccurate Voice Command	Speech recognizion might fail due to inaccurate user's voice or user's voice loss.
• Customize a specific function smart watch with more accurate speech recognition to fit the system.	
BLE Node Distribution	The node distribution and spacing determines the effectiveness of the user positioning.
• Place the nodes based in an equidistant fashion as possible.	
• Utilize the generated mathematical model to optimize node distribution.	
Number of Nodes	The number of nodes to cover a specific area affects the effectiveness of the user positioning.
• Cover the area with number of nodes that will ensure equidistant approach.	
• Utilize the generated mathematical model to optimize number of nodes.	
Shape of the room	The shape of the room determines the nodes distribution and number.
• Create mathematical model for most common shapes to optimize nodes distribution.	
• Test the system in different locations to ensure accuracy	

Fig. 9.17 Realistic Constraints List (RCL) of AmIE

different sizes and shapes. In addition, different navigation routes and algorithms will be exploited in the future to ensure optimal results for the BVI user. Testing the system's accuracy by varying the numbers of the location nodes is also a direction that we wish to explore more.

9.7 Conclusion

The development of an ambient intelligence and context-aware system, such as AmIE, is critical especially when it comes to assisting BVI people to become more integrated in the society. The system uses multiple nodes that are distributed around the building to assist and provide the user with relevant information about their surroundings. The sensor nodes are used to collect environment-related data and the location nodes facilitate the indoor positioning of the user. Furthermore, the system communicates with the user via voice commands in both English and Arabic languages received through the smart watch. In addition, the responses to the user's requests are audio messages that are played relative to the request. In comparison with similar work AmIE is effective and accurate in positioning the user and replying to their requests. Future work includes evaluating the system in more complex areas with different shapes to improve its accuracy and testing with actual blind and visually impaired people.

References

Abdullah, A., Enazi, S. A., & Damaj, I. (2016). AgriSys: A smart and ubiquitous controlled-environment agriculture system. In *Third MEC International Conference on Big Data and Smart City (ICBDSC), Muscat* (pp. 1–6). Washington, DC: IEEE.

Abu Doush, I., Alshatnawi, S., Al-Tamimi, A., Alhasan, B., & Hamasha, S. (2016). ISAB: Integrated indoor navigation system for the blind. *Interacting with Computers, 29*(2), 181–202.

Aladren, A., Lopez-Nicolas, G., Puig, L., & Guerrero, J. J. (2016). Navigation assistance for the visually impaired using RGB-D sensor with range expansion. *IEEE Systems Journal, 10*, 922–932.

Al-Chalabi, A., Shahzad, H., Essa, S., & Damaj, I. (2015). A weaable an ubiquitous NFC wallet. In *The IEEE Canadian Conference on Electrical and Computer Engineering (CCECE)*, Halifax, Nova Scotia (pp. 152–157).

Al-Fadhli, J., Ashkanani, M., Yousef, A., Damaj, I., & El-Shafei, M. (2014). RECON: A re-motely controlled drone for roads safety. In *International Conference on Connected Vehicles and Expo (ICCVE)*. Vienna (pp. 912–918).

Android Developers. (2017, December 12). Retrieved from Android: https://developer.android.com/reference/android/speech/SpeechRecognizer.html.

Angin, P., & Bhargava, B. K. (2011). Real-time mobile-cloud computing for context-aware blind navigation. *International Journal of Next-Generation Computing, 2*(2), 405–414.

Cheraghi, S. A., Namboodiri, V., & Walker, L. (2017). GuideBeacon: Beacon-based indoor wayfinding for the blind, visually impaired, and disoriented. In *IEEE International Conference on Pervasive Computing and Communications (PerCom)*, Kona, HI (pp. 121–130).

Damaj, I., & Kasbah, S. (2019). Integrated mobile solutions in an internet-of-things development. In S. Paiva (Ed.), *Mobile solutions and their usefulness in everyday life* (pp. 3–31). Netherlands: Springer.

Domingo, M. (2012). An overview of the Internet of Things for people with disabilities. *Journal of Network and Computer Applications, 35*(2), 584–596.

Dunai, L., Garcia, B. D., Lengua, I., & Peris-Fajarnés, G. (2012). 3D CMOS sensor based acoustic object detection and navigation system for blind people. In *The 38th Annual Conference on IEEE Industrial Electronics Society (IECON 2012)*, Montreal (pp. 25–28).

El-Shafei, M., Al Shalati, A., Rehayel, M., & Damaj, I. (2014). HOBOT: A customizable home management system with a surveillance RoBOT. In *IEEE 27th Canadian Conference on Electrical and Computer Engineering (CCECE)*, Toronto (pp. 1–7).

Hudec, M., & Smutny, Z. (2017). RUDO: A home ambient intelligence system for blind people. *Sensors, 17*(8), 1–45.

Pereira, A., Nunes, N., Vieira, D., Costa, N., Fernandes, H., & Barroso, J. (2015). An ultrasound sensor-based body area network for guiding blind people. *Procedia Computer Science, 67*, 403–408.

Prudhvi, B. R., & Bagani, R. (2013). Silicon eyes: GPS-GSM based navigation assistant for visually impaired using capacitive touch braille keypad and smart SMS facility. In *The 2013 World Congress on Computer and Information Technology (WCCIT)*, Sousse (pp. 22–24).

Raad, O., Makdessi, M., Mohamad, Y., & Damaj, I. (2018). SysMART indoor services: A system of connected and smart supermarkets. In *The 31st Canadian Conference on Electrical and Computer Engineering*, Quebec City (pp. 1–6).

Satan, A., & Toth, Z. (2018). Development of Bluetooth based indoor positioning application. In *IEEE International Conference on Future IoT Technologies (Future IoT)*, Eger (pp. 1–6).

Wafa, E., & Elleithy, K. (2017). Sensor-based assistive devices for visually-impaired people: Current status, challenges, and future directions. *Sensors, 17*, 565.

Wang, Y., Yang, X., Zhao, Y., Liu, Y., & Cuthbert, L. (2013). Bluetooth positioning using RSSI and triangulation methods. In *IEEE 10th Consumer Communications and Networking Conference (CCNC)*, Las Vegas (pp. 837–842.).

World Health Organization. (2018, December). Retrieved from World Health Organization: http://www.who.int/mediacentre/factsheets/fs282/en/.

Zhu, C., & Sheng, W. (2011). Wearable sensor-based hand gesture and daily activity recognition for robot-assisted living. *IEEE Transactions on Systems, Man, and Cybernetics – Part A: Systems and Humans, 41*, 569–573.

Chapter 10
Digital Enhancement of Cultural Experience and Accessibility for the Visually Impaired

Dimitris K. Iakovidis, Dimitrios Diamantis, George Dimas, Charis Ntakolia, and Evaggelos Spyrou

10.1 Introduction

Today, approximately 16% of the world's population lives with some form of visual impairment (WHO, 2018). Individuals with low or total absence of vision have to deal with various daily problems, struggling to fit in the modern way and rhythm of life. To address this important issue, researchers in the fields of medicine, smart electronics, computer science and engineering are joining their forces to develop assistive systems for the visually impaired individuals. To date, as a result of this effort, several designs and components of wearable camera-enabled systems for the visually impaired have been proposed.

A survey of relevant systems proposed until 2008 has been presented in Zhang, Ong, and Nee (2008). It identifies three categories of navigation systems: (a) based on positioning systems, including Global Positioning System (GPS) for outdoor positioning, and pre-installed pilots and beacons emitting signals, e.g., radiofrequency, infrared (IR), ultrasonic, etc., to determine the absolute position of the user in a local structured environment, (b) based on Radiofrequency Identification (RFID) tags with contextual information, such as surrounding landmarks, turning points; and vision-based systems exploiting the information acquired from digital cameras. In a more recent study performed in the beginning of 2017 (Elmannai

D. K. Iakovidis (✉) · D. Diamantis · G. Dimas · C. Ntakolia
Department of Computer Science and Biomedical Informatics, University of Thessaly, Lamia, Greece
e-mail: diakovidis@uth.gr; didiamantis@uth.gr; gdimas@uth.gr; cntakolia@uth.gr

E. Spyrou
Institute of Informatics and Telecommunications, National Center for Scientific Research "DEMOKRITOS", Athens, Greece
e-mail: espyrou@iit.demokritos.gr

© Springer Nature Switzerland AG 2020
S. Paiva (ed.), *Technological Trends in Improved Mobility of the Visually Impaired*,
EAI/Springer Innovations in Communication and Computing,
https://doi.org/10.1007/978-3-030-16450-8_10

& Elleithy, 2017), the state-of-the-art sensor-based assistive technologies were reviewed and assessed. The conclusions of that work indicate that most of the current solutions are still at a research stage, partially solving the problem of either indoor or outdoor navigation. It also suggests some guidelines for the development of relevant systems, which include: (a) real-time performance, i.e., fast processing for the exchanged information between the user and the sensors, and detection of suddenly appearing objects within a range of 0.5–5 m, regardless of the place and time; (b) wireless connectivity, (c) reliability, (d) simplicity, (e) wearability, and (f) low cost, affordable for most users.

Focusing on the most recent vision-based systems, their main, most critical functionalities include the detection of obstacles and provision of navigational assistance, whereas additional features include the recognition of objects, or scenes in general. A wearable mobility aid solution based on embedded 3D vision was proposed in Poggi and Mattoccia (2016). By wearing this device the users can perceive, be guided by audio messages and tactile feedback, receive information about the surrounding environment and avoid obstacles along a path. Another relevant system was proposed in Schwarze et al. (2016). That system was capable of perceiving the environment with a stereo camera, providing information about the obstacles and other objects to the user in the form of intuitive acoustic feedback (through sonification of objects/obstacles adjacent to the user). A system for joint detection, tracking and recognition of objects encountered during navigation in outdoor environments was presented in Tapu, Mocanu, and Zaharia (2017). The key principle considered for the development of that system was the alternation between tracking using motion information and prediction of the location of an object in time based on visual similarity. A project exploiting a smart-glass was presented in Suresh, Arora, Laha, Gaba, and Bhambri (2017). It investigated the development of a system that consists of a camera and ultrasonic sensors to recognize obstacles ahead, and assess their distance in real-time. The processing was performed on a portable computer. A wearable camera system proposed in Wang, Katzschmann, et al. (2017) was capable of providing also haptic-feedback to the user through vibrations. It was capable of identifying walkable spaces, planning a safe motion trajectory in the space, as well as recognition and localization of certain types of objects. A system called Sound of Vision was presented in Caraiman et al. (2017), aiming to provide the users with a 3D representation of the environment around them, conveyed by means of the hearing and tactile senses. The vision system was based on an RGB Depth (RGB-D) sensor, with an Inertial Measurement Unit (IMU) was used for tracking the head/camera orientation. In Lin, Lee, and Chiang (2017) a simple smartphone-based guiding system was proposed. That system included a fast feature recognition module running on the smartphone for fast processing of visual data. It also included remotely accessible modules, one for more demanding feature recognition tasks, and one for direction and distance estimation.

An augmented reality system, featuring obstacle localization was proposed in Yu, Yang, Jones, and Saniie (2018). That system was using predefined augment reality markers to identify specific accessible facilities, such as hallways, restrooms, staircases and offices within indoor environments. A scene perception system was proposed in Kaur and Bhattacharya (2018), based on a multi-modal fusion-based framework for object detection and classification. In Yang, Wang, et al. (2018) a unifying terrain awareness framework was proposed as an extension of a basic vision system based on an IR RGB Depth (RGB-D) sensor (Yang et al., 2017), aiming at attaining efficient semantic understanding of the environment. The approach was integrated into a wearable navigation system by incorporating a depth segmentation method. Another vision-based navigational aid based on an RGB-D sensor was presented in Lin, Wang, Yang, and Cheng (2018); however, that study was focusing on a specific component for road barrier recognition.

A relevant pre-commercial system promising both obstacle detection and audio-based user communication is investigated in the context of an H2020 funding scheme for Small Medium Enterprises (SMEs). The system, called EyeSynth (Audio-Visual System for the Blind Allowing Visually Impaired to See Through Hearing)[1], is based on a stereoscopic imaging system mounted on a pair of eye-glasses and the audio signals communicated to the user are non-verbal and abstract. The implementation details are not yet available. Other relevant commercially available solutions include ORCAM MyEye,[2] which is attachable to the users' eyeglasses and discreetly reads printed and digital text aloud from printed or digital surfaces, and recognizes faces, products, and money notes; eSight Eyewear,[3] which aims to enhance the vision of partially blind individuals by using a high-speed, high-definition camera that captures whatever the user is looking at, and then displays it on two near-to-eye displays; AIRA system,[4] which connects blind or low-vision people with trained, remotely located human agents who have access to what the user sees through a wearable camera, at the touch of a button, e.g., in the case of an emergency. These commercially available solutions do not yet incorporate any intelligent components for automated assistance.

The review performed reveals that during the last 2 years several studies and research projects have been initiated, setting higher standards toward a system for computer-assisted navigation of the visually impaired individuals. This chapter presents the concept of a novel vision-based system being developed in the recently initiated project ENORASI (Intelligent Audiovisual System Enhancing Cultural Experience and Accessibility, 2018–2021, funded by European Union and Greek national funds). It describes state-of-the-art (and beyond) methods considered for its development, and it investigates the user requirements based on the relevant literature.

The rest of this chapter consists of six sections. Section 10.2 presents the concept of the proposed system. Section 10.3 focuses on methods investigated for the implementation of a *Computer Vision* (*CV*) system capable of artificially perceiving the users' environment. Section 10.4 describes the concepts related to the methods

---

[1]https://eyesynth.com.

[2]https://www.orcam.com.

[3]https://www.esighteyewear.com.

[4]https://aira.io/.

considered for the implementation of its interactive intelligent user interface and decision-making modules. In Sect. 10.5, a set of user requirements are mined from the relevant literature. Section 10.6 discusses the technologies that better adapt to the goals of the proposed system, and the last section summarizes the conclusions of this study.

10.2 Vision-Based Navigation in Outdoor Cultural Environments

Museum (indoor) accessibility for the visually impaired individuals has been investigated in several studies (Alkhafaji, Fallahkhair, Cocea, & Crellin, 2016; Shah & Ghazali, 2018). However, the accessibility of outdoor sites of cultural interest has attracted less attention, although the experiences from visiting such sites can be equally significant. The ENORASI project aims to investigate and deliver a pre-commercial digital system to assist the visually impaired individuals on moving safely in external environments of cultural interest, e.g., of historic value, while providing them an enhanced touring experience. Besides the audible guidance and instructions for obstacle avoidance, the system provides also information about the sights in a descriptive way, through an emotionally aware, intelligent, speech user interface.

The main components of the proposed system include (Fig. 10.1): (a) stereo-scopic CV system for depth assessment, through visual sensors embedded on the users' eyeglasses; (b) emotion-aware speech interaction through a microphone and earphones that are also embedded to the users' eyeglasses in a way that it does not interfere with their hearing; (c) communication with a GPS-enabled Mobile Processing Unit (MPU), such as a smartphone or a tablet, customized for visually impaired individuals. A challenge is to enable robust performance in an energy-efficient way, based solely on visual sensors, without augmentation from additional sensors of the local environment such as ultrasound and IMU sensors. Also, to further increase autonomy, software optimizations, such as smart management of energy and computational resources are considered (Gubbi, Buyya, Marusic, & Palaniswami, 2013).

The proposed system is based on image/video and audio/speech processing and analysis methods. These include computer vision algorithms for automatic object recognition, e.g., obstacles, and the estimation of their distance from the user, and emotionally-aware speech recognition algorithms, which as well as algorithms for decision making based on the acquired multimodal data (images, audio, GPS). The analysis of the user experiences in relation to their emotions at different locations can be useful as a resource for feedback from the users to the system administrators, so as to enhance their services at these locations.

The processing and analysis of the acquired data is performed partially in the MPU, while more complex computational processes are performed in a remote

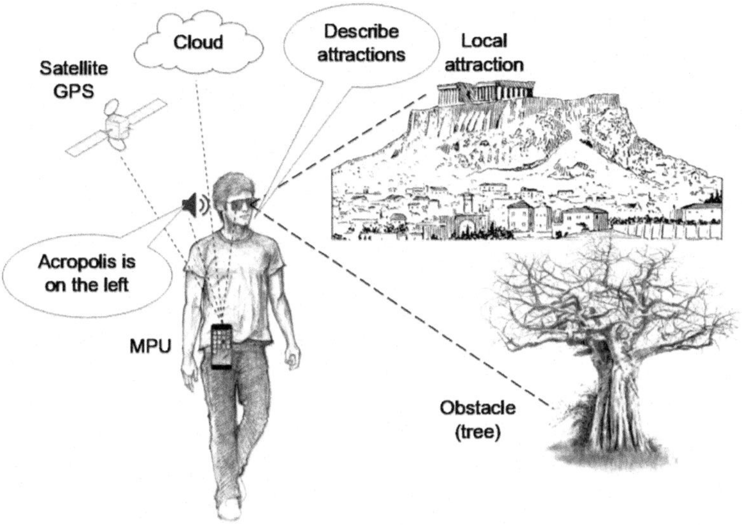

Fig. 10.1 The proposed system concept

server, through a computational cloud environment. Tasks performed in the MPU include obstacle detection, as it is the most critical task for the users' safety, as well as critical speech-based communication with the user, so as to enable basic functionalities even if the system is offline (i.e., the cloud is not accessible). More computationally demanding tasks, such as object or scene recognition, and decision making with respect to planning of the navigation route, or other higher-level inference such as route planning, complex speech and emotion recognition are performed on remote servers accessible through the cloud.

10.3   Human Vision Via Computer Vision

CV is a field of computer science that combines image processing and artificial intelligence to enable computers to recognize and assess the semantics within the images and video sequences. With its theoretical foundations back in the early sixties (Roberts, 1963), its developments have provided a variety of useful applications, spanning from everyday apps, such as the face detection feature of conventional cameras (Wang, Hu, & Deng, 2018), to specialized applications with social impact, such as image-guided anomaly detection in the medical domain (Iakovidis, Georgakopoulos, Vasilakakis, Koulaouzidis, & Plagianakos, 2018). The rapid evolution of parallel hardware architectures, such as the *Graphics Processing Units* (*GPUs*), has triggered unprecedented developments in *Artificial Neural Networks* (*ANNs*). These inherently parallel computational structures can bring us closer than ever to the development of systems that perceive the visual world like humans, and interpret it into auditory information for the visually impaired.

In this context, aspects investigated with respect to the perception of the visual world include the detection of obstacles, the recognition of objects, as well as the estimation of object sizes and distances.

10.3.1 Artificial Neural Networks for Computer Vision

Supervised ANN architectures, such as the *Multi-Layer Perceptron* (*MLP*) (Theodoridis & Koutroumbas, 2009), have been widely applied in the field of CV for object detection and recognition. In this context, usually shallow architectures, composed of three layers have been considered, with reference to their universal approximation capabilities (Hornik, Stinchcombe, & White, 1989). The input of these architectures was usually composed of so-called 'hand-crafted' image features, extracted using predefined methodologies. However, this imposed limitations in the generality of the CV approaches developed. To cope with such limitations, a revolutionary extension of the MLP for image classification, named *Convolutional Neural Network* (*CNN*), was presented in 1995 (LeCun, Bottou, Bengio, & Haffner, 1998). The core components of a CNN network are its convolutional layers, which contain a bio-inspired neuron connection arrangement mimicking the biological cells of visual cortex. In this layer, each neuron has pre-fixed connections to the input space, which form the so-called *receptive field* of the neuron. Multiple neurons span across the image with fixed receptive field and shared weights, which result into the extraction of the same feature across the entire input space, forming a *feature map*. Multiple feature maps are used to extract different features from the input space. This feature extraction process is applied over several convolutional layers. Also, pooling operations, such as maximum and average pooling, are performed after one or more convolutional layers, which facilitate dimensionality reduction. After this process, the resulting feature representations are classified by an MLP composed of three fully connected neuronal layers. The original CNN architecture proposed in LeCun et al. (1998) is known as LeNet. Due to the relatively large number of layers composing a CNN, its architecture is characterized as *deep*. This, along with the fact that such architectures are trainable, motivated the term *deep learning*, which is widely used to characterize machine learning using *Deep Neural Networks* (*DNNs*).

The CNN concept was revived in 2012, with an architecture named AlexNet (Krizhevsky, Sutskever, & Hinton, 2012), extending the original CNN approach (LeCun et al., 1998). This network won the ImageNet ILSVRC-2012 competition, which involved classification experiments on a large dataset, composed of one million images with over 10,000 object categories. That network had 62.3 million parameters, and its training became feasible by exploiting GPU computing. Since then, CNNs have been widely adopted in various applications, including object recognition (Szegedy, Ioffe, Vanhoucke, & Alemi, 2017), detection (Lin, Goyal,

Girshick, He, & Dollár, 2018), segmentation (He, Gkioxari, Dollár, & Girshick, 2017) and tracking (Held, Thrun, & Savarese, 2016). Considering their high computational requirements, a research branch is being developed toward the reduction of their complexity (Howard et al., 2017; Zhang, Zhou, Lin, & Sun, 2017), aiming to enable their introduction into mobile and embedded devices.

Unsupervised CNN architectures have been investigated as feature extractors in the form of *AutoEncoders (AE)* (Luo, Li, Yang, Xu, & Zhang, 2018). In principle, an AE consists of an input layer, called *encoder*, hidden layers, and an output layer, called the *decoder*. By training the network in an unsupervised manner, the resulting representation of the input space into its hidden layers form the image features, subsequently used for image classification. Another CNN type, called *Generative Adversarial Network (GAN)* (Goodfellow et al., 2014), is capable of generating image data by a reverse approach to that of AEs; instead of compressing a high-dimensional input space into its layers, it receives a low-dimensional vector which is subsequently used to generate a realistic output image. Useful applications in the context of CV include image resolution enhancement (Ledig et al., 2017) and visual saliency prediction (Pan et al., 2017), where the GAN is used to generate a saliency map, i.e., a map of regions within the images where objects of interest might be located.

Other ANN architectures that have been proved useful in the context of CV include the *Recurrent Neural Networks (RNNs)* and their extension, called *Long Short-Term Memory (LSTM)* (Hochreiter & Schmidhuber, 1997). RNNs maintain their internal hidden states to model the dynamic temporal behavior of sequences with arbitrary lengths through directed cyclic connections between its units. LSTMs extend RNNs by adding three gates to RNN neurons; namely, a so-called *forget gate* to control whether to forget the current state, an *input gate* to indicate if it should read the input, and an *output gate* to control whether to output the state. Recent approaches include combinations of these networks with CNNs for multi-label image classification (Wang et al., 2016), and video action recognition (Wang, Gao, Song, & Shen, 2017).

The following paragraphs provide further information on the state-of-the-art methods, including ANN architectures, considered in the context of this study.

10.3.2   Obstacle Detection

Obstacle detection addresses the detection of any object interfering with the motion trajectory of an agent, including a robot, a smart-vehicle, or a visually impaired person following the directions provided by a smart navigation system. In the following, an overview of the state-of-the-art object detection methods applicable in the context of obstacle detection for the visually impaired is provided.

Object Detection Methods

An integrated CNN-based framework for object detection was presented in Sermanet et al. (2013). That framework combined a CNN architecture for feature
extraction based on AlexNet (Krizhevsky et al., 2012), named OverFeat, and a
regression network to detect multiple bounding boxes around objects in images.
A *Region-based* CNN architecture for object detection was presented in Girshick,
Donahue, Darrell, and Malik (2014) with the name R-CNN. The methodology uses
selective search (Uijlings, Van De Sande, Gevers, & Smeulders, 2013) to extract
2000 class-agnostic region proposals from each image, which are then resized and
feed-forwarded into a pre-trained CNN model to extract features. The extracted
features are then used to train a linear *Support Vector Machine* (*SVM*) classifier
(Theodoridis & Koutroumbas, 2009) which classifies the extracted feature representations. Although R-CNN outperformed the OverFeat approach (Sermanet et
al., 2013) for object detection, it requires more computational resources. To reduce
its computational complexity, the Fast R-CNN (Girshick, 2015) was proposed, in
which feature maps are extracted from the entire input image. From these feature
maps, region proposals are extracted and reshaped into a fixed size, by a technique
called Region of Interest (RoI) pooling, so that they can be processed by a fully
connected layer. The Softmax function is used to predict the class of the RoI vector
while in parallel it computes the offset values for the bounding box of the object.

Another architecture, called *Spatial Pyramid Pooling Network* (*SPPNet*) (He,
Zhang, Ren, & Sun, 2015) aimed to cope with the problem of the fixed-size input
required by the CNNs which may impact the detection accuracy of the overall
model. This was done by implementing a novel spatial pyramid pooling which
enabled the network to generate fixed-length image representation regardless of the
image size. Compared with R-CNN, SPPNet relies on the same principles, yet it
does not have to process 2000 region proposals per image, as R-CNN does. Each
bounding box is classified by an SVM and bounding box regressor. A Faster R-CNN
(Ren, He, Girshick, & Sun, 2015) achieved real-time object detection capabilities,
by removing the selective search used by the previous methodologies.

A methodology for object detection that is fundamentally different from the
previous ones was presented in Redmon, Divvala, Girshick, and Farhadi (2016).
It is called *You Only Look Once* (*YOLO*) and it relies solely on a single forward pass
of an input image. The image is subdivided using a fixed-size grid, and entered
to a CNN that predicts bounding boxes and class probabilities for each box. A
saliency-inspired neural network model for object detection was proposed in Erhan,
Szegedy, Toshev, and Anguelov (2014). It predicts a set of class-agnostic bounding
boxes along with a single score for each box, corresponding to its likelihood of
containing any object of interest. In Liu, Anguelov, et al. (2016) an object detector
with name *Single Shot multibox Detector* (*SSD*) which achieved good balance
between computational performance and prediction accuracy. A region-based, *Fully
Convolutional Network* (*FCN*: a CNN without fully connected layers) was proposed
in Dai, Li, He, and Sun (2016). It relies on the generation of position-sensitive
score maps to cope with the dilemma between translation-invariance in image

classification and translation-variance in object detection. In Lin et al. (2017) an object detector for multi-scale object detection was proposed. That detector relies on a feature extractor, named *Feature Pyramid Network (FPN)*, which was designed to improve detection accuracy and speed. In Redmon and Farhadi (2017) YOLO9000, an extension of the YOLO approach (Redmon et al., 2016), was introduced for real-time object detection, considering 9000 object categories. A single-shot object detector, named *Deconvolutional SSD (DSSD)*, was presented in Fu, Liu, Ranga, Tyagi, and Berg (2017). It extended SSD by replacing the original VGGNet with a *Residual Network (ResNet)* (He, Zhang, Ren, & Sun, 2016) for feature extraction. ResNet architecture relies on small building blocks, named residual blocks, that feature skip connections and simple Convolutional-ReLu-Convolutional layers, which result in a network with 152 layers.

RetinaNet, proposed in Lin, Goyal, et al. (2018), is a single, unified network composed of a backbone network and two task-specific sub-networks. The backbone network is implemented by a ResNet architecture, used for feature extraction. The first sub-network performs the classification and the second one performs bounding box regression. A multi-scale extension of the DSSD network, called *Multi-Scale Deconvolutional SSD (MDSSD)*, has been proposed in Cui (2018), specifically for small object detection.

Obstacle Detection for the Visually Impaired

The ability to detect different types of objects in images is crucial for a system aiming to assist the navigation of the visually impaired. In the context of the project ENORASI, the user has to be able to trust the detection system to detect multiple types of obstacles/objects of different sizes in real-time, while in parallel the system should be able to accurately and reliably detect the surrounding area for potential cultural sights. Although some of the reviewed deep learning approaches are able to tackle the issue of real-time object detection, they are computationally demanding. This increases the need for a robust, multi-scale object detector, able to perform real-time object detection in mobile devices, so that the users will not have to rely on a client-server detection model that can degrade the overall performance due to network latency.

Among the various object detection methods that have been applied in the context of CV-based obstacle detection for the visually impaired, this paragraph focuses on the most recent ones. The obstacle detection module of the wearable mobility aid proposed in Poggi and Mattoccia (2016) was based on LeNet. The object detection in the DEEP-SEE framework presented in Tapu et al. (2017) was based on a YOLO CNN (Redmon et al., 2016). For the smart-glass approach presented in Suresh et al. (2017) three CNN architectures were encountered, namely Faster R-CNNs (Ren et al., 2015), YOLO (Redmon et al., 2016) and SSDs (Liu, Anguelov, et al., 2016). A Faster R-CNN (Ren et al., 2015) was used to detect and track objects in Kaur and Bhattacharya (2018). Motion, sharpening and blurring filters were used to enhance feature representation.

A state-of-the-art multi-scale FCN that we proposed in Diamantis, Iakovidis, and Koulaouzidis (2019) is presented as a candidate to cope with efficient obstacle detection. The proposed architecture, called Look-Behind FCN (LB-FCN), features multi-scale feature extraction capabilities with Look-Behind (LB) residual connections (Fig. 10.2a). The multi-scale feature extraction is bundled in a single block named Multi-scale Convolutional Block (MCB). Several MCBs are connected together forming a deep FCN (Fig. 10.2b). The LB connections aim to preserve the input volume, along with the extracted features per MCB. Each MCB input volume is feed-forwarded through the LB connection to the output of the MCB module where it is aggregated using an addition operation. The resulting network combines advantages of state-of-the-art architectures, including ResNet (He et al., 2016), ResNeXt (Xie, Girshick, Dollár, Tu, & He, 2017) and Inception-v4 (Szegedy et al., 2017) (discussed in the next section) but it features a lower number of free parameters, contributing to its time-efficiency over these and conventional CNNs,

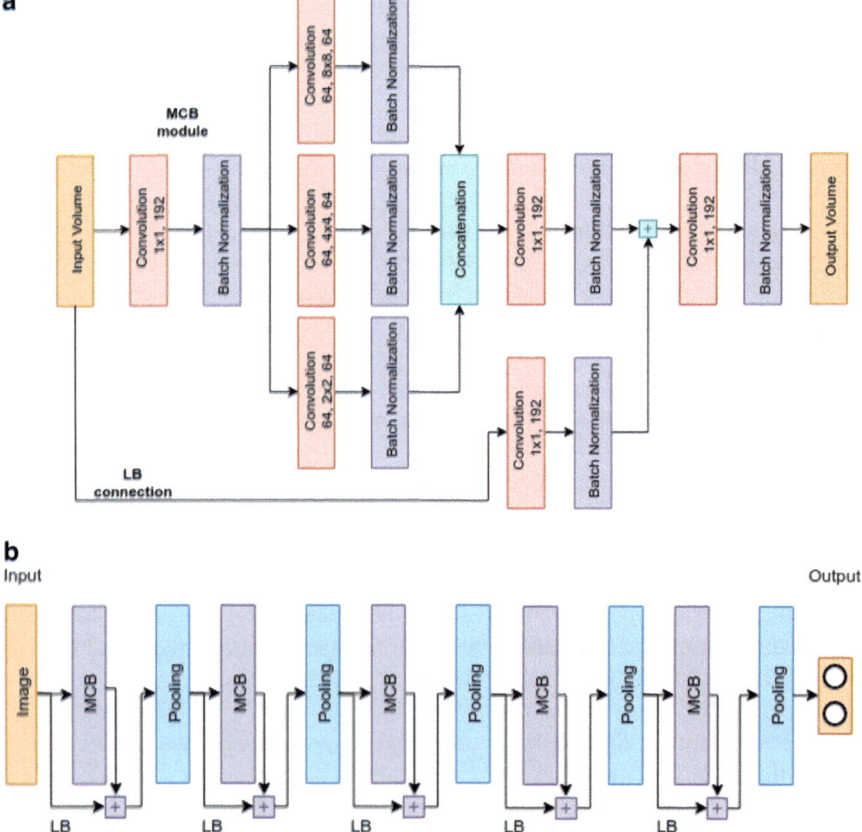

Fig. 10.2 The LB-FCN architecture. (**a**) The basic component of the architecture, formed by the MCB module and the LB connection. (**b**) An example LB-FCN with five MCB-LB components

such as VGGNet (Simonyan & Zisserman, 2014). Also, due to its multi-scale feature extraction capability it enables object detection at various scales. LB-FCN was benchmarked on open-access medical datasets, outperforming the state-of-the-art architectures and methods. Also, experiments using different datasets for training and testing of the architecture indicate its robustness against diversity of the objects to be detected and its generalization potentials (Diamantis, Iakovidis, & Koulaouzidis, 2018).

10.3.3   Object and Scene Recognition

Besides the detection of obstacles, which is critical for the safety of the visually impaired, object or scene recognition provides an additional quality in the visual perception of the world that can influence the decisions of the subjects during a guided tour. An object recognition system can provide information about the type of an obstacle, e.g., distinguish if the obstacle is a human or a tree, about the presence of a cultural sight within a scene and identify it, e.g., identify the Parthenon or the Caryatids of the Erechthion monuments in Acropolis. Object or scene recognition can be considered as a computationally more complex extension of object detection, since an intelligent system, such as an ANN, has to incorporate additional free parameters to encode additional knowledge about the different object types to be recognized. This means that most of the ANN-based object detection approaches reviewed in the previous subsection are extensible for object recognition. Similarly, ANN architectures proposed for object recognition can be simplified for object detection. In the following an overview of the most recent approaches to object recognition, applicable in the context of the proposed system, is provided.

Generic Recognition Approaches

Most of the state-of-the-art object recognition systems are also based on CNN architectures. Today, the Visual Geometry Group Network (VGGNet), and its variation VGG-16 (Simonyan & Zisserman, 2014), is considered as a baseline approach. VGGNet-16 is a CNN composed of 16 trainable layers with 138 million free-parameters. GoogLeNet CNN architecture (Szegedy et al., 2015), also known as Inception-v1, has a design that makes use of multiple Inception modules. An Inception module consists of parallel convolutional layers, with multi-scale feature extraction capabilities. Another CNN architecture that has been used for object recognition is ResNet (He et al., 2016). This architecture, which was also studied for object detection, won the ILSVRC-2015 challenge and for the first time, surpassing the human classification top-5 error rate by 5–10%.

A revised version of GoogLeNet architecture (Inception-v1) was presented in Szegedy, Vanhoucke, Ioffe, Shlens, and Wojna (2016) with name "Inception-v2", aiming to reduce the computational complexity by lowering the number of free parameters of the network. To achieve that, the network utilized factorized convolutions along with aggressive regularization. With primary focus on increasing the computational efficiency of DNN architectures, a recent study (Iandola et al., 2016) presented SqueezeNet architecture. The network was able to provide AlexNet-level accuracy on ImageNet dataset but with 50 times less number of free parameters. To formalize the Inception series architectures and to investigate if residual learning can benefit Inception-like architectures, a series of networks was presented in Szegedy et al. (2017). The result was the creation of three networks named Inception-v4, Inception-ResNet-v1 and Inception-ResNet-v2, with the first being a pure Inception architecture while the following Inception and ResNet hybrids. ResNeXt was presented in Xie et al. (2017) as an enhanced sequel of ResNet, expanding the original residual module with multiple parallel convolutional layers. The number of parallel convolutional layers in each ResNeXt building block, characterized as the *cardinality* of the network and after series of experiments it proved to be an equally important hyper-parameter when designing a network. ResNet was also the source of inspiration for the DenseNet (Huang, Liu, Van Der Maaten, & Weinberger, 2017) architecture. This architecture is based on a series of Dense Blocks which contain a series of convolutional layers, each one connected with all the following layers of the module in a feed-forward fashion. To battle the problem of long training time required by ResNet architecture Huang, Sun, Liu, Sedra, and Weinberger (2016) presented a Deep Network with Stochastic Depth. The network was trained utilizing a novel methodology similar to the dropout layer. Upon training, instead of disabling a percentage of neurons in a single layer, stochastic depth training disables entire layers of the network, vastly decreasing the training time. As an added benefit the authors found that training with stochastic depth can positively affect the classification accuracy of the network. To reduce the number of free parameters and allow CNN architectures to be used on mobile and embedded devices, Howard et al. (2017) presented a series of networks named *MobileNets*. The architecture utilizes depth-wise separable convolutions, instead of conventional convolutional layers which reduce the computational complexity. MobileNets expose two hyper parameters, named width and depth multipliers that balance the trade-off between the accuracy and the computational efficiency. Aiming to the same goal as MobileNets, Zhang, Zhou, et al. (2017) presented a CNN architecture with name *ShuffleNet*. The authors followed point-wise group convolution and channel shuffling to reduce the computational cost and maintain high classification accuracy. Experiments presented show ShuffleNet can achieve AlexNet classification accuracy on ImageNet dataset, increasing the speed by 13 times.

The semantic interpretation of scenes can also be considered as part of a scene recognition system. CNN architectures proposed for this purpose include encoder–decoder architectures, such as *SegNet* (Badrinarayanan, Kendall, & Cipolla, 2017).

Object or Scene Recognition for the Visually Impaired

Those of the recent vision-based navigation systems (Sect. 10.1) featuring object or scene recognition are based on CNN architectures as well. The mobility aid solution proposed in Poggi and Mattoccia (2016) uses a LeNet architecture for categorization of objects in eight classes. A kinetic real-time convolutional neural network for navigational assistance was presented by Lin, Wang, et al. (2018) with name *KrNet*. The system relies on a CNN architecture designed to provide navigational assistance for visually impaired individuals in the problem of road barrier recognition. The terrain awareness framework proposed in Yang, Wang, et al. (2018) was based on a CNN for semantic image segmentation. Various CNNs were tested including SegNet (Badrinarayanan et al., 2017).

Beyond the state-of-the-art approaches, the computational complexity of the multi-scale LB-FCN architecture that we proposed in Diamantis et al. (2019) (Sect. 10.3.2.2, can be further reduced by applying the depth-wise separable convolution approach proposed in Howard et al. (2017), and extended for multi-label classification of objects as described in Vasilakakis, Diamantis, Spyrou, Koulaouzidis, and Iakovidis (2018), so as to enable the recognition of multiple objects. Considering the benchmarks performed in Diamantis et al. (2019), it constitutes a promising alternative for the time-efficient object detection and recognition in the time-critical context of the system presented in this chapter.

10.3.4 Visual Distance Estimation

The research field tackling with the problem of the estimation of the traveled distance of a subject, based exclusively on visual cues, is known as Visual Odometry (VO). VO has been thoroughly investigated and approached by researchers from different perspectives (Forster, Zhang, Gassner, Werlberger, & Scaramuzza, 2017; Konda & Memisevic, 2015; Zhang, Kaess, & Singh, 2017) and on different application domains (Dimas, Spyrou, Iakovidis, & Koulaouzidis, 2017; Fang & Scherer, 2015; Maimone, Cheng, & Matthies, 2007). VO can be used to supplement or even replace other traditional navigation options, since it cannot be affected by GPS dropouts due to obstacles or other unfavorable conditions (Nistér, Naroditsky, & Bergen, 2004). VO methodologies can be rendered as an alternative navigational assistance method for the visually impaired individuals, since it can produce high-quality results with regard to the traveled distance approximation.

Quite a few works have been proposed, incorporating VO methods for the navigational assistance of the visually impaired. A framework involving multiple sensors for assistive navigation of the visually impaired was proposed in Xiao et al. (2015). That system features real-time localization by exploiting VO for the estimation of the location of the user with an RGB Depth (RGB-D) camera. The system proposed in Schwarze et al. (2016) was able to perceive the environment through a stereoscopic camera, using head tracking with visual odometry, an IMU sensor and sonification of objects/obstacles adjacent to the user. In another study (Aladren, López-Nicolás, Puig, & Guerrero, 2016) among multiple sensors tested, an RGB-D sensor was selected as sufficient. With the use of the RGB-D sensor both the depth and the visual information were sufficient for the detection of the main structural elements of a scene, in order to determine an obstacle-free path for the safe passage of a visually impaired individual.

The system proposed in Wang, Katzschmann, et al. (2017) segments the free space and maps it into free space motion instructions. In another study (Lin, Cheng, Wang, & Yang, 2018), robust visual localization (VO) is achieved via a GoogLeNet (Szegedy et al., 2016) and global optimization. To tackle the problem of accurate VO in crowded environments, an egocentric VO approach was proposed for crowd-resilient indoor assisted navigation (Yang, Duarte, & Ganz, 2018). A monocular VO approach for the assisted navigation of visually impaired individuals was proposed in Ramesh, Nagananda, Ramasangu, and Deshpande (2018). The aim of that work was to tackle the problem of real-time VO in indoor environments with a single camera. To achieve that, imaging geometry, VO, and object detection along with distance-depth estimation algorithms were combined.

Despite the interesting results reported by the afore-mentioned studies and the practical potentials of the deployment of the VO methodologies, there are still several challenges that need to be tackled. For example, the utilization of multiple sensors for better accuracy in navigation and distance estimation systems requires handling the synchronization among the sensors (Xiao et al., 2015). The positioning of the camera sensor is also important, since it can lead to unwanted noise in the collected data (Xiao et al., 2015). Another challenge to be tackled is the adaptability of the system in different environments, such as crowded, indoor and outdoor environments (Lin, Cheng, et al., 2018; Yang, Duarte, & Ganz, 2018). A direction toward coping with this issue is the use of machine learning algorithms, e.g., recently, *Recurrent CNNs (RCNNs)* have provided very good results in performing VO (Li, Wang, Long, & Gu, 2018; Wang, Clark, Wen, & Trigoni, 2017). CNNs have the capacity of learning optimal features for the task that they are trained to perform. Thus, a single RCNN may have the learning capability to extract features resilient to crowded, indoor and outdoor environments. Also, its recurrent nature enables making correlations between previous and next situations. However, using deep learning algorithms such as RCNNs, a lot of computational resources are needed, whereas real-time performance becomes also a challenge. Thus, further investigation and development of methodologies should include ways of handling computational payload on MPUs.

The proposed system exploits stereoscopic imaging for robust depth estimation, which can also contribute in more accurate VO, as compared with monocular VO. For this purpose the use of the state-of-the-art Intel® RealSense™ D435[5] sensor is investigated. This sensor is small enough ($90 \times 25 \times 25$ mm) to be mounted on the front side of the users' eyeglasses. It enables 3D depth sensing, with a maximum

[5]https://realsense.intel.com/intel-realsense-downloads/.

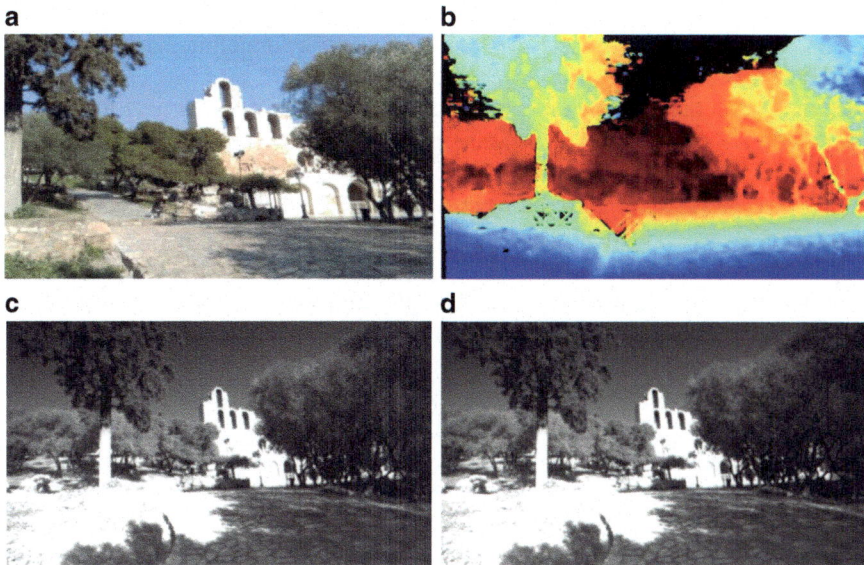

Fig. 10.3 Scene captured with the visual sensors of the proposed system near the Theatre of Herodes Atticus. (**a**) RGB image. (**b**) Depth map (more distant objects appear more reddish). (**c**) Left-stereo IR image. (**d**) Right-stereo IR image. The different visual sensors have different field of views

range of 10 m. It includes a stereoscopic system composed of two IR cameras, an IR projector and a high-resolution RGB camera. The infrared projector improves the depth estimation of the stereo camera system by projecting a static IR pattern on the scene. The IR pattern projection enables the texture enrichment of low texture scenes. An example of a scene captured with this sensor is illustrated in Fig. 10.3.

Visual Size Estimation

In the context of the proposed system, size estimation provides an added value in the assessment of obstacles and objects, which contributes in the enhancement of the users' experience. For example, it can be used as a cue to derive the level of deviation from a path, due to the presence of an obstacle, or as a quality to understand the size of a monument or a statue in a cultural environment.

The previous works in size estimation are limited. An object size measurement method that utilizes a stereo camera setup for the purposes of object identification has been proposed in Mustafah, Noor, Hasbi, and Azma (2012). That methodology includes object detection in the stereoscopic images, blob extraction and distance estimation. Another method aiming to both object localization and size measurement has been proposed in Liu, Yu, Chen, and Tang (2016). The algorithm used was based on the *Circle of Apollonius* for estimations without computing trigonometric functions. A review study on CV methodologies based on either monocular or stereo camera systems for size measurements was performed in Hao, Yu, and Li (2015). That review showed that the accuracy of the CV approach can be higher than traditional measurement methods. Another study (Pu, Tian, Wu, & Yan, 2016) proposed a novel framework to measure multiple objects in a scene using one or two photo shots.

More recently, we proposed a size measurement methodology that uses motion estimation over a video frame sequence in order to avoid the use of external references in size estimation (Iakovidis, Dimas, et al., 2018). This methodology exploits the distance estimated by an ANN toward the target object to be measured and then, the geometric model of the camera is used to estimate its dimensions.

There are still a lot of challenges to overcome toward accurate size measurements in the wild, using exclusively computer vision methodologies. As the authors of Hao et al. (2015) indicate in their review, the size estimation is prone to errors due to curved shape of the targeted object and to low/distorted image quality. In our work (Iakovidis, Dimas, et al., 2018), the size estimation is based on an accurate distance estimation from the camera to the target object, so the error is analogous to the distance estimation error. Also, the accurate object detection is of major importance for the good performance of size estimation methods (Mustafah et al., 2012).

In the proposed system, the visual size estimation via the method proposed by Iakovidis et al. (2018) can be augmented by the depth estimation provided by the use of the RGB-D sensor described in the previous subsection, as well as by the object detection methods discussed in Sect. 10.3.2. With the depth information and the accurate detection of the objects of interest, the geometric size measurement is possible after object segmentation.

10.4   Emotion-Aware Speech User Interface and Decision Making

In most mobile application human–machine interaction is performed through a visual user interface provided. In the case of visually impaired users, alternative, mainly auditory options, such as tactile and voice-enabled user interfaces, are preferable (Csapó, Wersényi, Nagy, & Stockman, 2015).

10.4.1   Voice User Interface

A Voice User Interface (VUI) aims to enable human–machine interaction through speech. Typically, VUIs are used to allow voice input as a means of controlling several types of devices or software applications. During the last few years, the advances of cloud services have led to the integration of VUIs in many popular mobile applications and smart environments. Smart assistants such as Apple's Siri, Amazon's Alexa, Samsung's Bixby, or Google Assistant have emerged. These are software agents integrated in smart mobile phones, smart-watches, or smart speakers. Their role includes performing tasks or services, e.g., managing emails/calendars using verbal commands, answering questions of users, e.g., regarding the news, or the weather and also controlling home automation, e.g., lights and thermostats. VUIs have also been playing a key role in several applications in call centers, where typically are used as interactive voice response systems, with limited natural language processing capabilities. Undoubtedly, VUIs have become very popular through their integration into devices of daily use, such as the smartphones.

10.4.2   Emotion Recognition

One of the most recent trends in the field of human–computer interaction is the recognition of the user's emotional state (Cowie et al., 2001). During the last few years, several approaches have been proposed, that are based on sensors, placed either within the users' environment such are cameras and microphones, or sensors that are wearable or embedded into devices carried by users, such as physiological or inertial sensors. In case of an approach based on the user's visual appearance, emotion recognition is based on facial, posture or motion features (Baltrusaitis et al., 2011; Piana, Stagliano, Odone, Verri, & Camurri, 2014). Body sensors may measure either physiological parameters, such as body temperature, heart and respiratory rate, muscle activity, skin conductance response or even brain activity (Haag, Goronzy, Schaich, & Williams, 2004) or extract inertial features (Tsatsou et al., 2018). Audio-based approaches are typically divided into two categories: (a) those that are based on the extraction of low- or mid-level features (Papakostas et al., 2017); and (b) those that are based on the processing of the spoken content, e.g., using a natural language understanding approach. It should be noted that each of these approaches has its own limitations, while user acceptance is typically low, e.g., in the case of cameras, the users may feel that their privacy is violated. Moreover, body sensors may cause discomfort when used for a long time. Totally non-invasive approaches are not yet available.

However, approaches that make use only of microphones are considered to be the least invasive. Sensors may be easily placed within the users' environment. Also, embedded microphones of mobile phones may be used. When assured that spoken content is not analyzed, and instead audio features are only used, people are less sensitive with privacy issues. Therefore, it should be clarified that the two discrete parts from which spoken content is composed. The *linguistic* content of speech includes the articulated patterns, as they are pronounced by the speaker. The *non-linguistic* content of speech may be described as the variation of the pronunciation of the aforementioned patterns, i.e., how the linguistic content has been pronounced (Anagnostopoulos, Iliou, & Giannoukos, 2015). When the goal is to classify spoken content to its underlying emotions based on its non-linguistic content, typical approaches are based on the extraction of low-level features. Common features include rhythm, pitch, intensity, etc. We should note that such non-linguistic methods easily provide language-independent models, yet they may be affected by cultural particularities.

Emotion recognition may be used for several reasons. Most popular fields of application include: (a) dynamical marketing, adaptive to the emotional reactions of users (i.e., potential customers) (Ren et al., 2015); (b) smart cars, recognizing the drivers' mood for prevention of accidents due to an unpleasant emotional state (Leng, Lin, & Zanzi, 2007); (c) evaluation of personality of candidates, e.g., during an interview (Lin, Kannappan, & Lau, 2013); (d) evaluation of employees and of user satisfaction in call centers (Petrushin, 1999); (e) enhancing gaming experience by understanding the players' emotional response, etc. (Psaltis et al., 2016). In previous work (Spyrou, Vretos, Pomazanskyi, Asteriadis, & Leligou, 2018) we have applied the assessment of the user affect based on the non-linguistic content of speech for personalization of a non-linear education process. For example, once the affect of a learner was detected to be out of the flow state tending to boredom, the system automatically increased the skill level of learner, while relaxed when she/he was detected in anxiety. In the context of the ENORASI project, the proposed system collects and maps user experiences by geographical region of interest, taking into account the users' emotional state, recognized while interacting with the VUI. This information will be used in analytics aiming to the enhancement of the provided services.

10.4.3   CNN-Based Speech and Emotion Recognition

The advantages of the CNN-based approaches discussed in the context of image analysis in Sect. 10.3 are also valid in the context of speech signal analysis. This motivated us to focus our research toward this direction. CNNs can be exploited visual feature extractors from spectrograms, which are 2D visual representations of the spectral content of the speech signals (Papakostas & Giannakopoulos, 2018). Spectrograms are extracted from fixed-length segments from a given audio sample. The Short-Time Fourier Transform (STFT) is then applied on the original signal. This way, pseudocolored images of spectrograms are generated. For robustness to noise and also for augmenting datasets we add a background sound (e.g., music). Thus, CNNs are trained on the extracted spectrograms. To provide a multilingual approach, the CNN model can be trained using datasets from different languages.

10.4.4   Higher-Level Decision Making

Besides the decision making implemented by ANN approaches, which resembles low-level cognitive processing, the proposed system considers higher-level decision-making approaches to provide feedback and guidance to the user through the VUI. Higher-level cognition can be modeled by artificial cognitive models capable of reasoning within a knowledge space of high-level, semantically relevant concepts. The knowledge about one or more domains can be described by a set of semantic, high-level, interrelated concepts forming a knowledge space. A cognitive model is a computational model capable of simulating human problem-solving and mental task processes within this knowledge space. In that sense, ENORASI investigates high-level cognitive models capable of reasoning based on multiple input concepts related to multiple recognized events (after low-level cognitive processing). The reasoning process results in inference of decisions, e.g., suggesting to the subject which direction to follow, situation assessment, e.g. risk assessment about an alternative, and control, e.g. regulate reaction and generate command for action.

The theory of fuzzy sets provides a sound mathematical framework for uncertainty modeling that has proved its effectiveness in a variety of applications. Fuzzy knowledge-based reasoning methods require that knowledge is represented in the form of rules between higher-level concepts, which can be represented as variables with linguistic values (Zadeh, 1983), e.g., the user interaction about the estimated distance from an obstacle can be based on expressions such as "the distance from the obstacle is small". The fuzzy cognitive map (FCM) approach can be the basis for enhanced networks for dynamic knowledge representation (Papageorgiou & Salmeron, 2013). An FCM is a fuzzy directed graph with causally interrelated nodes that correspond to the concepts involved in a knowledge domain. It is able to reason through an iterative algorithm updating the values of the graph nodes until a steady state is reached (Papageorgiou & Iakovidis, 2013). This approach is considered for navigation purposes according to the paradigm of Vaščák and Hvizdoš (2016), by also exploiting algorithms coping with the traveling salesman and shortest path problems (Kovács, Iantovics, & Iakovidis, 2018).

10.5 User Requirements

Requirements elicitation is the process of seeking, uncovering, acquiring and elaborating requirements for computer-based systems (Zowghi & Coulin, 2005). As a first step in this process, a literature review was performed for that purpose. A recommended approach to system design is the user-centered design process. This is based on an iterative and continuous update process interacting with the end users, analyzing their feedback and adopting their requirements until the final product is developed (Magnusson, Hedvall, & Caltenco, 2018). The human-centered process is currently well-defined and established as an ISO standard, namely, ISO 9241-210:2010 (Human-centered design for interactive systems) (International Organization for Standardization, 2010). The main axes of the human-centered process are the usability and the user experience. The usability is defined as the ability of the developed system, service or product used by specified users to achieve the defined goals effectively, efficiently and satisfactorily within a certain context of use. On the other hand, user experience is defined as the opinion and perception of the user on the system, service or product after their use (Magnusson et al., 2018).

The user requirements for assistive systems for visually impaired individuals were investigated from several studies in the literature. The most relevant ones, with the assistive system presented in this study, are summarized in Table 10.1. A total of ten studies were considered. Two of the studies investigated (Panchanathan, Black, Rush, & Iyer, 2003; Sosa-Garcia & Odone, 2017) have addressed elicitation of user requirements with respect to CV-based systems for low vision and blind individuals. Individuals with visual impairment have an acute auditory sense; therefore audio-based commands and alerts would make the use of an assistive system easier and more helpful. In the doctoral thesis of Fryer (2013), the effects of the quality of audio descriptions, with respect to the engagement of the visually impaired with the digital media were investigated. The findings of that research support the theory that language can be considered as multimodal, in the sense that it can replace vision within a framework of integrating sensory experience. Another study (Panchanathan et al., 2003) describes the user needs elicited during iCare project. That project was aiming to develop an assistive device that would help visually impaired individuals (mainly students) to 'pick up a book and read it', to get information about a person standing in front of them, and to have access to the internet by filtering all the unnecessary information.

Four studies on user requirements and design considerations for cloud/GPS-based information systems for the visually impaired individuals were considered. These include a study addressing an assistive system for urban mobility and transportation by using GPS navigation (Perakovic, Periša, & Prcic, 2015); another study for mobility on urban environments using a robotic guidance system (Hersh & Johnson, 2010); a study investigating various issues regarding outdoor mobility, including outdoor travel frequency, travel independency, different barriers, and shortcomings of GPS (Zeng, 2015); and, a study investigating the user requirements to support tactile mobility (Conradie, de Goedelaan, Mioch, & Saldien, 2014).

Three studies included relevant user requirements for designing a mobile service to enhance learning from cultural heritage. In Alkhafaji et al. (2016), which was focusing on the visually impaired individuals, the results indicated that a multi-service approach at cultural heritage sites should be able to cover services for navigation and directions, to spot nearby cultural heritage places, to receive historical information while touring about the place and the sites and to pre-organize a visit/guided tour. Furthermore, 62% of participants said they would like to customize their mobile application based on their interests. The second of the three studies (Asakawa, Guerreiro, Ahmetovic, Kitani, & Asakawa, 2018), was addressing indoor museum spaces, and it was not focusing to visually impaired individuals; however, some important aspects of museum experience for the visually impaired were mentioned, including purposes (socializing with friends and learning on-site while feeling the atmosphere of the museum), mobility issues, inaccessibility

Table 10.1 Summary of user requirements derived from the literature

#	Requirement	Ref.
1.	Real-time performance for detection/recognition tasks	Sosa-Garcia and Odone (2017)
2.	Ease of use, natural/intuitive user interface, acceptable by a broad user population, including senior citizens	Sosa-Garcia and Odone (2017)
3.	A simple training procedure, potentially scalable to new objects and personalization	Sosa-Garcia and Odone (2017)
4.	Tolerance to viewpoint variations	Sosa-Garcia and Odone (2017)
5.	Tolerance to illumination variations	Sosa-Garcia and Odone (2017)
6.	Tolerance to blur, motion blur, out of focus and occlusions	Sosa-Garcia and Odone (2017)
7.	Accuracy of directions and information	Panchanathan et al. (2003)
8.	Time-efficient access to information	Panchanathan et al. (2003)
9.	Alerts for unexpected events	Panchanathan et al. (2003)
10.	Information to help individuals to tour in an area of interest	Panchanathan et al. (2003)
11.	Audio descriptions of high quality	Fryer (2013)
12.	Automatic creation of return route	Perakovic et al. (2015)
13.	Voice navigation in native languages	Perakovic et al. (2015)
14.	Easy-to-use starting method and configuration	Perakovic et al. (2015)
15.	Use of alternative technologies to GPS for position tracking	Perakovic et al. (2015)
16.	Providing information on location, guidance and navigation	Perakovic et al. (2015)
17.	Providing information on facilities surrounding the user	Perakovic et al. (2015)
18.	Providing information about descending and ascending kerbstone	Perakovic et al. (2015)
19.	Providing information on the system operation	Perakovic et al. (2015)
20.	Providing information of arrival to the destination	Perakovic et al. (2015)
21.	Precise about the movement and location of the user 0.5 (m)	Perakovic et al. (2015)
22.	User-friendliness of the mobile terminal device	Perakovic et al. (2015)
23.	Ability of creating priority information	Perakovic et al. (2015)
24.	Economically affordable solution	Perakovic et al. (2015)
25.	Ability of creating pre-announcement prior to arriving to the destination	Perakovic et al. (2015)
26.	Ability of facility identification	Perakovic et al. (2015)
27.	Selection of the device operation mode offline–online	Perakovic et al. (2015)
28.	Personalization by giving the ability to the users to define their own level of disability	Perakovic et al. (2015)
29.	Minimize the dangers and errors by preventing consequences of incidental or unintentional activity	Perakovic et al. (2015)

(continued)

Table 10.1 (continued)

#	Requirement	Ref.
30.	Sharing information for accompanying contents of surroundings (coffee shops, hotels, hospitals, etc.)	Perakovic et al. (2015)
31.	Compatibility of the device with web applications	Perakovic et al. (2015)
32.	Keyboard as an additional component since visually impaired people are not familiar with touch screens	Perakovic et al. (2015)
33.	Integration with geo-location services with pre-defined SMS messaging	Perakovic et al. (2015)
34.	A multi-function device with GPS for orientation: Location and points of interest, such as 1-m GPS position accuracy, surroundings' description and information and identification of entrances	Hersh and Johnson (2010)
35.	Support and/or emergency: contacting police, ambulance, an emergency center and/or the user's family and giving them the user's location, as well as the provision of help in case the user gets lost	Hersh and Johnson (2010)
36.	A camera for detecting obstacles for also obstacle avoidance (moving and static objects/obstacles' shape, location, moving speed, etc.)	Hersh and Johnson (2010)
37.	Navigation and way-finding, such as finding a street name and safe route	Hersh and Johnson (2010)
38.	Distance and arrival time to the destination as well as the route properties, such as steps up or down, a bridge or a crossing	Hersh and Johnson (2010)
39.	A recording and/or memory function for routes to help the user retrace the route, learn from their mistakes and prepare for future journeys	Hersh and Johnson (2010)
40.	Weather conditions and terrain type notification to support long distance walking and walking in unknown or little known areas	Hersh and Johnson (2010)
41.	Recognizing the color of clothes	Hersh and Johnson (2010)
42.	Discreet and unobtrusive and not attract (undue or unwelcome) attention, including by making unnecessary sounds or noisy operation, or looking exotic, unusual or like medical equipment	Hersh and Johnson (2010)
43.	Attractive and elegant, possibly with a choice of different colors, but in an understated rather than attention grabbing way	Hersh and Johnson (2010)
44.	It should be robust, last a long time and not require maintenance, as well as resistant to damage, pressure, knocks and bumps, water and weather	Hersh and Johnson (2010)
45.	Simple and intuitive to use and look after, including by older people	Hersh and Johnson (2010)
46.	Extending battery life by the device only being powered for steering round obstacles and not for forward motion	Hersh and Johnson (2010)

(continued)

Table 10.1 (continued)

#	Requirement	Ref.
47.	A combination of methods for receiving information from and giving instructions to the robot, though one respondent felt that speech output was the most accessible to all blind and visually impaired people	Hersh and Johnson (2010)
48.	Both a loudspeaker and an earpiece should be available	Hersh and Johnson (2010)
49.	Instructions should be provided by speech and other ways, e.g., a joystick with a scrolling menu and push buttons	Hersh and Johnson (2010)
50.	Speech should be of good quality, sound human not mechanical and be pronounced clearly, with options to change the voice and regulate the volume and rate of delivery	Hersh and Johnson (2010)
51.	A security system to avoid theft, a connection to the user to avoid losing the robot, a manually operated brake, the avoidance of cables and metal parts and that the robot should have knowledge of self-defense	Hersh and Johnson (2010)
52.	An affordable price	Hersh and Johnson (2010)
53.	A USB port and/or wireless connection to update software and/or load data, text and music	Hersh and Johnson (2010)
54.	Software to automatically upgrade on contact with wireless internet but also an internet and/or PC connection to update data and the software	Hersh and Johnson (2010)
55.	The user should be able to move fast with the system, including upstairs and downstairs and in busy situations	Hersh and Johnson (2010)
56.	The design should have few crevices and bends where dirt accumulates and which are difficult to clean. White was considered a color to be avoided for this reason	Hersh and Johnson (2010)
57.	A barcode or RFID reader to read information from barcodes and RFID tags	Hersh and Johnson (2010)
58.	Any speech recognition system used should be of good quality and work well in noisy environments	Hersh and Johnson (2010)
59.	A small display to enable sighted people to read the information, as well as the use of large visual and tactile symbols	Hersh and Johnson (2010)
60.	User choice as to when they received information, particularly spoken information, to avoid irritation to them and other people and attracting attention	Hersh and Johnson (2010)
61.	The system should be re-programmable for the particular user, including accommodating the requirements of users with learning difficulties or other impairments	Hersh and Johnson (2010)
62.	Identification and information of buildings' entrances	Zeng (2015)
63.	Alert for irregular sidewalks	Zeng (2015)
64.	Identification and information of stairs	Zeng (2015)

(continued)

Table 10.1 (continued)

#	Requirement	Ref.
65.	Early alert for obstacles especially in a waist level	Zeng (2015)
66.	Position restore actions when the user gets lost	Zeng (2015)
67.	Roadside holes alert	Zeng (2015)
68.	Information about pedestrian crossings especially in complex forms	Zeng (2015)
69.	Environmental accessibly data	Zeng (2015)
70.	Up-to-date map data	Zeng (2015)
71.	High GPS location accuracy	Zeng (2015)
72.	Strong signal of GPS in urban environment	Zeng (2015)
73.	Notification of uneven floor surfaces such as loose street tiles, puddles or other small holes	Conradie et al. (2014)
74.	The assistive devices should take into account the people with a walking impairment	Conradie et al. (2014)
75.	Systems should reliably provide relevant information when needed, while also considering information accuracy	Conradie et al. (2014)
76.	Designers should also consider providing critical features such as re-location or re-positioning, to allow users to find their way back	Conradie et al. (2014)
77.	Users should be provided with system status information that is critical to use. This may include battery status or current system accuracy	Conradie et al. (2014)
78.	Devices that are used outdoor may need easy ways of recharging batteries, or make use of external batteries	Conradie et al. (2014)
79.	System complexity should also be avoided, to prevent long training times	Conradie et al. (2014)
80.	It should not interfere with other safety relevant interaction mechanisms	Conradie et al. (2014)
81.	Audio should not be the main mode of feedback, especially in situations where users rely heavily on sound to locate and orientate themselves	Conradie et al. (2014)
82.	Alternatives to in-ear earphones may be considered, but critical system information is best communicated via alternative means	Conradie et al. (2014)
83.	The types of obstacles that are communicated to the user should be restricted to those that are unexpected. This is especially important to limit information overload and reduce system complexity	Conradie et al. (2014)
84.	Different contexts may require different types of user interaction. Environments with many obstacles may require different types of notifications (i.e.: more frequent, closer in range)	Conradie et al. (2014)
85.	A balance between the wearing location of both the input sensors and the tactile feedback is needed to ensure the best user experience, while also providing the best results	Conradie et al. (2014)

(continued)

Table 10.1 (continued)

#	Requirement	Ref.
86.	Providing directions and navigation	Alkhafaji et al. (2016)
87.	Identify and give information for nearby cultural heritage places	Alkhafaji et al. (2016)
88.	Find the nearest services	Alkhafaji et al. (2016)
89.	Get historical information while people walk around, and finding out extra information about the sites	Alkhafaji et al. (2016)
90.	Pre-organize visits	Alkhafaji et al. (2016)
91.	Configuration options for personalized customization of the users' mobile app based on their interests	Alkhafaji et al. (2016)
92.	Providing services for cultural heritage information	Alkhafaji et al. (2016)
93.	Operation in parallel with guided tours and in respect to the cultural heritage place so the user will not be fully distracted from tour	Alkhafaji et al. (2016)
94.	Ability to operate offline to avoid poor network quality issues	Alkhafaji et al. (2016)
95.	User-friendly interface and easy operational menu	Alkhafaji et al. (2016)
96.	Weather proof devices in case of open space cultural heritage sites	Alkhafaji et al. (2016)
97.	Detailed audio content is necessary to gain new knowledge	Asakawa et al. (2018)
98.	To listen to the audio contents in front of the artworks, in order to have a similar experience to sighted people	Asakawa et al. (2018)
99.	To listen to human voices as long as they are neutral rather than too emotional	Asakawa et al. (2018)
100.	Concerning the content of the audio descriptions, an introduction/summary, the history, and a detailed visual description of the artwork, followed by detailed descriptions of the technique used should be provided	Asakawa et al. (2018)
101.	To be able to adjust the length of (or skip) the descriptions	Asakawa et al. (2018)
102.	Device functions to be in cooperation with sighted companions	Asakawa et al. (2018)
103.	Identified signs for stairs and toilets	Handa et al. (2010)
104.	Quality of service	Handa et al. (2010)
105.	Cultural information for original artwork	Handa et al. (2010)
106.	Pre-visit information on website and information from museum's website	Handa et al. (2010)
107.	Audio guides with additional information for those who want to get deeper knowledge	Handa et al. (2010)
108.	Assistive system to replace the staff's assistance by providing better quality of interpretation	Handa et al. (2010)

of artworks. The third study (Handa, Dairoku, & Toriyama, 2010) investigated priority needs in terms of museum service accessibility for visually impaired visitors.

10.6 Discussion

The surveys performed in Sects. 10.3–10.5 indicate that current imaging, computer vision, speech, emotion recognition, and decision-making technologies have the potentials to be evolved and integrated into an effective assistive system for the navigation and guidance of the visually impaired individuals. The ENORASI project investigates novel solutions to the challenges involved, aiming to deliver the integrated system described in Sect. 10.2, which should provide enhanced usability and accessibility.

Object detection and recognition are important features in the context of such a system. Object detection approaches, such as Overfeat (Sermanet et al., 2013) and R-CNN (Girshick et al., 2014) are based on two-stage detection approaches, which can be very accurate, yet they are generally computationally demanding. On the other hand, single shot detectors such as YOLO (Redmon et al., 2016) and SSD (Liu, Anguelov, et al., 2016) can provide real-time detection performance, while maintaining reasonable computational requirements; however, they tend not to be very competitive in terms of detection accuracy, as compared with the two-stage detectors. The need for real-time multi-scale obstacle detection for the guidance of the visually impaired increases the demand for the development of robust, light-weight multi-scale object detectors. The state-of-the-art LB-FCN (Diamantis et al., 2019) is considered as a solution toward multi-scale feature extraction and low computational requirements, as compared to conventional networks, such as VGGNet (Simonyan & Zisserman, 2014). Recent deep learning approaches for object recognition, such as GoogLeNet (Szegedy et al., 2015), ResNet (He et al., 2016) and DenseNet (Huang et al., 2017), have provided high object classification accuracies. These architectures require a large number of free parameters which increases their computational complexity, and thus their usage is limited to high-end workstations and servers. Recently, architectures, such as MobileNets (Howard et al., 2017) and ShuffleNets (Zhang, Zhou, et al., 2017), have been proposed aiming to solve this problem by using a fewer free parameters. These networks have been developed specifically to meet the needs of mobile and embedded computing, by making compromises between recognition accuracy and computational complexity. Such compromises may be acceptable in some object recognition applications; however, the guidance of the visually impaired requires real-time performance along with high classification accuracy. The benchmarks performed in Diamantis et al. (2019) suggest that LB-FCN can be considered as a solution to object detection in the proposed system, since it is characterized by smaller computational complexity than relevant architectures, which can be further reduced by utilizing approaches such as the depth-wise separable convolution (Howard et al., 2017). Recognition of multiple objects can be achieved by properly extending LB-FCN for multi-label classification (Vasilakakis et al., 2018).

The estimation of the distance traveled by the user through VO can be considered as a key element of a navigation system for the assistance of the visually impaired (Aladren et al., 2016; Lin, Cheng, et al., 2018; Ramesh et al., 2018; Schwarze et al., 2016; Wang, Katzschmann, et al., 2017; Xiao et al., 2015; Yang, Duarte, & Ganz, 2018). Even though interesting results have been reported in these studies, there are still a lot of challenges toward a reliable travel distance estimation methodology, based exclusively on visual cues. However, recent studies have shown that machine learning models, such as RCNNs (Li et al., 2018; Wang, Clark, et al., 2017), perform well in such tasks. Regarding the above, we opt to incorporate a state-of-the-art stereoscopic RGB-D sensor, namely Intel® RealSense™ D435 with machine learning models, in order to achieve accurate object distance estimation and enhance the performance and robustness of VO irrespectively of the environment, i.e., crowded, outdoor, indoor, etc. Another aspect of the visual measurement domain that could further contextualize the detected obstacles and objects toward enhanced users' experience is that of object/obstacle size measurement, based on visual cues. The research work on this domain is very limited. As reported in the studied literature, the accurate estimation of the size of an object depends on the shape of the object/obstacle, the quality of the image (Hao et al., 2015), the accurate distance estimation from the camera to the object to be measured (Iakovidis, Dimas, et al., 2018) and the accurate detection of the object (Mustafah et al., 2012). Taking into account all of the above, in the proposed system we consider the depth information acquired from the aforementioned RGB-D sensor, and the methodology we proposed in Iakovidis, Dimas, et al. (2018) alongside with the object detection methods discussed in Sect. 10.3.2. Since in the research domain of the visual size estimation there is wide space for improvement, extensions of our visual size estimation method are also investigated, along with the potentials of an ANN-based solution trained to estimate the size of an object/obstacle.

Undoubtedly, emotion recognition is a technology that has attracted the interest of numerous applications in the broader field of human–computer interaction and satellite research areas of computer science. Among these fields, emotion recognition from speech is expected to play an important role, since VUIs are continuously spreading in every part of daily life, i.e., within the home environment, the car, during interaction with computers, mobile phones, phone transactions, etc. It is considered as a slightly invasive approach, compared, e.g., to those using cameras or on-body sensors. The proposed non-linguistic approach uses a CNN, trained using raw speech information encoded as a spectrogram image, having potential to be effective even in cross-language situations. The determination of the users' emotional state during the interaction with the VUI may be used to provide a humanistic modality, able to enhance the process of collecting and mapping user experiences per geographical location visited by the users. In addition, near-natural human–machine interaction is complemented by the use of higher-level inference capabilities, through uncertainty-aware cognitive models, such as FCMs.

The human-centered design process is considered as an important process for setting and addressing the user and design requirements through the various stages of the system's development. For the elicitation of the user requirements for assistive systems focusing on visual impaired people's guidance, ten studies have been studied and in total 108 relevant user requirements have been identified, with respect to relevant CV-based systems, audio descriptions, cloud/GPS-based information systems, and services for learning from cultural heritage and museum accessibility. Most of the user requirements involve audio-based functions, tactile-functions, functions for guidance and description of the surrounding environment, requirements for addressing connectivity issues and design-oriented requirements like battery life and device size.

10.7 Conclusions

This chapter presented the concept of a novel system for computer-assisted navigation and guidance of visually impaired individuals to outdoor environments of cultural interest. The presentation of the system was supported by literature reviews targeted to identify state-of-the-art technological advancements and challenges toward its implementation.

The proposed system is wearable, in the form of smart-glasses, and fully intelligent, in the sense that it integrates components enabling both low and higher-level artificial cognitive processing of multimodal data, including audiovisual data acquired by a stereoscopic depth sensing camera and a microphone, and location data provided by a GPS. Core components that better adapt to the goals of the system include DNN architectures, such as LB-FCN and RNNs, which depending on the task, their design takes into account the tradeoff between the required accuracy and complexity. Features of the system include detection of obstacles, object recognition, emotion-aware voice-based interaction with the user, situation-awareness and decision making upon the users' responses and activities, while providing audio descriptions of the cultural sights of interest.

These capabilities render the system well-beyond the state-of-the-art with respect to: (a) conventional audiovisual aids that have been proposed mainly for navigation of indoor museum navigation, and (b) more general, commercially available solutions for outdoor navigation of the visually impaired. Novel features of the proposed system with respect to the state-of-the-art vision-based assistive technologies include: (a) critical object detection and human–machine interaction based on lightweight CNN architectures running on the MPU, aiming to real-time performance for the users' safety; (b) visual measurement capabilities enhanced with object size estimation; (c) recognition of the users' emotions.

Following the user-requirements analysis performed based on the literature, the most significant challenge is to maximize the system's usability, mainly with respect to:

- Real-time response times;
- Tolerance against various conditions related to the users' environment and activities;
- Natural, user-friendly and efficient human–machine interaction prohibiting cognitive overload;
- Accuracy with respect to navigation even in places where the information provided by the GPS is insufficient;
- Energy autonomy.

The proposed system is being developed in the scope of cultural sights accessibility; however, the vision is to provide an extensible solution that could be ultimately used as an everyday gadget that will improve the quality of life of the visually impaired.

Acknowledgments This research has been co-financed by the European Union and Greek national funds through the Operational Program Competitiveness, Entrepreneurship and Innovation, under the call RESEARCH—CREATE—INNOVATE (project code: T1EDK-02070).

References

Aladren, A., López-Nicolás, G., Puig, L., & Guerrero, J. J. (2016). Navigation assistance for the visually impaired using RGB-D sensor with range expansion. *IEEE Systems Journal, 10*, 922–932.

Alkhafaji, A., Fallahkhair, S., Cocea, M., & Crellin, J. (2016). A survey study to gather requirements for designing a mobile service to enhance learning from cultural heritage. In *European Conference on Technology Enhanced Learning* (pp. 547–550). Cham: Springer.

Anagnostopoulos, C.-N., Iliou, T., & Giannoukos, I. (2015). Features and classifiers for emotion recognition from speech: A survey from 2000 to 2011. *Artificial Intelligence Review, 43*, 155–177.

Asakawa, S., Guerreiro, J., Ahmetovic, D., Kitani, K. M., & Asakawa, C. (2018). The present and future of museum accessibility for people with visual impairments. In *Proceedings of the 20th International ACM SIGACCESS Conference on Computers and Accessibility* (pp. 382–384). New York, NY: ACM.

Badrinarayanan, V., Kendall, A., & Cipolla, R. (2017). SegNet: A deep convolutional encoder-decoder architecture for image segmentation. *IEEE Transactions on Pattern Analysis and Machine Intelligence, 39*, 2481–2495.

Baltrusaitis, T., McDuff, D., Banda, N., Mahmoud, M., el Kaliouby, R., Robinson, P., & Picard, R. (2011). Real-time inference of mental states from facial expressions and upper body gestures. In *Proceedings of 2011 IEEE International Conference on Automatic Face Gesture Recognition and Workshops (FG 2011)* (pp. 909–914). Washington, DC: IEEE.

Caraiman, S., Morar, A., Owczarek, M., Burlacu, A., Rzeszotarski, D., Botezatu, N., . . . Moldoveanu, A. (2017). Computer vision for the visually impaired: The sound of vision system. In *2017 IEEE International Conference on Computer Vision Workshop (ICCVW)* (pp. 1480–1489). Washington, DC: IEEE.

Conradie, P., Goedelaan, G. K. de, Mioch, T., & Saldien, J. (2014). Blind user requirements to support tactile mobility. In *Tactile Haptic User Interfaces for Tabletops and Tablets (TacTT 2014)* (pp. 48–53).

Cowie, R., Douglas-Cowie, E., Tsapatsoulis, N., Votsis, G., Kollias, S., Fellenz, W., & Taylor, J. G. (2001). Emotion recognition in human-computer interaction. *IEEE Signal Processing Magazine, 18*, 32–80.

Csapó, Á., Wersényi, G., Nagy, H., & Stockman, T. (2015). A survey of assistive technologies and applications for blind users on mobile platforms: A review and foundation for research. *Journal on Multimodal User Interfaces, 9*, 275–286.

Cui, L. (2018). MDSSD: Multi-scale Deconvolutional Single Shot Detector for small objects. arXiv preprint arXiv:1805.07009.

Dai, J., Li, Y., He, K., & Sun, J. (2016). R-fcn: Object detection via region-based fully convolutional networks. In *Advances in Neural Information Processing Systems* (pp. 379–387).

Diamantis, D., Iakovidis, D. K., & Koulaouzidis, A. (2018). Investigating cross-dataset abnormality detection in endoscopy with a weakly-supervised multiscale convolutional neural network. In *2018 25th IEEE International Conference on Image Processing (ICIP)* (pp. 3124–3128). Washington, DC: IEEE.

Diamantis, E. D., Iakovidis, D. K., & Koulaouzidis, A. (2019). Look-behind fully convolutional neural network for computer-aided endoscopy. *Biomedical Signal Processing and Control, 49*, 192–201.

Dimas, G., Spyrou, E., Iakovidis, D. K., & Koulaouzidis, A. (2017). Intelligent visual localization of wireless capsule endoscopes enhanced by color information. *Computers in Biology and Medicine, 89*, 429–440.

Elmannai, W., & Elleithy, K. (2017). Sensor-based assistive devices for visually-impaired people: Current status, challenges, and future directions. *Sensors, 17*, 565.

Erhan, D., Szegedy, C., Toshev, A., & Anguelov, D. (2014). Scalable object detection using deep neural networks. In *The IEEE Conference on Computer Vision and Pattern Recognition (CVPR)*.

Fang, Z., & Scherer, S. (2015). Real-time onboard 6dof localization of an indoor mav in degraded visual environments using a rgb-d camera. In *2015 IEEE International Conference on Robotics and Automation (ICRA)* (pp. 5253–5259). Washington, DC: IEEE.

Forster, C., Zhang, Z., Gassner, M., Werlberger, M., & Scaramuzza, D. (2017). Svo: Semidirect visual odometry for monocular and multicamera systems. *IEEE Transactions on Robotics, 33*, 249–265.

Fryer, L. (2013). Putting it into words: The impact of visual impairment on perception, experience and presence. Doctoral dissertation, Goldsmiths, University of London.

Fu, C.-Y., Liu, W., Ranga, A., Tyagi, A., & Berg, A. C. (2017). DSSD: Deconvolutional single shot detector. arXiv preprint arXiv:1701.06659.

Girshick, R. (2015). Fast r-cnn. In *Proceedings of the IEEE International Conference on Computer Vision* (pp. 1440–1448).

Girshick, R., Donahue, J., Darrell, T., & Malik, J. (2014). Rich feature hierarchies for accurate object detection and semantic segmentation. In *Proceedings of the IEEE Conference on Computer Vision and Pattern Recognition* (pp. 580–587).

Goodfellow, I., Pouget-Abadie, J., Mirza, M., Xu, B., Warde-Farley, D., Ozair, S., … Bengio, Y. (2014). Generative adversarial nets. In *Advances in Neural Information Processing Systems* (pp. 2672–2680).

Gubbi, J., Buyya, R., Marusic, S., & Palaniswami, M. (2013). Internet of Things (IoT): A vision, architectural elements, and future directions. *Future Generation Computer Systems, 29*, 1645–1660.

Haag, A., Goronzy, S., Schaich, P., & Williams, J. (2004). Emotion recognition using bio-sensors: First steps towards an automatic system. In *Tutorial and Research Workshop on Affective Dialogue Systems* (pp. 36–48). New York, NY: Springer.

Handa, K., Dairoku, H., & Toriyama, Y. (2010). Investigation of priority needs in terms of museum service accessibility for visually impaired visitors. *British Journal of Visual Impairment, 28,* 221–234.

Hao, M., Yu, H., & Li, D. (2015). The measurement of fish size by machine vision-a review. In *International Conference on Computer and Computing Technologies in Agriculture* (pp. 15–32). Cham: Springer.

He, K., Gkioxari, G., Dollár, P., & Girshick, R. (2017). Mask r-cnn. In *2017 IEEE International Conference on Computer Vision (ICCV)* (pp. 2980–2988). Washington, DC: IEEE.

He, K., Zhang, X., Ren, S., & Sun, J. (2015). Spatial pyramid pooling in deep convolutional networks for visual recognition. *IEEE Transactions on Pattern Analysis and Machine Intelligence, 37,* 1904–1916.

He, K., Zhang, X., Ren, S., & Sun, J. (2016). Deep residual learning for image recognition. In *Proceedings of the IEEE Conference on Computer Vision and Pattern Recognition* (pp. 770–778).

Held, D., Thrun, S., & Savarese, S. (2016). Learning to track at 100 FPS with deep regression networks. In *European Conference Computer Vision (ECCV)*.

Hersh, M. A., & Johnson, M. A. (2010). A robotic guide for blind people. Part 1. A multi-national survey of the attitudes, requirements and preferences of potential end-users. *Applied Bionics and Biomechanics, 7,* 277–288.

Hochreiter, S., & Schmidhuber, J. (1997). Long short-term memory. *Neural Computation, 9,* 1735–1780.

Hornik, K., Stinchcombe, M., & White, H. (1989). Multilayer feedforward networks are universal approximators. *Neural Networks, 2,* 359–366.

Howard, A. G., Zhu, M., Chen, B., Kalenichenko, D., Wang, W., Weyand, T., . . . Adam, H. (2017). Mobilenets: Efficient convolutional neural networks for mobile vision applications. arXiv preprint arXiv:1704.04861.

Huang, G., Liu, Z., Van Der Maaten, L., & Weinberger, K. Q. (2017). Densely connected convolutional networks. In *CVPR* (p. 3).

Huang, G., Sun, Y., Liu, Z., Sedra, D., & Weinberger, K. Q. (2016). Deep networks with stochastic depth. In *European Conference on Computer Vision* (pp. 646–661). Cham: Springer.

Iakovidis, D. K., Dimas, G., Karargyris, A., Bianchi, F., Ciuti, G., & Koulaouzidis, A. (2018). Deep endoscopic visual measurements. *IEEE Journal of Biomedical and Health Informatics.* https://doi.org/10.1109/JBHI.2018.2853987

Iakovidis, D. K., Georgakopoulos, S. V., Vasilakakis, M., Koulaouzidis, A., & Plagianakos, V. P. (2018). Detecting and locating gastrointestinal anomalies using deep learning and iterative cluster unification. *IEEE Transactions on Medical Imaging, 37,* 2196–2210.

Iandola, F. N., Han, S., Moskewicz, M. W., Ashraf, K., Dally, W. J., & Keutzer, K. (2016). Squeezenet: Alexnet-level accuracy with 50× fewer parameters and <0.5 mb model size. arXiv preprint arXiv:1602.07360.

International Organization for Standardization. (2010). ISO 9241-210:2010. https://www.iso.org/standard/52075.html.

Kaur, B., & Bhattacharya, J. (2018). A scene perception system for visually impaired based on object detection and classification using multi-modal DCNN. arXiv preprint arXiv:1805.08798.

Konda, K. R., & Memisevic, R. (2015). Learning visual odometry with a convolutional network. *VISAPP, 1,* 486–490.

Kovács, L., Iantovics, L., & Iakovidis, D. (2018). IntraClusTSP—An incremental intra-cluster refinement heuristic algorithm for symmetric travelling salesman problem. *Symmetry, 10,* 663.

Krizhevsky, A., Sutskever, I., & Hinton, G. E. (2012). Imagenet classification with deep convolutional neural networks. In *Advances in Neural Information Processing Systems* (pp. 1097–1105).

LeCun, Y., Bottou, L., Bengio, Y., & Haffner, P. (1998). Gradient-based learning applied to document recognition. *Proceedings of the IEEE, 86,* 2278–2324.

Ledig, C., Theis, L., Huszár, F., Caballero, J., Cunningham, A., Acosta, A., ... Twitter, W. S. (2017). Photo-realistic single image super-resolution using a generative adversarial network. In *CVPR* (p. 4).

Leng, H., Lin, Y., & Zanzi, L. (2007). An experimental study on physiological parameters toward driver emotion recognition. In *International Conference on Ergonomics and Health Aspects of Work with Computers* (pp. 237–246). Berlin, Heidelberg: Springer.

Li, R., Wang, S., Long, Z., & Gu, D. (2018). Undeepvo: Monocular visual odometry through unsupervised deep learning. In *2018 IEEE International Conference on Robotics and Automation (ICRA)* (pp. 7286–7291). Washington, DC: IEEE.

Lin, B.-S., Lee, C.-C., & Chiang, P.-Y. (2017). Simple smartphone-based guiding system for visually impaired people. *Sensors, 17,* 1371.

Lin, D. T., Kannappan, A., & Lau, J. N. (2013). The assessment of emotional intelligence among candidates interviewing for general surgery residency. *Journal of Surgical Education, 70,* 514–521.

Lin, S., Cheng, R., Wang, K., & Yang, K. (2018). Visual localizer: Outdoor localization based on convnet descriptor and global optimization for visually impaired pedestrians. *Sensors, 18,* 2476.

Lin, S., Wang, K., Yang, K., & Cheng, R. (2018). KrNet: A kinetic real-time convolutional neural network for navigational assistance. In *International Conference on Computers Helping People with Special Needs* (pp. 55–62). Berlin: Springer.

Lin, T.-Y., Dollár, P., Girshick, R. B., He, K., Hariharan, B., & Belongie, S. J. (2017). Feature pyramid networks for object detection. In *CVPR* (p. 4).

Lin, T.-Y., Goyal, P., Girshick, R., He, K., & Dollár, P. (2018). Focal loss for dense object detection. *IEEE Transactions on Pattern Analysis and Machine Intelligence.* https://doi.org/10.1109/TPAMI.2018.2858826

Liu, W., Anguelov, D., Erhan, D., Szegedy, C., Reed, S., Fu, C.-Y., & Berg, A. C. (2016). Ssd: Single shot multibox detector. In *European Conference on Computer Vision* (pp. 21–37). Cham: Springer.

Liu, Y., Yu, X., Chen, S., & Tang, W. (2016). Object localization and size measurement using networked address event representation imagers. *IEEE Sensors Journal, 16,* 2894–2895.

Luo, W., Li, J., Yang, J., Xu, W., & Zhang, J. (2018). Convolutional sparse autoencoders for image classification. *IEEE Transactions on Neural Networks and Learning Systems, 29,* 3289–3294.

Magnusson, C., Hedvall, P.-O., & Caltenco, H. (2018). Co-designing together with persons with visual impairments. In *Mobility of visually impaired people* (pp. 411–434). Switzerland: Springer.

Maimone, M., Cheng, Y., & Matthies, L. (2007). Two years of visual odometry on the mars exploration rovers. *Journal of Field Robotics, 24,* 169–186.

Mustafah, Y. M., Noor, R., Hasbi, H., & Azma, A. W. (2012). Stereo vision images processing for real-time object distance and size measurements. In *2012 International Conference on Computer and Communication Engineering (ICCCE)* (pp. 659–663). Washington, DC: IEEE.

Nistér, D., Naroditsky, O., & Bergen, J. (2004). Visual odometry. In *Proceedings of the 2004 IEEE Computer Society Conference on Computer Vision and Pattern Recognition, 2004 (CVPR 2004)* (pp. I652–I659). Washington, DC: IEEE.

Pan, J., Ferrer, C. C., McGuinness, K., O'Connor, N. E., Torres, J., Sayrol, E., & Giro-i-Nieto, X. (2017). Salgan: Visual saliency prediction with generative adversarial networks. arXiv preprint arXiv:1701.01081.

Panchanathan, S., Black, J., Rush, M., & Iyer, V. (2003). iCare-a user centric approach to the development of assistive devices for the blind and visually impaired. In *Proceedings. 15th IEEE International Conference on Tools with Artificial Intelligence, 2003* (pp. 641–648). Washington, DC: IEEE.

Papageorgiou, E. I., & Iakovidis, D. K. (2013). Intuitionistic fuzzy cognitive maps. *IEEE Transactions on Fuzzy Systems, 21,* 342–354.

Papageorgiou, E. I., & Salmeron, J. L. (2013). A review of fuzzy cognitive maps research during the last decade. *IEEE Transactions on Fuzzy Systems, 21,* 66–79.

Papakostas, M., & Giannakopoulos, T. (2018). Speech-music discrimination using deep visual feature extractors. *Expert Systems with Applications*. https://doi.org/10.1016/j.eswa.2018.05.016
Papakostas, M., Spyrou, E., Giannakopoulos, T., Siantikos, G., Sgouropoulos, D., Mylonas, P.,
& Makedon, F. (2017). Deep visual attributes vs. hand-crafted audio features on multidomain
speech emotion recognition. *Computation, 5*, 26.
Perakovic, D., Periša, M., & Prcic, A. B. (2015). Possibilities of applying ICT to improve safe
movement of blind and visually impaired persons. In C. Volosencu (Ed.), *Cutting edge research
in technologies*. London: IntechOpen.
Petrushin, V. (1999). Emotion in speech: Recognition and application to call centers. In *Proceed-
ings of Artificial Neural Networks in Engineering* (p. 22).
Piana, S., Stagliano, A., Odone, F., Verri, A., & Camurri, A. (2014). Real-time automatic emotion
recognition from body gestures. arXiv preprint arXiv:1402.5047.
Poggi, M., & Mattoccia, S. (2016). A wearable mobility aid for the visually impaired based
on embedded 3D vision and deep learning. In *2016 IEEE Symposium on Computers and
Communication (ISCC)* (pp. 208–213).
Psaltis, A., Kaza, K., Stefanidis, K., Thermos, S., Apostolakis, K. C., Dimitropoulos, K., &
Daras, P. (2016). Multimodal affective state recognition in serious games applications. In
2016 IEEE International Conference on Imaging Systems and Techniques (IST) (pp. 435–439).
Washington, DC: IEEE.
Pu, L., Tian, R., Wu, H.-C., & Yan, K. (2016). Novel object-size measurement using the digital
camera. In *Advanced Information Management, Communicates, Electronic and Automation
Control Conference (IMCEC), 2016 IEEE* (pp. 543–548). Washington, DC: IEEE.
Ramesh, K., Nagananda, S., Ramasangu, H., & Deshpande, R. (2018). Real-time localization and
navigation in an indoor environment using monocular camera for visually impaired. In *2018
Fifth International Conference on Industrial Engineering and Applications (ICIEA)* (pp. 122–
128). Washington, DC: IEEE.
Redmon, J., Divvala, S., Girshick, R., & Farhadi, A. (2016). You only look once: Unified, real-
time object detection. In *Proceedings of the IEEE Conference on Computer Vision and Pattern
Recognition* (pp. 779–788).
Redmon, J., & Farhadi, A. (2017). YOLO9000: Better, faster, stronger. arXiv preprint.
Ren, S., He, K., Girshick, R., & Sun, J. (2015). Faster r-cnn: Towards real-time object detection
with region proposal networks. In *Advances in Neural Information Processing Systems* (pp.
91–99).
Roberts, L. G. (1963). *Machine perception of three-dimensional solids*. Lexington, MA: Mas-
sachusetts Institute of Technology (MIT). Lincoln Laboratory.
Schwarze, T., Lauer, M., Schwaab, M., Romanovas, M., Böhm, S., & Jürgensohn, T. (2016). A
camera-based mobility aid for visually impaired people. *KI-Künstliche Intelligenz, 30*, 29–36.
Sermanet, P., Eigen, D., Zhang, X., Mathieu, M., Fergus, R., & LeCun, Y. (2013). Overfeat:
Integrated recognition, localization and detection using convolutional networks. arXiv preprint
arXiv:1312.6229.
Shah, N. F. M. N., & Ghazali, M. (2018). A systematic review on digital technology for enhancing
user experience in museums. In *International Conference on User Science and Engineering*
(pp. 35–46). Singapore: Springer.
Simonyan, K., & Zisserman, A. (2014). Very deep convolutional networks for large-scale image
recognition. arXiv preprint arXiv:1409.1556.
Sosa-Garcia, J., & Odone, F. (2017). "Hands on" visual recognition for visually impaired users.
ACM Transactions on Accessible Computing (TACCESS), 10, 8.
Spyrou, E., Vretos, N., Pomazanskyi, A., Asteriadis, S., & Leligou, H. C. (2018). Exploiting
IoT technologies for personalized learning. In *2018 IEEE Conference on Computational
Intelligence and Games (CIG)* (pp. 1–8). Washington, DC: IEEE.
Suresh, A., Arora, C., Laha, D., Gaba, D., & Bhambri, S. (2017). Intelligent smart glass for visually
impaired using deep learning machine vision techniques and robot operating system (ROS). In
International Conference on Robot Intelligence Technology and Applications (pp. 99–112).
Switzerland: Springer.

Szegedy, C., Ioffe, S., Vanhoucke, V., & Alemi, A. A. (2017). Inception-v4, inception-resnet and the impact of residual connections on learning. In *AAAI* (p. 12).

Szegedy, C., Liu, W., Jia, Y., Sermanet, P., Reed, S., Anguelov, D., ... Rabinovich, A. (2015). Going deeper with convolutions. In *Proceedings of the IEEE Conference on Computer Vision and Pattern Recognition* (pp. 1–9).

Szegedy, C., Vanhoucke, V., Ioffe, S., Shlens, J., & Wojna, Z. (2016). Rethinking the inception architecture for computer vision. In *Proceedings of the IEEE Conference on Computer Vision and Pattern Recognition* (pp. 2818–2826).

Tapu, R., Mocanu, B., & Zaharia, T. (2017). DEEP-SEE: Joint object detection, tracking and recognition with application to visually impaired navigational assistance. *Sensors, 17*, 2473.

Theodoridis, S., & Koutroumbas, K. (2009). *Pattern recognition* (4th ed.). Boston: Academic Press.

Tsatsou, D., Pomazanskyi, A., Hortal, E., Spyrou, E., Leligou, H. C., Asteriadis, S., ... Daras, P. (2018). Adaptive learning based on affect sensing. In *International Conference on Artificial Intelligence in Education* (pp. 475–479). Switzerland: Springer.

Uijlings, J. R., Van De Sande, K. E., Gevers, T., & Smeulders, A. W. (2013). Selective search for object recognition. *International Journal of Computer Vision, 104*, 154–171.

Vaščák, J., & Hvizdoš, J. (2016). Vehicle navigation by fuzzy cognitive maps using sonar and RFID technologies. In *2016 IEEE 14th International Symposium on Applied Machine Intelligence and Informatics (SAMI)* (pp. 75–80). Washington, DC: IEEE.

Vasilakakis, M. D., Diamantis, D., Spyrou, E., Koulaouzidis, A., & Iakovidis, D. K. (2018). Weakly supervised multilabel classification for semantic interpretation of endoscopy video frames. *Evolving Systems*, 1–13.

Wang, H., Hu, J., & Deng, W. (2018). Face feature extraction: A complete review. *IEEE Access, 6*, 6001–6039.

Wang, H.-C., Katzschmann, R. K., Teng, S., Araki, B., Giarré, L., & Rus, D. (2017). Enabling independent navigation for visually impaired people through a wearable vision-based feedback system. In *2017 IEEE International Conference on Robotics and Automation (ICRA)* (pp. 6533–6540). Washington, DC: IEEE.

Wang, J., Yang, Y., Mao, J., Huang, Z., Huang, C., & Xu, W. (2016). CNN-RNN: A unified framework for multi-label image classification. In *The IEEE Conference on Computer Vision and Pattern Recognition (CVPR)*.

Wang, S., Clark, R., Wen, H., & Trigoni, N. (2017). Deepvo: Towards end-to-end visual odometry with deep recurrent convolutional neural networks. In *2017 IEEE International Conference on Robotics and Automation (ICRA)* (pp. 2043–2050). Washington, DC: IEEE.

Wang, X., Gao, L., Song, J., & Shen, H. (2017). Beyond frame-level CNN: Saliency-aware 3-D CNN with LSTM for video action recognition. *IEEE Signal Processing Letters, 24*, 510–514.

WHO: World Health Organization. (2018). Blindness and visual impairment. http://www.who.int/news-room/fact-sheets/detail/blindness-and-visual-impairment.

Xiao, J., Joseph, S. L., Zhang, X., Li, B., Li, X., & Zhang, J. (2015). An assistive navigation framework for the visually impaired. *IEEE Transactions on Human-Machine Systems, 45*, 635–640.

Xie, S., Girshick, R., Dollár, P., Tu, Z., & He, K. (2017). Aggregated residual transformations for deep neural networks. In *2017 IEEE Conference on Computer Vision and Pattern Recognition (CVPR)* (pp. 5987–5995). Washington, DC: IEEE.

Yang, K., Wang, K., Bergasa, L. M., Romera, E., Hu, W., Sun, D., ... López, E. (2018). Unifying terrain awareness for the visually impaired through real-time semantic segmentation. *Sensors, 18*, 1506.

Yang, K., Wang, K., Zhao, X., Cheng, R., Bai, J., Yang, Y., & Liu, D. (2017). IR stereo realsense: Decreasing minimum range of navigational assistance for visually impaired individuals. *Journal of Ambient Intelligence and Smart Environments, 9*, 743–755.

Yang, Z., Duarte, M. F., & Ganz, A. (2018). A novel crowd-resilient visual localization algorithm via robust PCA background extraction. In *2018 IEEE International Conference on Acoustics, Speech and Signal Processing (ICASSP)* (pp. 1922–1926). Washington, DC: IEEE.

Yu, X., Yang, G., Jones, S., & Saniie, J. (2018). AR marker aided obstacle localization system for assisting visually impaired. In *2018 IEEE International Conference on Electro/Information Technology (EIT)* (pp. 271–276). Washington, DC: IEEE.

Zadeh, L. A. (1983). A computational approach to fuzzy quantifiers in natural languages. *Computers & Mathematics with Applications, 9*, 149–184.

Zeng, L. (2015). A survey: outdoor mobility experiences by the visually impaired. In *Mensch und Computer 2015–Workshopband*.

Zhang, J., Kaess, M., & Singh, S. (2017). A real-time method for depth enhanced visual odometry. *Autonomous Robots, 41*, 31–43.

Zhang, J., Ong, S., & Nee, A. (2008). Navigation systems for individuals with visual impairment: A survey. In *Proceedings of the Second International Convention on Rehabilitation Engineering & Assistive Technology* (pp. 159–162). Singapore: Singapore Therapeutic, Assistive & Rehabilitative Technologies (START) Centre.

Zhang, X., Zhou, X., Lin, M., & Sun, J. (2017). ShuffleNet: An extremely efficient convolutional neural network for mobile devices. ArXiv e-prints.

Zowghi, D., & Coulin, C. (2005). Requirements elicitation: A survey of techniques, approaches, and tools. In *Engineering and managing software requirements* (pp. 19–46). Berlin, Heidelberg: Springer.

Part III
Case Studies and Applications

Chapter 11
Toward Sustainable Domestication of Smart IoT Mobility Solutions for the Visually Impaired Persons in Africa

Abdulazeez Femi Salami, Eustace M. Dogo, Nnamdi I. Nwulu, and Babu Sena Paul

11.1 Introduction

According to projections of the World Health Organization, a considerably large proportion (more than 80%) of the world's visually impaired or blind population are in developing countries where capital needed for development and industrialization is inadequately very low (Pascolini & Mariotti, 2012; Resnikoff et al., 2004; World Health Organization, 2010, 2011). Unfortunately, Africa has a higher visual impairment or blindness burden in comparison with other developing economies as Africa is having about 10% of the global visually impaired and 15% of blind people while contributing only around 12% to the world's population (Pascolini & Mariotti, 2012; Resnikoff et al., 2004; Thylefors, Négrel, Pararajasegaram, & Dadzie, 1995). This visual impairment burden is exacerbated by the shortage of orthoptists, optometrists, ophthalmologists, orientation and mobility specialists, eye care facilities and eye health infrastructure in many African countries (Cooke, 2010; Smith, Frick, Holden, Fricke, & Naidoo, 2009).

A. F. Salami (✉)
Computer Engineering Department, Faculty of Engineering & Technology, University of Ilorin, Ilorin, Nigeria
e-mail: salami.af@unilorin.edu.ng

E. M. Dogo · N. I. Nwulu
Department of Electrical and Electronics Engineering Science, Faculty of Engineering and the Built Environment, University of Johannesburg, Johannesburg, South Africa
e-mail: eustaced@uj.ac.za; nnwulu@uj.ac.za

E. M. Dogo · B. S. Paul
Institute for Intelligent Systems, Faculty of Engineering and the Built Environment, University of Johannesburg, Johannesburg, South Africa
e-mail: eustaced@uj.ac.za; bspaul@uj.ac.za

© Springer Nature Switzerland AG 2020
S. Paiva (ed.), *Technological Trends in Improved Mobility of the Visually Impaired*,
EAI/Springer Innovations in Communication and Computing,
https://doi.org/10.1007/978-3-030-16450-8_11

Visually impaired people in Africa are therefore faced with impediments and high costs of accessing primary eye care services (AMD Alliance International, 2010; Kuper et al., 2008). Due to the challenging economic situation in most African countries, most of the visually impaired cannot afford these basic services and are thus socially excluded while in most cases, relying heavily on volunteers, human guides and crude navigation aids like walking sticks/canes for their daily routines and movements (Cooke, 2010; Kuper et al., 2008; Smith et al., 2009). It is therefore manifestly clear that mobility needs of the visually impaired in Africa are unique, pressing and demanding a paradigmatic shift from the manual to the technological.

A viable technological solution that can fill this void and meet these mobility needs is the Internet of Things (IoT) or Internet of Objects. IoT is the third wave of internet evolution concerned with the connection of objects with sensors, electronic devices, software and other network components in an intelligent/smart manner (Harvard Business Review, 2014; Mattern & Floerkemeier, 2010). The ubiquity of internet connectivity coupled with the miniaturization of sensors, actuators, and electronic devices have facilitated this revolutionary transition into IoT (Harvard Business Review, 2014; Vermesan & Friess, 2012). The abilities, benefits, potentials, promises, and prospects of this explosive technology are immense, limitless, and most especially, the successful implementation of IoT can significantly improve the standard/quality of living for people with disabilities and special needs (Mattern & Floerkemeier, 2010; Vermesan & Friess, 2012).

Moreover, the Internet of Everything (IoE) is another pertinent emerging technology which aims to connect things with data, people, and processes in order to achieve richer and more meaningful information, more effective and powerful capabilities, and more fruitful economic opportunities for citizens, corporations, and countries (Mitchell, Villa, Stewart-Weeks, & Lange, 2013; Vermesan & Friess, 2012). A number of IoT-based smart assistive technologies have already been designed and deployed for the visually impaired in developed ICT economies (Daugherty, Negm, Banerjee, & Alter, 2015; Vermesan & Friess, 2012). However, the African ICT economy still needs to dynamically transform from being consumers of IoT solutions relying on technology transfer to genuine prosumers who can use technology domestication and innovation to harness the full benefits of smart IoT mobility solutions.

This chapter provides an assessment of smart IoT-based mobility solutions, potential applications, and implementation instances pertinent to the African context. Section 11.2 of this chapter discusses relevant key background concepts as IoT, IoE, cloud computing, big data, and data mining by shedding light on the relevant technical definitions, characteristics, and features. This section also elucidates the IoT/IoE models, architectures, and components together with the general benefits of adopting this revolutionizing technology. This section also discusses the prospects, promises, and potentials of this emerging technology. Furthermore, the landscape of IoT/IoE in Africa is overviewed.

The specific applications of IoT as smart mobility solutions for the visually impaired together with pertinent implementation instances and examples of smart IoT mobility solutions in Africa are discussed in Sect. 11.3. In Sect. 11.4, technology transfer and domestication are discussed with respect to their technical definitions, selected characteristics, and salient features. Subsequently, the vital importance and urgent need for technology domestication in African countries is explained. Subsequently, selected models, factors, and relevant strategies for domesticating technology in Africa are examined. The section lastly analyses the important topic of sustaining domestication in order to achieve the vital goal of sustainable domestication.

In Sect. 11.5, an outline of the state of sustainable domestication in Africa is discussed. Adoption challenges and implementation barriers to the sustainable domestication of smart IoT mobility solutions for the visually impaired in Africa are discussed. Subsequently, facilitation factors and growth catalysts for sustainable domestication of smart IoT mobility solutions for the visually impaired in the African context are examined. This section lastly proffers implementable, practical, and technical recommendations as a solution to the existing challenges in order to shed more light on feasible avenues for sustainable technology domestication of smart IoT mobility solutions for the visually impaired in Africa. Section 11.6 concludes this chapter.

11.2 Overview of Key Background Concepts

This section explains the concepts of IoT, IoE, cloud computing, big data, and data mining by shedding light on the relevant technical definitions, characteristics, and features. The section also elucidates the IoT and IoE models, architectures, and components together with the general benefits of adopting this revolutionizing technology and the prospects, promise, and potentials of IoE are discussed. Furthermore, the landscape of IoT/IoE in Africa is overviewed.

11.2.1 Internet of Things (IoT)

IoT is a vast and complex area of research that encompasses enabling hardware, software, middleware components, and associated protocols and operating system that enable it to function as a complete system, its impact on society including security and privacy, legal and regulatory frameworks and the information expected to be derived from the generated data. It is also a representation of the convergence of several domains. This makes defining IoT holistically a very challenging task, due to these different perspectives. In Minerva, Biru, and Rotondi (2015) two definitions are proffered depending on the IoT deployment scale as:

Small-scaled IoT deployment: *"An IoT is a network that connects uniquely identifiable "Things" to the Internet. The "Things" have sensing/actuation and potential programmability capabilities. Through the exploitation of unique identification and sensing, information about the "Thing" can be collected and the state of the 'hing' can be changed from anywhere, anytime, by anything."*

Large-scaled IoT deployment: *"Internet of Things envisions a self-configuring, adaptive, complex network that interconnects 'things' to the Internet through the use of standard communication protocols. The interconnected things have physical or virtual representation in the digital world, sensing/actuation capability, a programmability feature and are uniquely identifiable. The representation contains information including the thing's identity, status, location or any other business, social or privately relevant information. The things offer services, with or without human intervention, through the exploitation of unique identification, data capture and communication, and actuation capability. The service is exploited through the use of intelligent interfaces and is made available anywhere, anytime, and for anything taking security into consideration."*

IoT now finds application in every spheres of life which includes smart cities and environmental monitoring, smart grids, Industry 4.0, smart transportation and logistics, critical infrastructure and remote monitoring, healthcare and assistive living, agriculture and recently for IP-based interconnection of Nano-scale devices known as Internet of Nano-Things (IoNT) and in so many other domains (Gardašević et al., 2017).

The following are characteristics and features of IoT:

- Interconnection of Things/Devices
- Connection of things/devices to the internet
- Uniquely identifiable things/devices
- Ubiquity, sensing & actuation capability
- Embedded intelligence
- Interoperable communication capability
- Self-configurability and programmability.

Smart devices or things are physical or virtual objects with the ability to collaborate and network within the IoT ecosystem. Since these smart devices are broad and diverse, ranging from sensor/actuators, RFID tags, smartphone and people, and anything with the capability to interact and communicate with each other, it becomes challenging to have a single reference IoT architecture that is applicable to all scenarios and domains (Gardašević et al., 2017). Moreover, the common IoT architectures that have been proposed do not take into consideration the specific requirements of visually impaired segment of the society; hence a four-layer architecture is proposed in Vasco Lopes, Pinto, Furtado, and Silva (2014). Comprising: device/perception, network, service and application layers, depicted in Fig. 11.1, as against the five-layer TCP/IP stack of physical, data link, network, transport, and application layers.

IoT is an enabling technology found in all aspects of our life, across several industries and application domain. When properly implemented, IoT has great potential to improve our lives in several ways, including the visually impaired segment of the society. Generally, the benefits of IoT specific to visually impaired application will include (1) Reduced human interventions, (2) Cost reduction and efficiency, (3) Better data-driven decision support, (4) Increased productivity and social, economic, political and cultural inclusion, (5) Improved safety and

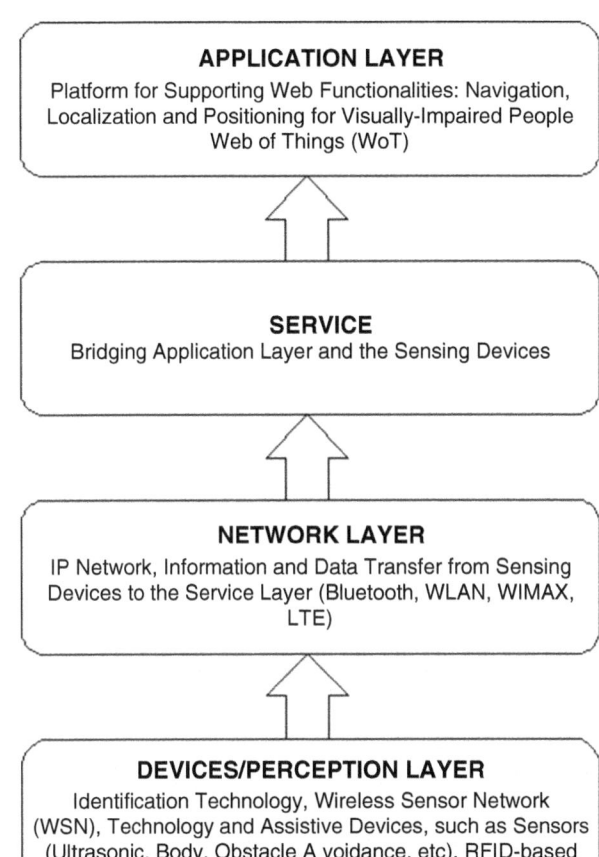

Fig. 11.1 IoT architecture (Domingo, 2012; Vasco Lopes et al., 2014)

situational-awareness, and (6) Independency and self-confidence (Domingo, 2012). Despite, all the benefits that IoT offers, security and privacy, coupled with legal liabilities that may arise due to implementation of IoT solutions, example will be a mishap due to error or cyber-attack on the IoT infrastructure leading to loss of life, are still the major concerns (Weber, 2010; Yang, Wu, Yin, Li, & Zhao, 2017).

11.2.2 Internet of Everything (IoE)

IoE is originally a Cisco concept and perspective of IoT in terms of the complex networked connection of people, data, processes, and things. Cisco defines IoE as (Cisco Systems, 2013): *"Bringing together people, process, data and things*

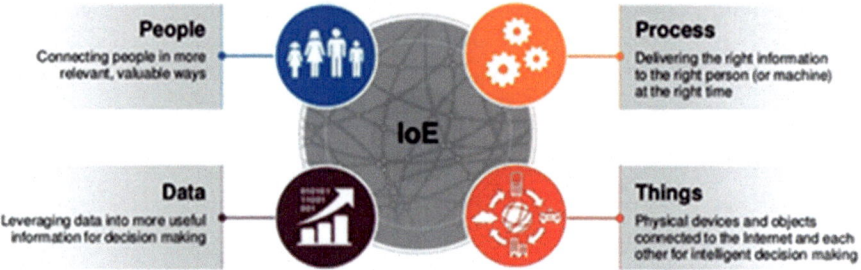

Fig. 11.2 IoT networked connection of people, processes, data, and things (Cisco)

to make networked connections more relevant and valuable than ever before, turning information into actions that create new capabilities, richer experiences and unprecedented economic opportunity for businesses, individuals and countries." IoE extends the scope of IoT beyond communications between machine-to-machine (M2M) communications to include machine-to-people (M2P) or people-to-machine (P2M) and technology-enabled user-generated people-to-people (P2P) communications and interactions, it envisions a scenario where people, information, and devices are interconnected (Evans, 2012), with advances in Artificial Intelligences (AI) and cognitive computing as enabling factors (Snyder & Byrd, 2017).

The IoE model is built on the convergence of four components of people, data, process, and things as conceptualized and depicted in Fig. 11.2, aimed at enriching the lives of people, businesses, and countries through industrial and business processes in numerous ways (Evans, 2012). People will be connected to the internet in diverse ways, data generated by devices or things like sensors will be transformed into information for better decision support. This process determines how people, data, and things relate with one another. In addition to this, advanced functionalities will be incorporated into this process to ensure that correct information gets to the right person at the right time in a secured manner (Evans, 2011, 2012).

Prospects, Promises, and Potentials of IoE

According to Cisco systems, IoE is an evolving concept that is going to find application and incredible impact in virtually all spheres of society, such as application in smart cities, smart grids (water, energy, etc.), business and commerce, manufacturing and Industry 4.0, healthcare and in security and emergency situations. It also has the potential to tackle numerous challenges facing humanity by analyzing heterogenous data in real-time from a vast number of interconnected sensors for the benefit of people and society. However, this comes with a considerable amount of risks and vulnerabilities (Evans, 2011, 2012), which must be addressed in order to realize the full potential of IoT.

Landscape of IoT and IoE in Africa

IoT in Africa is developing at a fast rate due to its practical application and potential to better the lives of people in the region. Applications such as internet and mobile banking help for easy payment of utilities and other services. IoT solutions in Africa are making life easier and more meaningful to the population through provisioning of the necessity of life, hence its quick adoption. An important enabling factor is the growth and penetration of mobile communication in Africa, perhaps due to its wireless transmission characteristics. Reliable network connectivity is a key ingredient for IoT and IoE to thrive. However, unlike the developed western economies, Africa still has challenges, ranging from unreliable power supply, governments hesitant to invest in IoT infrastructure due largely to dwindling financial incomes, and overdependence on unwilling foreign investors due to the complexities and risks involved. Despite these challenges, the region must find a way to invest in this critical and important technological trend due to the tremendous benefits that can be reaped now and in the future.

11.2.3   Cloud Computing

Cloud computing is a model for the delivery of on-demand computing resources and services over the internet through virtualization and multi-tenancy arrangement (Mell & Grance, 2011). Cloud computing architecture design is key to ensuring that assistive technology for visually impaired persons is accessible both technologically and financially as against standalone implementations in developing economies, by reducing hardware requirement, providing enhanced data analytics and heterogenous services (Temuçin, Keçeli, Kaya, Yaliç, & Tekinerdogan, 2018). Readers are referred to (Dogo, Salami, Aigbavboa, & Nkonyana, 2019; Dogo, Salami, & Salman, 2013) for details on cloud computing concepts, its analysis and how it relates to Africa.

11.2.4   Big Data and Data Mining

The rate of deployment and proliferation of IoT-connected devices and sensors is a major source of data being generated and transmitted over the cloud. It is a consensus by the majority of researchers that the number of these connected devices will grow exponentially in the near future, with Cisco predicting over 50 billion by 2020. It must be mentioned that data generated in this manner should meet the "big data" criteria, namely; volume, variety, velocity, veracity, and value (Neves &

Bernardino, 2015). Deep learning algorithms would play a crucial role in processing and providing better and faster decision support services as it relates to smart IoT solutions (Temuçin et al., 2018).

11.3 Smart IoT Mobility Solutions for the Visually Impaired Persons

This section looks at the specific applications of IoT as smart mobility solutions for the visually impaired and with the pertinent implementation instances and examples of smart IoT mobility solutions in Africa.

11.3.1 Specific Applications of IoT as Smart Mobility Solutions

The main aim of IoT-based smart mobility solutions is to ensure safety and high level of independency to the visually impaired persons, which will enhance their quality of life, improve productivity and social inclusiveness. Visual assistive technology which is a technological solution that provides blind persons the ability to navigate their physical environment with easy using IoT sensors can be broadly categorized into three broad categories: vision enhancement, vision substitution, and vision replacement (Elmannai & Elleithy, 2017). Vision enhancement is based on the visually displayed output from processed camera inputs, while vision substitution is non-visual display, based on hearing and touch senses. The vision replacement is a medical and technology-related solution (Elmannai & Elleithy, 2017). Vision substitution is further subdivided into Electronic Travel Aids (ETA), Electronic Orientation Aids (EOA), and Position Locator Devices (PLD) which are well detailed in Elmannai and Elleithy (2017).

Assistive devices can also be categorized based on their use such as computer and electronic aids, household and domestic activities aids, educational aids, mobility aids, reading aids, sports and outdoor leisure aids, writing and printing aids, signpost and currencies recognition aids and reading glasses as vision correction aid and other purposes (Disability Info South Africa, 2016).

11.3.2 Implementation Instances and Application Examples in Africa

In comparison with developed ICT economies, the African region has fewer application instances of IoT devices for the visually impaired. The most common

Fig. 11.3 Google glass with camera for zoom in

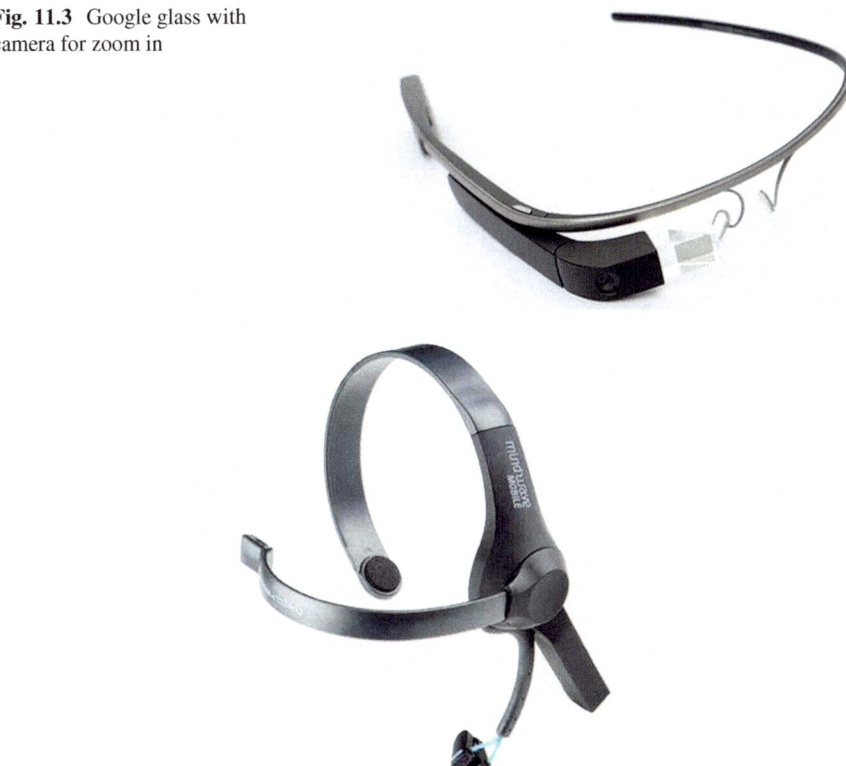

Fig. 11.4 Neurosky mindwave EEG headset with biosensors

and affordable navigation aids for visually impaired are walking cane and trained guide dogs. Nevertheless, over the past few years, African inventors are proffering technological-based solutions for the visually impaired which fall into vision enhancement, vision substitution or vision replacement, which are all visual assistive-based technologies. These implementation examples are based on smartphones, mobile phone applications, and sensors technologies. A few of these implementations of assistive technology and their technical contents are further discussed as follows:

ThinkAndZoom is a brain control-based blind assistive technology application designed by an African inventor that leverages on wearable technology and able to run on Google Glass (Fig. 11.3) or similar product built on Android to tackle visual impairment through performing visual magnification through zooming as soon as it receives focus brainwave signals from an *Electroencephalography* (EEG) reader, in this case *Neurosky Mindwave* biosensor (Fig. 11.4) (IT News Africa, 2015; ThinkandZoom, 2018).

GSM Communication Enabled Walking Cane Robot (GWCR) (FUTMinna, 2016; Okpanachi, 2018), designed by researchers at the Federal University of Technology

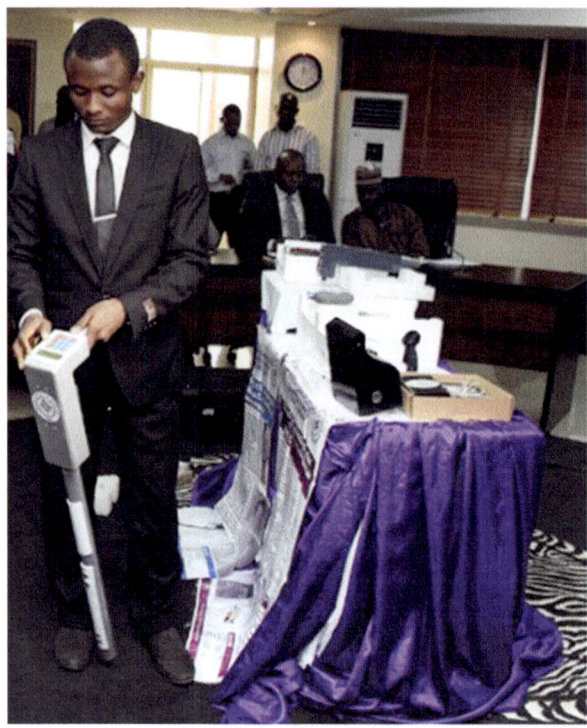

Fig. 11.5 GWCR prototype demonstration (Okpanachi, 2018)

Minna (FUTMinna), is equipped with mobile phone communication, fall and obstacle detection algorithm, flashlight for easy of navigation in dark environment, monitoring vital signs of individual and real-time transmission of the vital signals to a remote health care center. The system was developed with aged people in mind to enhance their ambulation, they also form a substantial number in the society that are visually impaired. A prototype demonstration of GWCR is depicted in Fig. 11.5 (Okpanachi, 2018).

Mobility Support Smart Walking Stick (MSSWS) (Onwuka, Oladepo, John, & Mark, 2017) for obstacle avoidance with a mobile phone incorporated to initiate calls in case of a fall or emergency situation. Are other assistive devices based on microcontrollers, GSM module to enable mobile communication, sensors as ultrasonic, light and collision avoidance sensor; and actuators as buzzer and vibrator, in addition to system control and power buttons source that are currently being developed. Figure 11.6 shows a block diagram of such a design's consideration.

BeSpecular (BeSpecular, 2016) is an app where the visually impaired people seek help from sighted people in the BeSpecular community, by taking a photo of what they need help with and with an accompanying voice message. The sighted people reply either in the form of a text or voice message to the inquiring of the

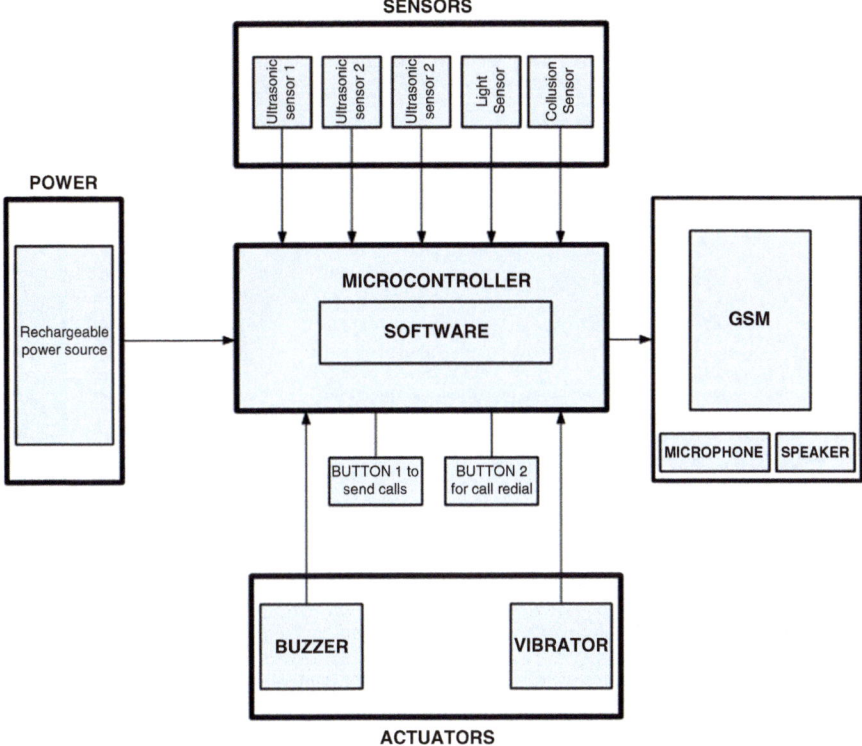

Fig. 11.6 Block diagram of mobility support smart walking stick

visually impaired person, who in turn rates the helpfulness of the response received from the sighted persons.

Mali-Bhala developed by blind SA (BlindSA, 2017) is a low-cost assistive device (Fig. 11.7) used to differentiate between the five South African bank notes as well as a signature guide, thereby enabling the visually impaired person to independently sign documents and count money.

Table 11.1 shows a summary of the highlighted assistive technology implementation instances in Africa. We could conclude that, due to the economic and peculiar situation in Africa, focus should be in developing innovative, indigenous, and low-cost assistive devices to cover a large spectrum of society. This is because high-tech devices would either be expensive to acquire or/and complex to use especially for the elderly or non-literate persons.

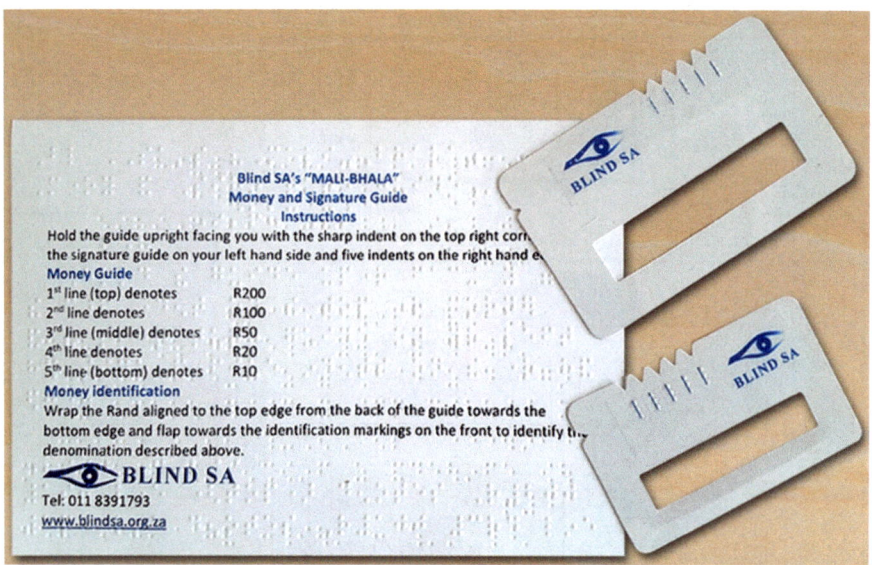

Fig. 11.7 Mali-Bhala money counting and signature aid

Table 11.1 Comparative summary of assistive technology implementations

	Assistive technology				
Feature	Think&Zoom	GWCR	MSSWS	BeSpecular	Mali-Bhali
Vision aid category	Vision enhancement	Vision substitution	Vision substitution	Vision substitution	Vision substitution
IoT enabled	Yes	Yes	Yes	Yes	No
Mobility features	No	Yes	Yes	No	No
Country developed	United States	Nigeria	Nigeria	South Africa	South Africa
Research institution	Private Company	Public University	Public Universities	Private Company	NGO
Country deployed	United States	Nigeria	Nigeria	South Africa	South Africa
Domestication status	Exogenous innovation; Patented R&D product prototype	Indigenous innovation; R&D product prototype	Indigenous innovation; R&D product prototype	Indigenous innovation; Commercialized product	Indigenous innovation; Commercialized product

11.4   Technology Transfer, Domestication, and Sustainability

In this section, technology transfer and domestication are discussed with respect to their technical definitions, selected characteristics, and salient features. Subsequently, the vital importance and urgent need for technology domestication in African countries is explained. Then, selected models, factors, and relevant strategies for domesticating technology in Africa are examined. The section lastly analyses the important topic of sustaining domestication in order to achieve the vital goal of sustainable domestication.

11.4.1   Technical Definitions and Characteristic Features

Technology can be conceptually viewed as the penta-partite combination of software, hardware, management, know-how, and maintenance support (Jafarieh, 2001; Saad, 2000). Based on this definition, hardware, production plants, manufacturing processes, industrial machineries, specialized equipment, and other tangible forms of technology can be broadly termed as hard technology while software, management skills, technical know-how, innovative ideas, conceptual models, and other intangible forms of technology can be generally categorized as soft technology (Jafarieh, 2001; Redor & Saadi, 2011). However, technology transfer has a rather unusual meaning and unconventional understanding in the African ICT economy. From the African perspective, technology transfer entails the procurement and introduction of foreign technology from developed ICT economies into African countries for the purpose of industrial development and meeting other socio-economic needs (Davidson, 2001; Du Toit, 2002; United Nations, 1995). In this technology transaction model, transferees in African countries are reduced to mere consumers of technology since they do not actively participate and effectively contribute to the modeling, design, manufacturing, and production process (Patel, 1972, 1974). The key characteristic features of this approach to technology transfer are the strong dependence on learning by apprenticeship and the heavy reliance on foreign technology suppliers and turnkey projects for the rapid acquisition of ready-made services, products, equipment, and machineries from advanced ICT economies that are ready to be easily used upon delivery in African countries (Maskus, Hoekman, & Saggi, 2004; Patel, 1974).

On the other hand, technology domestication is the absorption, adaptation, and reinvention of foreign technology from developed ICT economies using local resources to suit local socio-economic conditions and requirements for the purpose of technological advancement, knowledge improvement, and industrial development (Berker, 2006; Lie & Sørensen, 1996). In this technology transaction model, recipients in African countries will assume the role of prosumers who can actively engage in production choices and the manufacturing process by customizing and indigenizing the foreign technology to suit local needs and requirements. The key characteristic features of this form of technology domestication are incremental innovation, capacity development, skills acquisition, personnel training, and mutual collaboration between indigenous and foreign experts (Lie & Sørensen, 1996; Silverstone & Haddon, 1996).

11.4.2 The Need and Significance of Technology Domestication

In the era of the fourth industrial revolution, the growth and advancement of nations are no more judged by ideals and ideologies but based on the yardstick of innovative technologies, smart solutions, pragmatic policies, and judicious practices (Akubue, 2000; Sachs, 2015). African ICT economy is uniquely complex as the constituent countries have different economic conditions, cultural inclinations, social orientations, and political situations. This reinforces the evident fact that a localized approach to technology adoption is needed in the African case in order to ensure innovations and technological solutions match the prevailing local challenges. In addition to this, there is also the urgent need for Africans to produce the technologies they consume by facilitating the establishment of a robust, specialized, and indigenous production market for home-grown solutions, innovations, and technologies (Akubue, 2000; Du Toit, 2002; Saad, 2000; United Nations, 1995).

This prosumer approach will strengthen and revive indigenous technology firms across African countries and most especially, entrench the culture of technology reuse, waste reduction, quality management, local capacity development, preventive maintenance, low-cost repair, and protection of data/information sensitive to homeland security (Sachs, 2015; United Nations, 2016). The ultimate benefit of the practical implementation of technology domestication is that it is a potent economic instrument for breaking the prevailing vicious cycle of unemployment, poverty, economic dependency, unsustainable consumption, energy inadequacies, infrastructural failures, technological backwardness, non-competitive market performance, and a plethora of other socio-economic challenges (United Nations, 2016; Zelenika & Pearce, 2014).

11.4.3 Domestication Factors and Strategic Process

The key detrimental factors of domestication in the context of African ICT economy are information penetration, fiscal justification, environmental condition, socio-economic situation, local competition, regional cooperation, foreign intervention, human considerations, government regulations, political will, local readiness, and other pertinent domestication factors (Du Toit, 2002; Patel, 1972). In order to ensure an effective and meaningful implementation of technology domestication, a number of vital steps and procedures need to be taken. These procedures are subsequently explained in the succeeding paragraphs with respect to the aforementioned domestication factors. It should be mentioned that this domestication process is adaptive, cyclic, and continuous as real-life events are inherently nonlinear, nonstationary, and nondeterministic (Davidson, 2001; Golomski & Golomski, 2002; Wallace, 2005; World Bank, 2008).

- *Needs Identification, Evaluation, and Concretization*: Environmental impact assessment needs to be carried out first by prospective recipients of foreign technology in African countries in order to unambiguously ascertain the real environmental consequences of adopting the technology of interest. Then, systematic gap analysis needs to be conducted in order to clearly identify technological gaps and actual needs based on local capacity, conditions and requirements and most importantly, to determine the right steps and decisions to be taken in order to achieve the desired level of technological advancement by putting the potential technology into good service. In addition to this, concretization research is needed to ensure that the technology acquisition plan and all associated estimations, projections, formulations, recommendations, and evaluations are solidly backed up and supported with convincing investment layouts, realistic schedules, feasible milestones, and demonstration of relevance to the local socio-economic needs.
- *Information, Knowledge, and Skills Acquisition*: In this stage, local research, training and development (RTD) centers; science, technology and innovation (STI) institutions; and other concerned stakeholders need to be galvanized into action in order to create enabling environments and equip the project team with the requisite sensitization, technical knowledge, managerial skills, resources, capacity and methods of conducting performance monitoring and obtaining quality feedback. Furthermore, there is the need for local stakeholders and foreign technology suppliers to synergize in order to establish a reliable technical support network and gain regular first-hand information and updates on the technology.
- *Agreement, Acquisition, and Assimilation*: After establishing a win-win synergy and understanding between local stakeholders and foreign technology suppliers, the technology transaction is properly and officially sealed through a contractual agreement that is enforceable by law. The technology is thereafter acquired through a mutually agreed means which is in line with the terms and conditions of the contract. Upon acquisition and meticulous inspection, a comprehensive technology assimilation plan needs to be developed in order to qualitatively stipulate and quantitatively measure all efforts needed for the full-scale adoption and domestication of the technology.
- *Value Engineering, Reverse Engineering and Re-engineering*: After cementing the technology assimilation plan, an incisive practical study of the different functionalities of the acquired technology needs to be conducted with the aim of value enhancement and performance improvement. Value engineering will

also take into consideration the cost of utilizing local resources in performing this practical investigation. The technological product needs to be disassembled afterwards in order to make the system architecture, structural organization, and detailed design layout accessible for the discovery and extraction of vital technical knowledge. Reverse engineering is followed by the replicative process of contriving a new technological product with similar operational performance and functionalities as the acquired technology.

- *Innovation, Valuation, Commercialization, and Competition*: After completing series of satisfactory checks and tests on the re-engineered technology, enhancements, improvements, and modifications are carefully and gradually included to suit local conditions with the objective of adding real and sustainable value to the technology. Valuation is subsequently carried out by authenticators, appraisers, valuators, and valuers in order to come up with a trustworthy report on the genuine worth, quality, validity, and authenticity of the innovation. Upon successful valuation, the domesticated technology is prepared for large-scale production, distribution, promotion, and sale for competition in the local, regional, and international ICT market.

11.4.4   Support for a Sustainable Domestication

Technology domestication is a very delicate process that involves the absorption, adaptation, and reinvention of an exogenous technology with indigenous resources to suit local conditions and meet socio-economic challenges (Berker, 2006; Lie & Sørensen, 1996; Silverstone & Haddon, 1996). However, domestication needs to be adequately sustained first before expecting domestication in return to sustain the local ICT economy and tackle socio-economic challenges. In order to sustain domestication, respective governments and stakeholders in different African countries need to address the following existing issues (Akubue, 2000; Davidson, 2001; Golomski & Golomski, 2002; Patel, 1974; World Bank, 2008; Zelenika & Pearce, 2014):

- Entering into lopsided, restrictive, exclusive, and inhibitive contracts and agreements
- Acquisition of readymade technologies having many complexities and intricacies
- Lack of lasting cordial relationship with foreign technology suppliers
- Dearth of local capacity and technical skills
- Low utilization of acquired technologies due to operational bottlenecks
- Long production intervals and significantly low productivity
- Out-of-date operation handbooks, cryptic documentations, and substandard manuals
- Reliance on quick fixes due to poor and reactive maintenance culture
- Management process is monotonous, highly bureaucratic, largely manual-based and too dependent on paper-works

- Critical delays resulting from faults, failures, breakdowns, and malfunctions
- Long waiting period for foreign fixtures, spare parts, extra components, and adjustment tools
- Unreliability and low quality of local equipment, facilities, infrastructures and raw materials coupled with high rate of electronic waste and scrap deposition
- Fragile internal linkage strategies and weak project planning, monitoring and control schemes
- Lack of political will and effective policies to drive sustainable consumption and production of technology
- Lack of commitment to total quality management and negligence of global best practices in ensuring safety and managing risks/disasters
- Lack of flexible and continuous training/learning process in accordance with frequent advancements and recent global technological trends

By tackling the aforementioned issues head-on, domestication will be properly sustained in order to ensure that the domesticated technology will meet the socio-economic needs of the present African generation without jeopardizing the local wants, demands, and requirements of future generations.

11.5 Sustainable Domestication of Smart IoT Mobility Solutions

In this section, an outline of the state of sustainable domestication in Africa is discussed. Afterwards, adoption challenges and implementation barriers to the sustainable domestication of smart IoT mobility solutions for the visually impaired in Africa are explained. Subsequently, facilitation factors and growth catalysts for sustainable domestication of smart IoT mobility solutions for the visually impaired in the African context are examined. This section lastly proffers practicable, practical, and technical recommendations as solution to the existing challenges in order to shed more light on feasible avenues for sustainable technology domestication of smart IoT mobility solutions for the visually impaired in Africa.

11.5.1 Sustainable Domestication of Technology in Africa

The world is now technically entering the fourth industrial age which is typified by and tightly linked to innovative technologies, smart solutions, advanced automation, accelerated globalization, rapid industrialization, and sustainable urbanization (Sachs, 2015; United Nations, 2016). In developed ICT economies, investments in these technological advancements have generated billions of dollars in revenue for recent years. Furthermore, statistics have shown that this high rate of return on technology investment is projected to follow a positively increasing trend

(Daugherty et al., 2015; Future Market Insights, 2018). However, the African ICT economy is still yet to maximize the potentials of smart technological solutions and reap these financial benefits.

Unfortunately, the current policy of consumerism is further widening this digital and economic divide and most importantly, it has made Africa's domestication of smart innovations and technological solutions relatively very slow in most instances (Patel, 1972, 1974). This undesirably slow rate of sustainable domestication has further worsened Africa's foreign technology reliance, economic dependency, declining production, rising unemployment, and pervading inequality. It is worthy of note that many foreign technology firms are already operating in Africa by bringing in expert services and selling their products to local consumers. The worrisome aspect of such foreign business interventions is that investment returns, generated revenues, and profits are not locally retained in most cases but transferred back to developed countries (Davidson, 2001; Patel, 1974; United Nations, 1995).

Consequently, most African countries are genuinely not in control of these business transactions and sadly, cannot derive maximum benefits from taxes and enforce equitable re-investment of generated revenues to serve local needs and requirements (Du Toit, 2002; Maskus et al., 2004; Saad, 2000). In addition to this, the present inadequacy of indigenous manufacturing capacity and homemade technological solutions is aggravating the situation and making consumption of readymade foreign innovations indispensable for African countries (Akubue, 2000; Patel, 1974; United Nations, 2016). It is therefore undoubtedly clear that African countries need to urgently shift focus from short-term gains to the practical implementation of sustainable domestication in order to reap the maximum long-term benefits of sustainable technological development.

11.5.2 Adoption Challenges and Implementation Barriers

The adoption challenges and implementation barriers to sustainable domestication of smart IoT mobility solutions for the visually impaired in Africa are (Abdul, 2015a, 2015b; Belay, 2005; Dogo et al., 2013, 2019):

- *Socio-Cultural Perception and Socio-Economic Exclusion*: Most African societies view this special group (blind and visually impaired) as burdens/liabilities and as a result, treat them with stigmatization, discrimination, and marginalization. This negative view changed with time into strong habits and hardened belief and unfortunately, due to frequent repetition and exposure, this special group are gradually yielding and beginning to accept these demoralizing perceptions and limiting beliefs about them as truths and facts resulting in the erroneous feeling of guilt, shame, withdrawal, introversion, weakness, dependence, inactivity, and incapability. The implication of these limiting beliefs is the exclusion of this special group from mundane functions/responsibilities and socio-economic activities. This means their wants, thoughts, needs, perspectives, views, demands, and opinions are mostly not considered in devising socio-economic solutions, formulating national policies, and implementing fiscal plans. In addition to what has been mentioned, most of those who fall into this special group are downtrodden, disadvantaged and in a state of poverty and vulnerability. This makes effective social participation extremely difficult for them and most importantly, it cuts them off from actively and productively contributing in the process of domesticating smart IoT mobility solutions by participating in experimental trials, prototype testing, actual deployments, product assessments, specifying design requirements, and providing useful feedbacks for sustainable innovation.

- *Market Restrictions and Financial Constrictions*: Most governments of African countries impose local regulations and support oligopolistic practices and back-door arrangements that block the transaction channel between willing foreign technology suppliers and local prosumers, start-ups, and entrepreneurs. In addition to restricting free interaction, another barrier is the unstable and erratic market situations which frightens and discourages foreign technology suppliers from investing in many African countries. Other barriers relevant to this research context are the undesirably small market size; unsatisfactorily low level of capital, competitiveness, credit access, incentives, income, and productivity; tight trade barriers; and high investment risks/costs. In addition to this, most African countries are battling with huge national debts, resource deficits, and financial doldrums. These challenges make it difficult for the wholesale adoption and practical implementation of sustainable domestication of smart IoT mobility solutions for the support of the visually impaired in Africa.

- *Weak Institutions and Inconsistent Regulations*: Volatile policies, incompatible laws, and uncertain standards are very common with African countries. These problems are as a result of ineffective governance, political nonchalance, weak public mechanisms, legal sloppiness, negotiation deadlocks, government opacity and distrust, little understanding of local needs and demands, lack of vision, incoordination among local STI institutions, non-conformance with global best practices, and refusal to assume responsibilities and share liabilities. These existing issues discourage foreign technology investment that can foster sustainable domestication of smart IoT mobility technologies that will assist the visually impaired in Africa.

- *Crippled Backbone Infrastructure*: The core and critical infrastructure needed for the sustainable domestication of smart IoT mobility solutions for the visually impaired are in a very fragile, deplorable, and obsolete state in most African countries. In addition to this, another associated barrier is the lack of technical records and documentation on how infrastructural obsolescence have led to the failure of past foreign technology investments and agreements. This infrastructural failure is worsening due to institutionalized and systemic corruption, low funding of local engineering research and development (R&D) and mismanagement of national assets.

- *Limited Awareness and Low Capacity*: One of the key barriers to sustainable domestication of smart IoT mobility solutions for the visually impaired in Africa is the inadequacy of local capacity, training, materials, information resources, technical data, skills, and skilled personnel. Furthermore, another associated barrier is the low level of awareness with respect to emerging technologies, global technological trends, new/credible offers in the technology market and potential foreign technology suppliers/partners. In addition to this, the dearth of orientation and mobility (O&M) specialists is also a serious impediment as they are the ones with first-hand knowledge and experience regarding the mobility needs of the visually impaired and most importantly, the O&M specialists are key stakeholders whose practical opinions and recommendations are constantly needed by the system designers and engineers during the domestication process.

11.5.3 Facilitation Factors and Growth Catalysts

The facilitation factors and growth catalysts to sustainable domestication of smart IoT mobility solutions for the visually impaired in Africa are (Dogo et al., 2013, 2019; Mutele & Odeku, 2013; Omede, 2015):

- *Rural Innovations and Local Improvisations*: Most dwellers of rural areas in Africa are forced to improvise in order to survive and meet the minimum living standard. Basic guideposts, traditional home retrofits, walking frames, indigenous orientation aids, and simple crane/crutch modifications are some of the many interesting rural innovations used to facilitate the movement and navigation of the visually impaired within and outside the home. These helpful rural innovations are favorable and big drivers to sustainable domestication because the technological upgrades and tweaks needed to transform and adapt these local improvisations to smart IoT mobility solutions are relatively cheaper and requiring lesser complexity and sophistication.
- *Growing Advocacy for Disability Rights and Diversity*: Respective governments of most African countries are now realizing and becoming aware of the fact that sustainable technological development for addressing socio-economic challenges cannot be achieved without paying genuine attention to and taking care of diversity, social inclusion, and rights of people with special needs. Consequently, many non-governmental organizations (NGOs) are now vigorously campaigning for the rights of the blind and visually impaired in the rural areas of Africa. These movements and campaigns are gradually forcing the government to respect, recognize, and cater for the needs of this marginalized group.
- *Booming Millennials*: One of the strongest drivers for the sustainable domestication of smart IoT mobility solutions for the visually impaired in Africa is the large and growing population of millennials who are entrepreneurial, industrious, resourceful, trainable, technologically immersed, and more open-minded. These confident youths are tech-savvy, have high expectations and are much more eager to learn and comply with sustainable technology practices. This makes it very easy, quick and less costly for these vibrant African youths to be trained on global

best practices for domesticating and managing smart IoT mobility solutions for the visually impaired.

- *Upsurge of Internet and Mobile Penetration*: The continuing rise and success of internet service providers, mobile telecommunication industries, and wireless data players in Africa has practically made it possible for connecting, communicating, and reaching out to people with special needs in the outskirts, remote regions, and rural areas of Africa. By taking advantage of this rapid internet access and mobile penetration rate, Africa can strategically collaborate with global IoT leaders and leading innovators around the world to catalyze the sustainable domestication of smart IoT mobility solutions for the visually impaired in different African countries.
- *Boost from Local Industries*: Indigenous companies are gradually moving toward automated systems, IoT, and smart solutions in order to improve service delivery and achieve better customer satisfaction in urban and rural areas. This genuine interest from local industries to revolutionize their business with the power of smart IoT solutions is a strong facilitation factor and growth catalysts for the sustainable domestication of this technology. Furthermore, this positive industrial focus will open up fruitful opportunities and create enabling environments and receptive atmosphere for the seamless implementation of sustainable domestication of smart IoT mobility solutions for the visually impaired in Africa.

11.5.4 Technical Recommendations

The technical recommendations for sustainable domestication of smart IoT mobility solutions for the visually impaired in Africa are (Agarwal & Steele, 2016; Dogo et al., 2013, 2019; UNESCO, 2013):

- *Systematic Policy Reforms for Inclusion and Diversity*: Smart IoT mobility solutions for the visually impaired in Africa need solid support and backing from the government in order for sustainable domestication of this technology to survive and thrive. Consequently, there is the pressing need for strategic policy reforms in African countries at federal, state and local government levels in order to effectively make enforcements and provisions that will ensure the rights and needs of the visually impaired are respected and sufficiently met.
- *Smart Incentives and Investment-Friendly Regulations*: Respective governments of African countries need to promote fair competition, stable market systems, open economy, level playing field, fiscal integrity, and financial transparency. In addition to this, there is the need to provide incentives, relax trade barriers, and minimize investment risks/costs in order to attract global innovators and leading technology suppliers that will speed up the sustainable domestication of smart IoT mobility solutions for the visually impaired in Africa.
- *Forming Networks of Harmonized and Cohesive Institutions*: In order to ensure sustainable domestication of smart IoT mobility solutions for the visually

impaired in Africa, there is urgent need to ensure harmony, cohesion, and coordination among local STI institutions, corporate bodies, and all levels of government. This will lead to robust policies, impactful regulations, and sustainable practices that reflect strong vision and genuine understanding of the needs of visually impaired and people with special needs in the rural communities.

- *Massive Investment in Infrastructure*: Respective governments of African countries need to urgently devise and implement smart infrastructure financing strategies for the core and critical facilities needed for sustainable domestication of smart IoT mobility solutions for the visually impaired. Furthermore, there is the need to be committed to sustainable development and total quality management, urgently curb corrupt procurement practices, and continuously and adequately fund local science, engineering, and ICT research and development.
- *Propagate Intensive and Extensive STEM Skills*: There is an urgent need for infusing multidisciplinary and associative thinking skills in Africa at elementary, secondary, vocational, post-secondary, and postgraduate educational levels. This will inculcate the culture of curiosity, creativity, ingenuity, innovation and most importantly, ability to independently conduct multidisciplinary research for solutions to pressing socio-economic challenges. This will also be a fast track to the sustainable domestication of smart IoT mobility solutions for the visually impaired in Africa.

11.6   Conclusion

Sustainable development and domestication of smart IoT mobility solutions for the visually impaired are still in the budding phase in most African countries. However, it is highly imperative and urgent for respective governments of different African countries to make practical and bold steps for sustainable IoT transition in order to be a relevant/key player in the global ICT landscape and a major competitor in the global technology market. The present global technological trend is focused on contriving smart/intelligent networks of physical objects with data, devices, people, process, sensors, and software in order to achieve richer and more meaningful information, more effective and powerful capabilities, and more fruitful economic opportunities for citizens, corporations, and countries. The abilities, benefits, potentials, promises, and prospects of IoT/IoE are immense, limitless and most importantly, the sustainable development and domestication of this explosive technology can address the current socio-economic challenges and mobility needs of the visually impaired by positively improving their standard/quality of living. This strategic advantageous position can only be gained through the judicious acquisition, absorption, adaptation, and reinvention of existing and novel IoT solutions such as electronic orientation aids, wireless wearable navigation guides, position locator devices, electronic travel aids, and other forms of smart IoT mobility solutions for the visually impaired. By adopting this smart IoT mobility solutions for the visually impaired, the African ICT economy will be effectively equipped with home-grown innovative solutions that can appropriately and sustainably tackle a plethora of recurrent problems such as foreign technology reliance, unsustainable consumption, economic dependency, technological laggardness, declining production, deepening poverty, rising unemployment, pervading inequality, non-competitive market performance, and other forms of socio-economic challenges embattling the African continent.

References

Abdul, B. (2015a). How to harness mobile technology for services of persons with visual impairment in Africa. Beyond 2015: Delivering on the agenda for persons with visual impairment in Africa. In *Proceeding of Sixth Africa Forum*, Kampala, Uganda (pp. 325–330).

Abdul, B. (2015b). Technology transfer as a vehicle of ICT accessibility for all. Beyond 2015: Delivering on the agenda for persons with visual impairment in Africa. In *Proceeding of Sixth Africa Forum*, Kampala, Uganda (pp. 325–330).

Agarwal, A., & Steele, A. (2016). *Disability considerations for infrastructure programmes*. Retrieved December 9, 2018, from https://assets.publishing.service.gov.uk/media/57a08954ed915d3cfd0001c4/EoD_HDYr3_21_40_March_2016_Disability_Infrastructure.pdf.

Akubue, A. (2000). Appropriate technology for socioeconomic development in third world countries. *The Journal of Technology Studies, 26*(1), 33–43. https://doi.org/10.21061/jots.v26i1.a.6

AMD Alliance International. (2010). *The global economic cost of visual impairment*. Retrieved May 19, 2018, from http://www.icoph.org/dynamic/attachments/resources/globalcostofvi_finalreport.pdf.

Belay, T. E. (2005). African perspective on visual impairments – ICT's and policies: A personal experience, a variety of perspectives and technological solution. A paper presented to UNESCO at the World Summit on the Information Society Workshop on ICT and persons with disabilities.

Berker, T. (2006). *Domestication of media and technology* (1st publ. ed.). UK: Open University Press.

BeSpecular. (2016). *What is BeSpecular.* Retrieved December 6, 2018, from http://www.bespecular.com/en/.

BlindSA. (2017). *Breakthrough in assistive devices by blind sa.* Retrieved December 9, 2018, from http://blindsa.org.za/mobility/.

Cisco Systems. (2013). *The internet of everything: Global private sector economic analysis.* Cisco.

Cooke, J. G. (2010). Public health in Africa – A report of the CSIS global health policy center. *Journal of Public Health in Africa, 1*(1). https://doi.org/10.4081/jphia.2010.e8

Daugherty, P., Negm, W., Banerjee, P., & Alter, A. (2015). *Driving unconventional growth through the industrial internet of things.* Retrieved May 17, 2018, from https://www.accenture.com/mz-en/_acnmedia/Accenture/next-gen/reassembling-industry/pdf/Accenture-Driving-Unconventional-Growth-through-IIoT.pdf.

Davidson, O. R. (2001). *CDM and technology transfer: African perspectives.* Point de Vue, issue 14.

Disability Info South Africa. (2016). *Assistive devices & equipment.* Retrieved December 9, 2018, from http://disabilityinfosa.co.za/visual-impairments/assistive-devices-equipment/.

Dogo, E. M., Salami, A., & Salman, S. (2013). Feasibility analysis of critical factors affecting cloud computing in Nigeria. *International Journal of Cloud Computing and Services Science, 2*(4), 276–287. https://doi.org/10.11591/closer.v2i4.4162

Dogo, E. M., Salami, A. F., Aigbavboa, C. O., & Nkonyana, T. (2019). Taking cloud computing to the extreme edge: A review of mist computing for smart cities and industry 4.0 in Africa. In F. Al-Turjman (Ed.), *Edge computing*. Cham: Springer.

Domingo, M. C. (2012). An overview of the internet of things for people with disabilities. *Journal of Network and Computer Applications, 35*(2), 584–596. https://doi.org/10.1016/j.jnca.2011.10.015

Du Toit, A. S. A. (2002). The information economy in Africa: Putting the power into the hands of the individual. In L. Banwell & M. Collier (Eds.), *Human aspects of the Information Society: An international collection of papers* (pp. 61–69). Newcastle upon Tyne: Information Management Research Institute, Northumbria University.

Elmannai, W., & Elleithy, K. (2017). Sensor-based assistive devices for visually-impaired people: Current status, challenges, and future directions. *Sensors (Basel, Switzerland), 17*(3), 565. https://doi.org/10.3390/s17030565

Evans, D. (2011). *The internet of things: How the next evolution of the internet is changing everything.* Document, Retrieved December 5, 2018, from http://parlinfo.aph.gov.au/parlInfo/ search/display/display.w3p;query=library/jrnart/4327029.

Evans, D. (2012). *The internet of everything: How more relevant valuable connections will change the world.* Cisco Systems.

FUTMinna. (2016). *Development of GSM communication-based walking cane robot (GWCR) for enhancing ambulation.* Retrieved December 6, 2018, from https://seet.futminna.edu.ng/ departments/Mechatronics_Engineering/index.php/about-us/major-achievements.

Future Market Insights. (2018). Internet of things security product market to register a staggering expansion at 14.9% CAGR through 2027. *Web News Wire,* SyndiGate Media Inc.

Gardašević, G., Veletić, M., Maletić, N., Vasiljević, D., Radusinović, I., Tomović, S., & Radonjić, M. (2017). The IoT architectural framework, design issues and application domains. *Wireless Personal Communications, 92*(1), 127–148. https://doi.org/10.1007/s11277-016-3842-3

Golomski, W. A. J., & Golomski, W. A. (2002). A review of: "Methodological and technological issues in technology transfer: A special report of the intergovernmental panel on climate change" Bert Metz et al. (editors). Cambridge University Press. *IIE Transactions, 34*(6), 587–589.

Harvard Business Review. (2014). *Internet of things: Science fiction or business fact?* Retrieved May 13, 2018, from https://hbr.org/resources/pdfs/comm/verizon/ 18980_HBR_Verizon_IoT_Nov_14.pdf.

IT News Africa. (2015). *African inventor tackles visual impairment with ThinkAndZoom.* Retrieved June, 20, 2018, from http://www.itnewsafrica.com/2015/07/exclusive-african-inventor-tackles-visual-impairment-with-thinkandzoom/.

Jafarieh, H. (2001). Technology transfer to developing countries: A quantitative approach. University of Salford. Retrieved from ProQuest Dissertations & Theses Full Text: The Humanities and Social Sciences Collection database. Retrieved from https://search.proquest.com/docview/ 301583265.

Kuper, H., Polack, S., Eusebio, C., Mathenge, W., Wadud, Z., & Foster, A. (2008). A case-control study to assess the relationship between poverty and visual impairment from cataract in Kenya, the Philippines, and Bangladesh. *PLoS Medicine, 5*(12), e244. https://doi.org/10.1371/journal.pmed.0050244

Lie, M., & Sørensen, K. H. (1996). *Making technology our own?* Oslo: Scandinavian University Press. Retrieved from http://libris.kb.se/resource/bib/7168670

Maskus, K. E., Hoekman, B., & Saggi, K. (2004). *Transfer of technology to developing countries: Unilateral and multilateral policy options.* Policy Research Working Paper Series, issue 3332. Retrieved from http://econpapers.repec.org/paper/wbkwbrwps/3332.htm.

Mattern, F., & Floerkemeier, C. (2010). From the internet of computers to the internet of things. In *From active data management to event-based systems and more* (pp. 242–259). Berlin, Heidelberg: Springer Berlin Heidelberg.

Mell, P., & Grance, T. (2011). *The NIST definition of cloud computing.* Gaithersburg, MD: Computer Security Division, Information Technology Laboratory, National Institute of Standards and Technology.

Minerva, R., Biru, A., & Rotondi, D. (2015). Towards a definition of the internet of things (IoT). *IEEE Internet of Things.* Retrieved from iot.ieee.org.

Mitchell, S., Villa, N., Stewart-Weeks, M., & Lange, A. (2013). *The internet of everything for cities: Connecting people, process, data, and things to improve the 'livability' of cities and communities*. Cisco Systems.

Mutele, N. P., & Odeku, K. O. (2013). The role of an instructor in managing orientation and mobility of students with visual impairments at the University of Limpopo, South Africa. *Journal of Social Sciences, 36*(2), 165–173. https://doi.org/10.1080/09718923.2013.11893185

Neves, P. C., & Bernardino, J. (2015). Big data in the cloud: A survey. *Open Journal of Big Data (OJBD), 1*(2), 1–18.

Okpanachi, M. (2018, Researchers and students of FUT Minna develop multiple operator-enabled SIM card and digital walking stick. *TechNext*. Retrieved from https://technext.ng/2018/05/24/researchers-students-fut-minna-develop-simless-operator-digital-walking-stick/.

Omede, A. A. (2015). The challenges of educating the visually impaired and quality assurance in tertiary institutions of learning in Nigeria. *International Journal of Educational Administration and Policy Studies, 7*(7), 129–133. https://doi.org/10.5897/IJEAPS2015.0407

Onwuka, I. E., Oladepo, O., John, A., & Mark, A. (2017). A mobility support device (smart walking stick) for the visually impaired. *International Journal of Computer and Information Technology, 6*(4), 196–202.

Pascolini, D., & Mariotti, S. P. (2012). Global estimates of visual impairment: 2010. *The British Journal of Ophthalmology, 96*(5), 614–618. https://doi.org/10.1136/bjophthalmol-2011-300539

Patel, S. J. (1972). UNCTAD-III and the transfer of technology to developing countries. *Foreign Trade Review, 7*(3), 262–279. https://doi.org/10.1177/0015732515720305

Patel, S. J. (1974). The technological dependence of developing countries. *The Journal of Modern African Studies, 12*(1), 1–18. https://doi.org/10.1017/S0022278X00008946

Redor, D., & Saadi, M. (2011). International technology transfer to developing countries: When is it immiserizing? *Revue D'Économie Politique, 121*(3), 409–433. Retrieved from EconLit database. Retrieved from https://www.jstor.org/stable/43859919

Resnikoff, S., Pascolini, D., Etya'ale, D., Kocur, I., Pararajasegaram, R., Pokharel, G. P., & Mariotti, S. P. (2004). Global data on visual impairment in the year 2002. *Bulletin of the World Health Organization, 82*(11), 844. Retrieved from MEDLINE database. Retrieved from http://www.ncbi.nlm.nih.gov/pubmed/15640920

Saad, M. (2000). *Development through technology transfer: Creating new organisational and cultural understanding*. Intellect. Retrieved from http://www.vlebooks.com/vleweb/product/openreader?id=none&isbn=9781841508207&uid=none.

Sachs, J. D. (2015). *Age of sustainable development*. New York: Columbia University Press.

Silverstone, R., & Haddon, L. (1996). *Design and the domestication of information and communication technologies: Technical change and everyday life*. Oxford: Oxford University Press.

Smith, T. S. T., Frick, K. D., Holden, B. A., Fricke, T. R., & Naidoo, K. S. (2009). Potential lost productivity resulting from the global burden of uncorrected refractive error. *Bulletin of the World Health Organization, 87*(6), 431. Retrieved from MEDLINE database. Retrieved from http://www.ncbi.nlm.nih.gov/pubmed/19565121

Snyder, T., & Byrd, G. (2017). The internet of everything. *Computer, 50*(6), 8–9. https://doi.org/10.1109/MC.2017.179

Temuçin, H., Keçeli, A. S., Kaya, A., Yaliç, H. Y., & Tekinerdogan, B. (2018). A cloud-based big data system to support visually impaired people. In *Computational intelligence for multimedia big data on the cloud with engineering applications*. Elsevier Academic Press. Retrieved from http://www.narcis.nl/publication/RecordID/oai:library.wur.nl:wurpubs%2F540636

ThinkandZoom. (2018). *ThinkandZoom – Hands free visual magnification powered by the human mind*. Retrieved Jun 20, 2018, from http://thinkandzoom.com/.

Thylefors, B., Négrel, A. D., Pararajasegaram, R., & Dadzie, K. Y. (1995). Global data on blindness. *Bulletin of the World Health Organization, 73*(1), 115. Retrieved from MEDLINE database. Retrieved from http://www.ncbi.nlm.nih.gov/pubmed/7704921

UNESCO. (2013). *The ICT opportunity for a disability-inclusive development framework: New action-oriented report.* Retrieved December 6, 2018, from https://en.unesco.org/news/ict-opportunity-disability-inclusive-development-framework-new-action-oriented-report.

United Nations. (1995). Technology transfer, negotiation and acquisition in the context of promoting the African Economic Community. In *ECA African Regional Conference on Science and Technology Meeting.* Addis Ababa, Ethiopia: UN.

United Nations. (2016). *Global sustainable development report.* New York. Retrieved December 9, 2018, from https://sustainabledevelopment.un.org/globalsdreport/.

Vasco Lopes, N., Pinto, F., Furtado, P., & Silva, J. (2014). IoT architecture proposal for disabled people. In *2014 IEEE 10th International Conference on Wireless and Mobile Computing, Networking and Communications (WiMob)* (pp. 152–158). https://doi.org/10.1109/WiMOB.2014.6962164.

Vermesan, O., & Friess, P. (2012). *Internet of things: Converging technologies for smart environments.* Aalborg: River Publishers.

Wallace, B. (2005). *Becoming part of the solution: The engineer's guide to sustainable development.* Reston, VA: ASCE Publications.

Weber, R. H. (2010). Internet of things – New security and privacy challenges. *Computer Law and Security Review: The International Journal of Technology and Practice, 26*(1), 23–30. https://doi.org/10.1016/j.clsr.2009.11.008

World Bank. (2008). *Global economic prospects 2008: Technology diffusion in the developing world.* Washington, DC: World Bank Group. Retrieved 12 December 2018 from http://documents.worldbank.org/curated/en/827331468323971985/Global-economic-prospects-2008-technology-diffusion-in-the-developing-world

World Health Organization. (2010). *Global data on impairments 2010.* Retrieved May, 17, 2018, from http://www.who.int/blindness/GLOBALDATAFINALforweb.pdf.

World Health Organization. (2011). *World health statistics 2011.* Retrieved May, 19, 2018, from http://www.who.int/whosis/whostat/2011/en/index.html.

Yang, Y., Wu, L., Yin, G., Li, L., & Zhao, H. (2017). A survey on security and privacy issues in internet-of-things. *IEEE Internet of Things Journal, 4*(5), 1250–1258. https://doi.org/10.1109/JIOT.2017.2694844

Zelenika, I., & Pearce, J. (2014). Innovation through collaboration: Scaling up solutions for sustainable development. *Environment, Development and Sustainability, 16*(6), 1299–1316. https://doi.org/10.1007/s10668-014-9528-7

Chapter 12
Large-Scale Interactive Environments for Mobility Training and Experience Sharing of Blind Children

Marcella Mandanici and Antonio Rodà

12.1 Introduction

The problem of supporting blind people's navigation through the use of electronic devices has been widely studied and many technological solutions have been proposed for delivering environmental data such as obstacle detection, local and global landmarks, written information and so on (Giudice & Legge, 2008). Particularly, with the development of portable and light technological devices, spatial audio cues useful for an accurate representation of the environment have been employed for both local mobility and navigation aids (Spagnol et al., 2018). Independently from the technology employed, all these systems rely on the blind person's ability to perceive, analyze and decode complex sensory inputs. This ability is called "sensory efficiency" and is very important for blind people, as their active senses are the main channel through which they can get information about the world and the environment.

12.1.1 Sensory Integration

Sensory efficiency is one of the qualifying points of the Expanded Core Curriculum, a series of guidance principles for the educational program of blind children

M. Mandanici (✉)
Department of Information Engineering, University of Padova, Padova, Italy

Department of Music Education, Music Conservatory "L. Marenzio", Brescia, Italy

A. Rodà
Department of Information Engineering, University of Padova, Padova, Italy
e-mail: roda@dei.unipd.it

© Springer Nature Switzerland AG 2020   301
S. Paiva (ed.), *Technological Trends in Improved Mobility of the Visually Impaired*,
EAI/Springer Innovations in Communication and Computing,
https://doi.org/10.1007/978-3-030-16450-8_12

("The Expanded Core Curriculum", 2018). Also if it has been proved that congenitally blind people improve other senses by using the visual brain area for tactile, auditory or other sensory data ("People Blind from Birth", 2010), sensory efficiency cannot be taken for granted for every blind person.

The process through which the brain organizes the input coming from the various senses (touch, sound, smell, taste, proprioception, balance, and so on) is called sensory integration (Ayres & Robbins, 2005). It provides a framework for understanding how our senses cooperate to deliver coherent information to the brain. Sensory integration usually develops from early childhood and feeds many cognitive processes and motor skills. As much of the sensory information is coordinated by vision (Gori, 2015), sensory integration may be compromised in blind children and particularly can affect negatively the tactile, proprioceptive and vestibular system. As a consequence blind children can suffer of difficulties with fine motor skills, sound articulations, exaggerate reactions of fear, clumsy movements, loss of balance and muscle tone. The proposed therapy consists of tactile activities (manipulation of water, beans and various textures of clothes), proprioceptive activities (prone weight bearing, adding weights to items for more feedback, climb and lie on large pillows) and vestibular activities (using rocker and spin boards, bouncy shoes, etc.), all aiming at the solicitation of automatic sensory responses during the goal-directed exercises ("Ricketts, OTR", 2008). From this analysis clearly emerge that orientation and mobility training depend on the blind child's ability of processing sensory data and of coping with any sensory integrative dysfunction. This level of sensory efficiency can be achieved with long exposures to various environmental stimuli, which can attract children's attention and interest.

12.1.2 Chapter Organization

Starting from these premises, this book chapter begins with analyzing the state of art of the existing games for blind children with a focus on orientation and mobility (Sect. 12.2). The case of "Following the Cuckoo Sound", a large-scale interactive environment designed to train blind children in walking straight, is presented and evaluated in Sect. 12.3 both for its design and for quantitative and qualitative data resulting from assessment. The important peculiarities of full-body interaction, which characterizes this kind of environment, are outlined and the potentials of haptic and kinesthetic senses to help orientation and mobility are analyzed. Interactive audio has strong emotional outcomes, which, in the case of blind children, can go from rejection or fear to curiosity and fascination. Thus, the psychological impact of sound must be thoroughly evaluated, together with its power of motion redirection. This background is the core of Sect. 12.4, where the possibilities of designing an environment that can provide a rich and stimulating experience are illustrated. The effectiveness of audio to build a narrative has been widely exploited in interactive storytelling and in soundscape composition, where the listener can imagine places and routes by processing auditory information. In the same way it is possible to organize sound environments where the blind child can navigate through the audio rendering of natural or artificial soundscapes, such as woods, beaches, mountains, harbors or factories. Children can imagine their own narrative by exploring the environment and by building a cognitive map where sound and sensory information about the spatial location of the various elements are joined together. They can move along their own sound sequence inside the environment, and by doing so they can dwell in the active space and train in directing motion for a long time. This is not only an orientation and mobility practice, but involves also sensory efficiency, emotion, cognition and self-confidence. Socialization activities may be arranged by sharing the experience in the interactive soundscape with other children sitting at the borders of the active area and listening to the audio result of the exploration of their peers. Children can invent games such as reaching a sound, walking a determined sound sequence, sonorize a story invented by the group with the elements of the soundscape and so on.

12.2 Gaming Activities for Blind Children

The conditions necessary for an effective training of blind children cited above (long exposures to various environmental stimuli, attention and interest) can be met in the practice of gaming. According to Juul (2011), the game is a formal system characterized by six main features: rules, variable and quantifiable outcome, valorization of outcomes, player effort, player attached to outcome and negotiable consequences. This is a general framework for structured games, where users pursue a goal defined by rules and are engaged in the activity because they feel rewarded by a score achievement. This framework has been widely used and enhanced in the video games, which, leveraging on the possibilities offered by interactive sound and graphics, exert a strong attraction on users ranging from total immersion to addiction. While some attempts have been done for adapting popular video games to the necessities of blind people Buaud, Svensson, Archambault, and Burger (2002) and Carvalho, Guerreiro, Duarte, and Carriço (2012), a deeper analysis of blind children needs reveals that they prefer to play tactile-auditory or exploratory games rather than symbolic, and that they require more auditory games and more similarity between play action and reality (Tröster & Brambring, 1994). Moreover, they tend to demonstrate atypical social participation skills and individual play behavior (Celeste & Grum, 2010). Thus, also if some cognitive content and leisure can be derived from video games, for sure they do not fully respond to blind children requirements, which focus mainly on exploration, curiosity, and on the acquisition of social competence.

12.2.1 3D Sound Virtual Environments Games

Many computer games have been developed with the aim of training navigation skills of blind children. These systems rely upon 3D sound virtual environments, which are based on the reconstruction of the spectral properties that characterize sound sources in everyday-life environments. They can also provide multimodal training through haptic feedback in order to increase sound localization abilities (Balan et al., 2017). Children can thus navigate the virtual environment with keyboard and mouse commands or with head-tracking devices and joysticks (Allain et al., 2015). Receiving the interactive audio feedback from the virtual environment through headphones, they can locate the various sounds exploiting the ability of the human ear to decode sound spectral information. Thus they can play first-person shooter games (Merabet & Sánchez, 2009) or accomplish virtual world navigation tasks for improving their geographical knowledge (Sánchez & Sáenz, 2006). Also if Connors, Yazzolino, Sánchez, and Merabet (2013) obtained positive evidence that spatial data and orientation skills learned with the training in such environments can effectively be transferred in the reality, the very limited physical interaction employed deprives this experience of all the proprioceptive and kinaesthetic cues that characterize orientation and mobility in the physical world. Moreover, the games are played individually and no social activity is provided.

12.2.2   Orientation and Mobility Games with Physical Interaction

With the development and diffusion of cheap motion capture systems and wearables, physical interaction has become much easier to implement. A first example is the *Digital Clock Carpet*, a sensorized round surface where children can move to indicate the perceived direction of the sound (Sánchez, Sáenz, & Garrido, 2010). Another example is *VI-Tennis*, an application where blind children can simulate the tennis game by interacting with the sound of a virtual ball through a *Wiimote* controller ("Wii Remote", 2018) used as if it was racket (Morelli, Foley, Columna, Lieberman, & Folmer, 2010). Also Lee, Huang, and Sheu (2013) propose an audio game where blind children have to recognize and to skip the various car sounds in a busy road. All the cited games employ physical interaction, also if only for the upper limbs as in the case of *VI-Tennis* or in a very small portion of space as in the case of *Digital Clock Carpet*. A completely different approach is followed by Coroama and Röthenbacher (2003) who propose a free navigation in a space where each object delivers audio information (spoken text and sound) about its existence. A similar approach is proposed by Freeman et al. (2017), who combine sound from a wearable bracelet and from the environment to give to children information about nearby people, places and activities. This solution aims at providing children in the first school years with the opportunity to be confident with the environment, to train movement and social skills and to be independent from external guidance. Based on very similar principles is the *ABBI* bracelet, a wearable device that outputs audio signals when moving and keeps silent when still. Its very simple design allows a lot of orientation and mobility games for blind children including a very high degree of social activities. Games such as "find the sound" (i.e. finding the child with the same sound) or "hide and seek" (i.e. remaining still not to be chased by a seeker) are very funny activities that foster sensorimotor training and social interrelationship (Magnusson et al., 2015). This short review of orientation and mobility games clearly shows the benefits of physical interaction and of moving without constraints in large spaces for blind children. These characteristics inform a new approach to orientation and mobility training, which considers the problem of blindness in the wider range of sensory integration and social interrelationship.

12.3 "Following the Cuckoo Sound": An Interactive Physical Environment to Train Children to Avoid Veering

In 2015 we were required by the Robert Hollman Foundation of Padova (Italy) (http://fondazioneroberthollman.it/index.html) to design an application for helping blind children to avoid veering. Veering is a great problem for blind people, who are at permanent risk of missing their target when trying to reach a point. Veering is a complex phenomenon whose causes are still unclear. It has been attributed to a natural tendency to walk in circles due to accumulating noise of the sensorimotor system (Souman, Frissen, Sreenivasa, & Ernst, 2009), to deviations in single step orientation (Kallie, Schrater, & Legge, 2007), to encoding errors in path integration (Loomis, Klatzky, Golledge, & Philbeck, 1999) or to slight asymmetries in the two limbs (Boyadjian, MariN, & Danion, 1999). In any case, when the quick spatial updating allowed by vision is missing, the blind child must rely on kinaesthesia, proprioception and haptic cues to walk straight. It is clear that all this sensory input is possible only when the blind child has a high degree of sensory efficiency and self-consciousness and that this must be carefully trained linking bodily interaction with sensory input. Technology offers a good way of doing this through the use of large-scale interactive environments.

12.3.1 Large-Scale Interactive Environments for Therapy and Rehabilitation

Many commercial interactive systems are available for therapy and rehabilitation. Such environments combine tactile surfaces with lighting, smell and music effects to help sensory integration by producing various outputs useful in the care of dementia and for other clinical applications (Chung, Lai, Chung, & French, 2002). Kinaesthetic interaction and movement sonification have also been experimented in therapies for motor and cognitive impairment rehabilitation (Ghisio et al., 2015). Bergsland and Wechsler (2016) outline the positive psychological effects of kinaesthetic interactive sonification and of musical creativity for the rehabilitation and socialization of participants with severe disabilities with their non-disabled peers.

Large-scale interactive environments can provide both sensory integration and interactive sonification. These environments are similar to any other touch-sensitive surface, such as smartphones or touch-screens. But, thanks to their dimensions (usually ranging from 1.5×2 m to 3×4 m or more), they allow children to walk inside the interactive space. Large-scale interactive environments applications usually employ interactive graphics and sound to engage children in sensory games such as touching running objects or animals or playing matches with their peers (https://activefloor.com/en/frontpage/) and (https://www.vertigo-systems.de/en/). Full-body interaction is much more complex than common touch-screen gestural interaction such us tip, drag, rotate and so on, because it involves the use of the whole body. This means that factors such as weight, speed, fatigue, orientation, proprioception and self-confidence are brought into play and that the impact on the sensorimotor system is much greater and engaging. When used in learning environments full-body interaction meets different learning styles and can include impaired children together with all the members of the class in the activities (Mandanici, Altieri, Rodà, & Canazza, 2018). Moreover, children have no device to wear and can enjoy the sonification experience in full freedom.

12.3.2 Application Design

With the cooperation of Giulia Cavagnoli, a trainee of the University of Padova, we proposed the use of a large-scale interactive environment where the blind children could be trained in walking straight with the use of interactive sonification. We employed AILearn (Amico, 2012) a very light and portable motion tracking system composed by a camera hanging from the ceiling and a software component for RGB data processing. AILearn can easily fit any room or closed space, is light sensitive and provides a tracking area of 3×4 m when the distance between floor and camera is 3 m. Our idea was to exploit the properties of interactive audio to guide children along a corridor of 0.6×4 m running from one side to the other of the rectangular area. An intermittent audio signal coming from a speaker put just in front of the corridor indicates that the child is inside the corridor area. As soon as the child veers to the right the signal is transposed to a higher frequency or to a lower frequency if the child veers toward the left. To make the experience of traveling along the corridor a little bit funny, we added some soundscape elements to the interactive environment. Particularly, as soon as the child enters the active area, the sounds of a wood are played. A cuckoo sound was chosen as the intermittent sound that characterizes the corridor, at the end of which a final jingle notifies that the end point has been correctly reached. Further description of the system can be found in Mandanici, Rodà, Canazza, and Cavagnoli (2017). A video with the demonstration of the interactive walk is also available at https://youtu.be/yUkPcD1M-OQ.

12.3.3 Assessment

To verify if the walk along the corridor with interactive audio could help children in walking straight, we planned a pilot experiment with pre-test, test and post-test phases. Six children (five congenitally blind) aged from 5 to 8 years were chosen for assessment. Before beginning the assessment, the educator explained the procedure and allowed the children to make some exploratory walk inside the interactive environment. After this, three pre-test walks were performed with the aim of measuring and observing the children's ability to walk straight. The interactive environment was kept silent and only the motion tracking system was working. Children started at the beginning of the corridor positioned in the direction of the end, where the educator remained waiting. The trial began with the call of the educator and ended when the child reached the end point or exited the active area. In the test children performed the walk in the same way but with interactive audio. Post-test was performed exactly in the same way as pre-test.

12.3.4 Method

After each trial a log with the coordinates of the participants' movement has been recorded. We employed these data to plot the path of the participants during the trials. Figure 12.1 depicts the application's active space with the middle corridor inside which the cuckoo sound remains unaltered (the rectangle within the thin black line). The participant's path is represented by the little empty circles curve that begins exactly in the middle of the corridor. Following the findings of Kallie et al. (2007), we evaluated participants' veering as the result of two components: the initial orientation error and the systematic errors in step direction. The initial orientation error (constant error, CE) is expressed by the deviation angle, calculated between the perpendicular straight line from the start to the end point (solid black line in Fig. 12.1) and the trajectory line from the start to the last point of the veering path (dashed line in Fig. 12.1). As each participant repeated the trial three times, we calculated also the variable error (VE) as the standard error among the trials, which expresses the participants' stability in the error (Guth & LaDuke, 1994). The errors in the step direction are calculated by means of orthogonal linear regression. The SSE statistic (Sum of Squared Errors) represents a measure of how much the subject's veering path differs from the best-fitting line (the line with little points in Fig. 12.1).

For qualitative assessment, after a discussion with the Robert Hollman Foundation educators and trainee, we focused our observation on a grid formed by four behavioral indicators that were supposed to be meaningful for understanding blind children's reactions to the interactive environment (confidence, enjoyment, curiosity and reaction to sound). Plus or minus signs are used to express our evaluation as defined in the grid of Table 12.1.

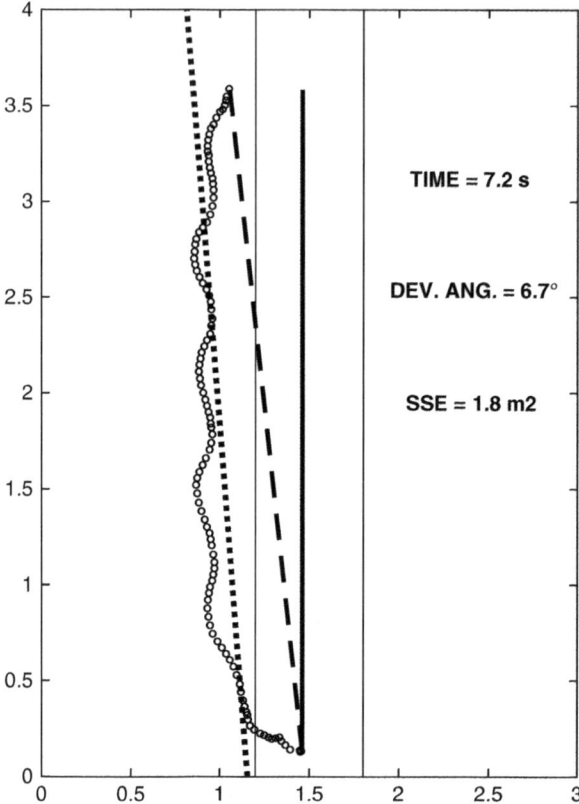

Fig. 12.1 Participant's A post-test. In this example are reported the time employed to walk from the starting point to the end, the deviation angle (between the solid and the dashed line) and sum of squared errors (SSE)

Table 12.1 Grid for qualitative assessment of children's behavior during the trials

Indicators	+	−
Confidence	The child shows sensorimotor and psychological maturity while moving in the interactive space	The child is shy, unsecure and fearful
Enjoyment	The child declares to enjoy the experience and appears emotionally engaged	The child declares not to like the experience
Curiosity	The child explores the environment and tries to understand how it reacts	The child does not show any interest about the interactive environment
Reaction to sound	The child listens carefully to the interactive soundscape	The child shows nuisance or has exaggerated responses to the sound

Table 12.2 Quantitative results of the assessment trials, with pre- and post-test means of constant and variable errors and SSE

	Constant error CE (°)		Variable error VE (°)		Sum of squared errors SSE (m^2)	
Participant	Pre	Post	Pre	Post	Pre	Post
A	3.89	3.73	3.82	1.52	0.31	1.07
B	13.67	5.85	7.06	2.74	0.88	1.49
C	25.67	6.59	18.92	1.71	0.72	0.31
D	7.55	25.38	7.26	8.08	0.87	0.66
E	3.98	4.52	1.91	1.29	0.09	0.69
F	11.34	11.30	1.58	2.98	4.39	0.44
Mean	11.67	9.14	6.76	3.06	1.30	0.77
SE	1.40	2.43	2.22	0.88	0.73	0.18

12.3.5 Quantitative and Qualitative Results

The quantitative results are summarized in Table 12.2, with the means of constant error (CE), variable error (VE) and sum of squared errors (SSE). These values show a general decrease of veering, also if veering data vary a lot depending on participants. Participant C is the only one who really reduces veering, as she decreases in all the three values of CE, VE and SSE.

Table 12.3 is a summary where quantitative and qualitative results are compared. Age, sex, ophthalmic disease and participants' particular conditions have been added for a general evaluation. The quantitative results are expressed with a minus or plus to express decrease or increase from pre- to post-test. The signs are assigned to indicators following the criteria presented in the grid of Table 12.1, while the empty cells indicate that nothing relevant has been noticed for that indicator.

12.3.6 Discussion

The blind children who took part to the "Following the Cuckoo Sound" assessment showed a general reduction of veering after the sound walk in the interactive environment. This can be simply the effect of test repetition: each participant did the walk along the corridor nine times one after the other during the test, thus acquiring or improving the necessary information to accomplish the task. Unfortunately no other training session was allowed, preventing us from collecting data about the long-term effects of the experiment. Moreover, the very low number of participants makes any statistical analysis unwise. In this study, we focus on participants' behavior in the light of the considerations about the difficulties in sensory integration to which blind children are subject. Particularly, in the following analysis we try to outline individual results in relation to the level of emotional and psychomotor confidence shown by children, combining thus quantitative and qualitative data.

Table 12.3 Quantitative results and indicators recorded during the trials, compared to age, sex, ophthalmic disease and participants' particular conditions

Participant		A	B	C	D	E	F
Age		5	6	5	6	8	8
Sex		F	M	F	F	M	F
Disease		Retinal dystrophy	Retinopathy of preterm (ROP)	Retinal dystrophy of Leber's amaurosis and exudative retinopathy (Coats' disease)	ROP	Bilateral congenital glaucoma	ROP
Particular conditions		Already experienced in the use of the long cane	Perceives the light in a dark environment			Not congenitally blind	
Quantitative results	CE	−	−	−	+	+	−
	VE	−	−	−	+	−	+
	SSE	+	+	−	−	+	−
Indicators	Confidence	+	−	+	−	+	−
	Enjoyment	+		+	+	+	+
	Curiosity			+		+	+
	Reaction to sound	+	+	+	−	+	−

Minus and plus signs in the quantitative results indicate a decrease or an increase from pre- to post-test. For indicators the signs are used to express our evaluation as defined in the grid of Table 12.1

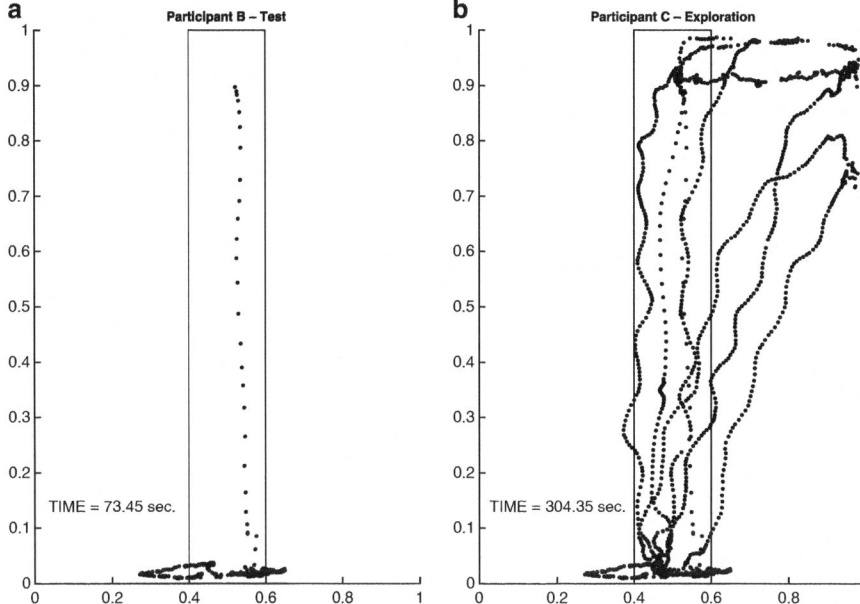

Fig. 12.2 (**a**) Example of fearful behavior, with participant lingering for a long time in the start position and then running quickly towards the end. (**b**) Example of a very long and free exploration of the environment after having completed the trials

Participant A: she was one of the youngest participants and showed great self-confidence. Probably because already trained in the use of the long cane, she obtained very low constant and variable errors both in pre- and post-test.

Participant B: this child was very unsecure in the test phase, lingering for a long time in the start area and then running suddenly very quickly towards the end point (see Fig. 12.2a). Proceeding in the experiment, he became more and more secure. Reactions of fear in front of new situations are one of the symptoms of the lack of sensory integration (Gori, 2015). In this case, the interactive environment seems to have helped this child to recover confidence. In the post-test he decreased constant and variable errors, but not SSE.

Participant C: this child was fascinated by the sound of the interactive environment. She wanted to touch the speaker to check the origin of the sound and refused to correct her position during the test because she was much most interested to the changes in the cuckoo frequency than in accomplishing the task of walking straight. After the end of the trials the educator allowed her a long exploratory phase (see Fig. 12.2b). This child gained the best improvement from the experience, diminishing a lot constant, variable error and SSE in post-test.

Participant D: this child veered a lot during pre-test, showing exaggerated reaction to an accidental sound from the environment (see Fig. 12.3a). She veered

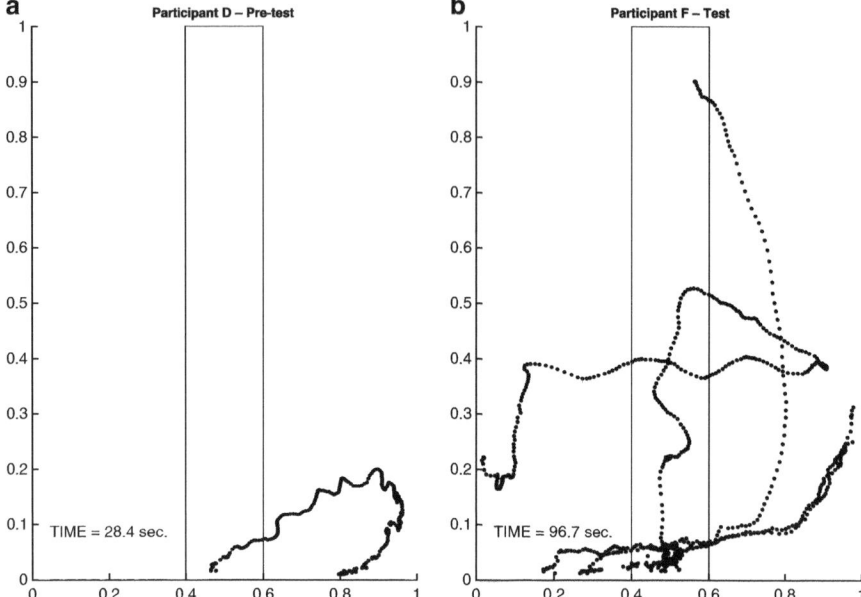

Fig. 12.3 (**a**) Participant D suddenly changes the walking direction during pre-test because of unexpected environmental noise. (**b**) Participant F exploring the limits of the active area during the test

much less during the test and enjoyed a lot the cuckoo sound. However in post-test she increased a lot the initial orientation error.

Participant E: this child was confident in the movements and walked the corridor with nearly no veering in the pre-test trials. He explored a lot after completing the trials, moving quickly from the lower to the higher zone of the cuckoo. He exited and entered the active zone to play and stop the sounds of the wood. He tried to crawl and to jump in search of new reactions from the environment. Similarly to participant A, he was very low in constant, variable error and SSE already from pre-test, perhaps due to the fact that he was not congenitally blind.

Participant F: this child showed hypersensitivity to sound and asked to lower the volume of the sound. She did not enjoy the jingle and in general did not like the experience in the interactive environment. She walked on all fours and explored the limits of the active area during the test (see Fig. 12.3b). The post-test results were nearly the same as the pre-test for constant error, while she improved SSE.

From this analysis clearly emerges that the child who performed best (participant C) obtained a plus in all the four indicators. This means that these are the ideal conditions for achieving results in an interactive environment such as "Following the Cuckoo Sound", where the children are solicited by the sonic interaction obtained by walking inside the active area. The resulting engagement is not only emotional (4 participants out of 6 with a plus for enjoyment) but also cognitive (3 participants out of 6 with a plus for curiosity), because as soon as these children realize the mechanism of the sonic interaction, they are eager to discover all the tricks that could have been hidden in the environment. Also participants F and A obtained respectively 4 and 3 plus, but they improved much less or decreased their performance because they were already able to walk straight and fully confident in the movements. Bad reaction to sound seems to be the most significant indicator to evaluate children's sensory efficiency and openness. Participant D showed sudden and exaggerated reaction to sound, that, together with a very scarce self-confidence, prevented her from a positive reaction to the environment. Also participant F had a very bad reaction to sound, showing annoyance and disappointment. However, unexpectedly, she was also curious and explored the environment for a long time after the end of the trials.

12.4 Conclusion

In Sect. 12.2 we examined the advantages of using games for an effective training of blind children, with a particular focus on attention and interest. The employment of the game framework for a precise purpose beyond pure entertainment defines the category of "serious games" (Djaouti, Alvarez, & Jessel, 2011). Serious games are employed in military training, business, advertising and many other fields (Michael & Chen, 2005).

"Following the Cuckoo Sound" was created with the aim of helping children to avoid veering. Its design can provide a prize for the child who does not exit the area of the corridor, and a penalty for the child who exits it, causing the change in the cuckoo sound. This structure could have placed "Following the Cuckoo Sound" in the category of serious games, but children's behavior observed during the test disclosed other perhaps more interesting possibilities. In fact, when considering two important application fields (education and therapy), the requirements of a structured game may result too complex for young children or disabled people. Thus, other less structured approaches may be required. Deterding, Dixon, Khaled, and Nacke (2011) provided a general framework to define all these different systems and tools, classifying them inside a two-dimensional space delimited by two axes. One is the *game-play* vertical axis, which describes the various states between the *game* (the most structured one) and the *playing* (a free serendipitous approach based on exploration and discovery). The other is the *whole systems-parts* axis, which describes the various degrees from a fully structured game to systems that can include only some game elements. Serious games are positioned in the upper left part of the space, in the area between *whole-systems* and *game*. The area opposite to *game* is *playing*, which indicates a less systematic and free approach, characterized by exploration and improvisation and corresponding to the ancient Greek term of "paidia" (Caillois, 2001). This was exactly the behavior of the blind children who took part in the "Following the Cuckoo Sound" assessment. In fact they were not so much interested to reach the proposed goal but rather preferred

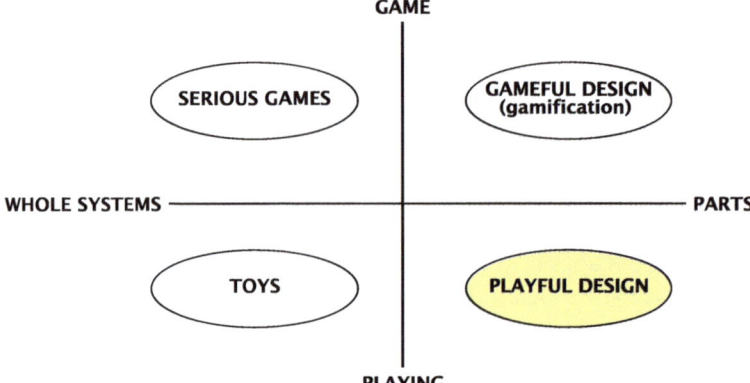

Fig. 12.4 The game-playing and whole systems-parts two-dimensional space for the classification of serious games, gamification, toys and playful design (adapted from Deterding et al., 2011). The area of playful design is highlighted as the most promising for blind children training

to discover the changes in the sound of the cuckoo, thus satisfying their curiosity. Hence their behavior ranks "Following the Cuckoo Sound" in the playful design area (highlighted in Fig. 12.4) rather than in the serious games area.

12.4.1 Lesson Learned from Blind Children While Testing "Following the Cuckoo Sound"

This unexpected reaction of blind children together with the analysis presented in Sect. 12.3.6 suggested the following reflections:

1. Interactive sound is a tool of great impact for blind children, capable of redirecting their movements and of provoking not only emotional but also cognitive processes.
2. The task of walking straight is a kind of absolute requirement that does not fit well children capabilities and expectations. We observed two cases: or the task was too easy because the subject had already developed all the sensorimotor and perceptual cues which permitted a straight walk; or the child showed shyness, exaggerated reactions or perceptual immaturity such as to make the requirement a little bit unwise.
3. The shift from serious game to playful design suggests the creation of an interactive environment much more rich in sounds which can be organized as a localized soundscape to be explored by occupying the various parts of the active surface.

4. Many different activities may be organized in an environment such as this: from simple exploration, to directed soundwalks, from search games to sound map reconstruction.
5. These activities, beyond fostering sensory efficiency and self-confidence, may also reinforce children's social interrelationship and cooperation.

12.4.2 Interactive Virtual Soundscapes for Blind Children

The attention to environmental sound originates from the experience of the World Soundscape Project at Simor Fraser University (Canada). In the early 70s Murray Schafer and Barry Truax began to study urban soundscapes, developing techniques and theories aimed at understanding sound ecology. Sound carries with it a lot of information about its place of origin, the materials or the gestures that produced it (Gaver, 1993). This great communicative quality is the base of soundscape composition, where environmental sounds lead the listener through an imaginary journey, rich of memories and emotional involvement (Truax, 2001). For these properties soundscape recordings are also used in the context of environmental music therapy, where listening can promote relaxation and wellbeing (Viega, 2014) and (Nazemi, 2014). In the case of blind children, listening to soundscapes can provide a substitution of real travels, as they can reproduce every single aspect of an environment. Thus, following the project already developed by Lionello, Mandanici, Canazza, and Micheloni (2017) we propose the use of an interactive soundscape to promote sensory efficiency and orientation and mobility skills of blind children. A simulation of this can be found at https://vimeo.com/146137215, where various sounds of a harbor are scattered on the interactive surface. Blind children can enter the interactive space and make a real soundwalk through it. They can be stimulated in discovering all the sounds of the harbor, in following a determined sound track and in plotting the sound map of their sonic travel. The flexibility of such environment can fit various degrees of self-confidence and sensibility to sound and can promote higher levels of sensory integration in blind children.

References

Allain, K., Dado, B., Van Gelderen, M., Hokke, O., Oliveira, M., Bidarra, R., . . . Kybartas, B. (2015, March). An audio game for training navigation skills of blind children. In *2015 IEEE Second VR Workshop on Sonic Interactions for Virtual Environments (SIVE)* (pp. 1–4). Washington, DC: IEEE.

American Foundation for the Blind. (2018). *The expanded core curriculum for blind and visually impaired children and youths.* Retrieved July 29, 2018, from http://www.afb.org/info/programs-and-services/professional-development/education/expanded-core-curriculum/the-expanded-core-curriculum/12345.

Amico, L. (2012). *La Stanza Logo-Motoria. Un Ambiente multimodale interattivo per l'insegnamento a bambini in situazione di multi-disabilità* (Master's thesis). Dipartimento di Ingegneria dell'Informazione, Università di Padova.

Ayres, A. J., & Robbins, J. (2005). *Sensory integration and the child: Understanding hidden sensory challenges*. Torrance, CA: Western Psychological Services.

Balan, O., Moldoveanu, A., Moldoveanu, F., Nagy, H., Wersenyi, G., & Unnporsson, R. (2017). Improving the audio game-playing performances of people with visual impairments through multimodal training. *Journal of Visual Impairment & Blindness, 111*(2), 148–164.

Bergsland, A., & Wechsler, R. (2016). Turning movement into music: Issues and applications of the MotionComposer, a therapeutic device for persons with different abilities. *SoundEffects – An Interdisciplinary Journal of Sound and Sound Experience, 6*(1), 23–47.

Boyadjian, A., Marin, L., & Danion, F. (1999). Veering in human locomotion: The role of the effectors. *Neuroscience Letters, 265*(1), 21–24.

Buaud, A., Svensson, H., Archambault, D., & Burger, D. (2002, July). Multimedia games for visually impaired children. In *International Conference on Computers for Handicapped Persons* (pp. 173–180). Berlin, Heidelberg: Springer.

Caillois, R. (2001). *Man, play, and games*. Champaign, IL: University of Illinois Press.

Carvalho, J., Guerreiro, T., Duarte, L., & Carriço, L. (2012, July). Audio-based puzzle gaming for blind people. In *Proceedings of the Mobile Accessibility Workshop at MobileHCI (MOBACC)*.

Celeste, M., & Grum, D. K. (2010). Social integration of children with visual impairment: A developmental model. *İlköğretim Online, 9*(1), 11–22.

Chung, J. C., Lai, C. K., Chung, P. M., & French, H. P. (2002). Snoezelen for dementia. *Cochrane Database of Systematic Reviews*, (4), CD003152.

Connors, E. C., Yazzolino, L. A., Sánchez, J., & Merabet, L. B. (2013). Development of an audio-based virtual gaming environment to assist with navigation skills in the blind. *Journal of Visualized Experiments: JoVE*, (73). https://doi.org/10.3791/50272.

Coroama, V., & Röthenbacher, F. (2003, October). The chatty environment—Providing everyday independence to the visually impaired. In *Workshop on Ubiquitous Computing for Pervasive Healthcare Applications at UbiComp*.

Deterding, S., Dixon, D., Khaled, R., & Nacke, L. (2011, September). From game design elements to gamefulness: Defining gamification. In *Proceedings of the 15th International Academic MindTrek Conference: Envisioning Future Media Environments* (pp. 9–15). New York, NY: ACM.

Djaouti, D., Alvarez, J., & Jessel, J. P. (2011). Classifying serious games: The G/P/S model. In *Handbook of research on improving learning and motivation through educational games: Multidisciplinary approaches* (pp. 118–136). IGI Global.

Freeman, E., Wilson, G., Brewster, S., Baud-Bovy, G., Magnusson, C., & Caltenco, H. (2017, May). Audible beacons and wearables in schools: Helping young visually impaired children play and move independently. In *Proceedings of the 2017 CHI Conference on Human Factors in Computing Systems* (pp. 4146–4157). New York, NY: ACM.

Gaver, W. W. (1993). What in the world do we hear?: An ecological approach to auditory event perception. *Ecological Psychology, 5*(1), 1–29.

Georgetown University Medical Center. (2010, October 10). People blind from birth use visual brain area to improve other senses: Can hear and feel with greater acuity. *ScienceDaily*. Retrieved June 20, 2018, from www.sciencedaily.com/releases/2010/10/101006131203.htm.

Ghisio, S., Coletta, P., Piana, S., Alborno, P., Volpe, G., Camurri, A., ... Bergamaschi, V. (2015, June). An open platform for full body interactive sonification exergames. In *2015 Seventh International Conference on Intelligent Technologies for Interactive Entertainment (INTETAIN)* (pp. 168–175). Washington, DC: IEEE.

Giudice, N. A., & Legge, G. E. (2008). Blind navigation and the role of technology. In *The engineering handbook of smart technology for aging, disability, and independence* (pp. 479–500). New York, NY: John Wiley & Sons.

Gori, M. (2015). Multisensory integration and calibration in children and adults with and without sensory and motor disabilities. *Multisensory Research, 28*(1–2), 71–99.

Guth, D., & LaDuke, R. (1994). The veering tendency of blind pedestrians: An analysis of the problem and literature review. *Journal of Visual Impairment & Blindness, 88*, 391–400.

Juul, J. (2011). *Half-real: Video games between real rules and fictional worlds.* Cambridge, MA: MIT Press.

Kallie, C. S., Schrater, P. R., & Legge, G. E. (2007). Variability in stepping direction explains the veering behavior of blind walkers. *Journal of Experimental Psychology: Human Perception and Performance, 33*(1), 183.

Lee, H. P., Huang, Y. H., & Sheu, T. F. (2013). *An interactive training game using 3D sound for visually impaired people.* International Association for Development of the Information Society.

Lionello, M., Mandanici, M., Canazza, S., & Micheloni, E. (2017). Interactive soundscapes: Developing a physical space augmented through dynamic sound rendering and granular synthesis. In *Proceedings of the 14th Sound and Music Computing Conference.*

Loomis, J. M., Klatzky, R. L., Golledge, R. G., & Philbeck, J. W. (1999). Human navigation by path integration. In *Wayfinding behavior: Cognitive mapping and other spatial processes* (pp. 125–151). Baltimore, MD: Johns Hopkins University Press.

Magnusson, C., Rydeman, B., Finocchietti, S., Cappagli, G., Porquis, L. B., Baud-Bovy, G., & Gori, M. (2015, August). Co-located games created by children with visual impairments. In *Proceedings of the 17th International Conference on Human-Computer Interaction with Mobile Devices and Services Adjunct* (pp. 1157–1162). New York, NY: ACM.

Mandanici, M., Altieri, F., Rodà, A., & Canazza, S. (2018). Inclusive sound and music serious games in a large-scale responsive environment. *British Journal of Educational Technology, 49*, 620–635. https://doi.org/10.1111/bjet.12630

Mandanici, M., Rodà, A., Canazza, S., & Cavagnoli, G. (2017, November). Following the cuckoo sound: A responsive floor to train blind children to avoid veering. In *International Conference on Smart Objects and Technologies for Social Good* (pp. 11–20). Cham: Springer.

Merabet, L., & Sánchez, J. (2009). Audio-based navigation using virtual environments: Combining technology and neuroscience. *AER Journal: Research and Practice in Visual Impairment and Blindness, 2*(3), 128–137.

Michael, D. R., & Chen, S. L. (2005). *Serious games: Games that educate, train, and inform.* New York, NY: Muska & Lipman/Premier-Trade.

Morelli, T., Foley, J., Columna, L., Lieberman, L., & Folmer, E. (2010, June). VI-Tennis: A vibrotactile/audio exergame for players who are visually impaired. In *Proceedings of the Fifth International Conference on the Foundations of Digital Games* (pp. 147–154). New York, NY: ACM.

Nazemi, M. M. (2014). Affective soundscape composition for evoking sonic immersion. *Journal of Sonic Studies, 7.* Retrieved June 17, 2018, from https://www.researchcatalogue.net/view/88052/88052/11/1762.

Ricketts, L. (2008, Fall). OTR, Texas School for the Blind and Visually Impaired. *Texas Sense Abilities.* Retrieved July 29, 2018, from http://www.tsbvi.edu/deaf-blind-project/3159-occupational-therapy-and-sensory-integration%2D%2Dvisual-impairment.

Sánchez, J., & Sáenz, M. (2006). 3D sound interactive environments for blind children problem solving skills. *Behaviour & Information Technology, 25*(4), 367–378.

Sánchez, J., Sáenz, M., & Garrido, J. M. (2010). Usability of a multimodal video game to improve navigation skills for blind children. *ACM Transactions on Accessible Computing (TACCESS), 3*(2), 7.

Souman, J. L., Frissen, I., Sreenivasa, M. N., & Ernst, M. O. (2009). Walking straight into circles. *Current Biology, 19*(18), 1538–1542.

Spagnol, S., Wersényi, G., Bujacz, M., Bălan, O., Herrera Martínez, M., Moldoveanu, A., & Unnthorsson, R. (2018). Current use and future perspectives of spatial audio technologies in electronic travel aids. *Wireless Communications and Mobile Computing, 2018*, 3918284.

Tröster, H., & Brambring, M. (1994). The play behavior and play materials of blind and sighted infants and preschoolers. *Journal of Visual Impairment & Blindness, 88*(5), 421–432.

Truax, B. (2001). *Acoustic communication* (Vol. 1). Westport, CT: Greenwood Publishing Group.

Viega, M. (n.d.). Listening in the ambient mode: Implications for music therapy practice and theory. Retrieved from https://doi.org/10.15845/voices.v14i2.778

Wii Remote. (2018, December). Retrieved December 18, 2018, from https://en.wikipedia.org/wiki/Wii_Remote.

Chapter 13
HapAR: Handy Intelligent Multimodal Haptic and Audio-Based Mobile AR Navigation for the Visually Impaired

Ahmad Hoirul Basori

13.1 Introduction

Augmented Reality tries to combine digital contents into the real world. By adding additional media to the world, it enables human as the user to enhance their perception of reality. When a user sees the world through a camera, the system tracks the captured environment and augments it with digitally generated data such as 3D model. Ideally, when the user moves the camera, the model will move together, as if it registers seamlessly with the real world. Although current technology explored generally aims for visual augmentation, some AR application has been utilized to also give a sensation of sound, scent or touch. With the tremendous growth of interest in AR, Azuma published a survey in 1997, in which he proposed a commonly acknowledged definition of AR as a system that has to comply with the following features Azuma (1997):

- Combines virtual and real objects.
- Registers three-dimensionally.
- Has a real-time interactivity.

The term Augmented Reality itself was coined by aeroplane engineers Caudell and Mizell, they introduce their study of see-through Head-Mounted Display (HMD) google that displays CAD models to help engineers in aeroplane manu-facturing process (Caudell & Mizell, 1992). The google generates an Augmented Reality that will improve worker's visual perception of aeroplane parts. Milgram introduced a continuum of the real-virtual environment to define the relationship

A. H. Basori (✉)
Faculty of Computing and Information Technology Rabigh, King Abdulaziz University, Rabigh, Makkah, Saudi Arabia
e-mail: abasori@kau.edu.sa

© Springer Nature Switzerland AG 2020
S. Paiva (ed.), *Technological Trends in Improved Mobility of the Visually Impaired*,
EAI/Springer Innovations in Communication and Computing,
https://doi.org/10.1007/978-3-030-16450-8_13

between real and virtual environment (virtual reality). Virtual Reality is an entity where laws governing real worlds such as physics of matter and gravity can be completely replaced with a new, synthetic one (Milgram, Takemura, Utsumi, & Kishino, 1994). Users can immerse in this reality as if the real world does not exist in their current perception. As such, Milgram placed Virtual Environment in the farthest distinction with Real Environment. If AR defined as a process to complement real world with virtual objects, inversely, Augmented Virtuality (AV) is an artificial entity with added reality inside. The objective of Augmented Reality is to provide stronger information into the environment and integrate it seamlessly in real-time. Apprehending this concept, paramount of AR mainly lies in computer vision and computer graphics research field. Concatenation of artificial data to real world requires the system to be able to see and track the viewed environment with the computer vision. When the world has been tracked, computer graphics will construct and render realistic models that can be interacted by the user in real-time.

This manuscript presents an innovative solution for helping visually impaired user with a unique navigation system based on predefined geo-location of the destination and current user location. Users only need to point out their mobile devices in a particular direction, and then audio and haptic aid will guide them carefully. The structure of the paper can be explained as follows: The literature review and critical analysis of current work are presented in the next section. Next, the methodology of the research is given and then followed by a test and evaluation for the upcoming section. Finally, the last part describes the conclusion and future direction of the research.

13.2 Problem Analysis and Literature Review

A number of elements act as a fundamental part of developing Augmented Reality system (Zhou, Duh, & Billinghurst, 2008):

1. Tracking techniques to calculate and track the user's position and orientation with respect to the environment.
2. Tools for registering the tracker to support the tracking technique alignment.
3. Graphics processing unit and program to render the desired 3D augmentation.
4. Virtual interaction system to enable interactivity with the AR content.
5. Display hardware (HMD, monitor) to view the synthetic contents together with the real environment.
6. Computer processing unit to run the system and support the input/output interfaces.

All of the mentioned elements are involved together to form a framework illustrated in Fig. 13.1. The real-world scene is captured by the capturing module through the device's eye, typically a camera. In the meantime, the tracking module calculates the camera pose, which is the coordinate and orientation of the camera relative to the real world. When a user moves the camera view from the original

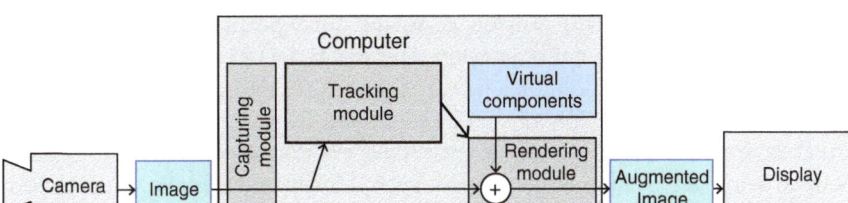

Fig. 13.1 A typical AR system framework. Image courtesy of Siltanen (2012)

position, the tracking module will track the movement and calculate the new camera pose so that the system can keep the integration with the environment.

Moreover, some researcher has studied wayfinding an approach with location-based augmented reality for the pilgrim in Makkah, while the other focus on studying the markerless tracking on the planar environment with combination with a special sensor to augment tracking features (Afif, Basori, & Saari, 2013; Albaqami, Allehaibi, & Basori, 2018; Basori et al., 2015). The rendering module is responsible for augmenting virtually generated components into the captured scene and rendering to become augmented image. Lastly, the display device (monitors, see-through Head Mounted Displays, etc.) will show the augmented image to the user along with the real-world view. There are various tracking techniques that have been researched. Generally, these can be categorized into three: sensor-based, vision-based and hybrid techniques. The sensor-based technique relies on transducers to measure camera pose of the system. On the other hand, computer vision technique attempts to calculate camera pose based on the scene captured by a camera. A hybrid technique exploits both sensor-based and vision-based tracking to achieve the goal, Afif, Basori, & Saari, (2013).

The other researchers have mentioned that the need for assistive technology is increasing rapidly along with the growth of wearable computing. The mobile device has equipped with sensors and camera as well as a powerful computing processor. So, an application that builds in small device becomes an intuitive technology that chosen for impaired people (Bhowmick & Hazarika, 2017; Tapu, Mocanu, & Zaharia, 2018). Coughlan and Miele (2017) have produced AR4VI that designed for low vision or blind people by creating augmented reality menu through relief map and a fiducial marker board for their destination. The other innovative solution is handsight, a project initiated by Findlater et al. (2015). It has been used as a tool for reading by installing the microcamera at the subject's finger. NAVIG provides a spatial database for guiding visually impaired user toward their destination. They used semantic audio guidance and bio-inspired vision system to recognize traffic or any road sign then convey the message to the user (Katz et al., 2012).

ShahSani, Ullah, and Rahman (2017) used mobile phones and fiducial marker to generate path automatically. This path is editable and stored in the database. Their solution is mainly focused on the large indoor environment. Perrois, Laviole, Briant, and Brock (2018) work intensely over 6 months to design an augmented reality map that has audio and tactile feedback to guide the low vision and blind persons. Zhao et al. (2018) provide gears for blind people that consist of VR Headset, Controller as a haptic controller. This device has a brake instrument when it gets in touch with an object, then it will generate the vibrotactile and audio effect as a message to the user. The design has successfully navigated the persons in a virtual environment. Whilst, there are researchers that focused on generating audio footnote using geolocation as predefined marked location and audio. Furthermore, augmentation of AR technology is being used for impaired or low vision. The collected image will be stored and to be used later for navigation headed to their destination (Gleason, Fiannaca, Kneisel, Cutrell, & Morris, 2018; Stearns, Findlater, & Froehlich, 2018).

Based on the observation of previous work, there is a research gap that brings an opportunity for the proposed solution. This paper initiates the Point of Interest (POI) by rendering the 3D icon which is location-based calculation through mobile phone with GPS and gyroscope sensor. The orientation of mobile devices will be considered as an initial position for the tracking location according to inertial sensors reading. Then the distance between the current position and destination will be updated in real time.

In modern devices such as Smartphone or tablets, the mechanical version of the sensor is not used. Instead, the engineers use the digital chip version called micromachined inertial sensors, such as a microelectromechanical system (MEMS), piezoresistive sensor or capacitive sensors (Yazdi, Ayazi, & Najafi, 1998). Even though the physical shape and material are different, they are still working on the same basic principle. Typically, accelerometers and gyroscopes work together. Both the resultant outputs are then integrated to provide a total of 6-DOF measurement of the orientation of position (Welch & Foxlin, 2002), with the workflow illustrated in Fig. 13.2.

Aside from AR application, accel-gyro sensors have been used as a control scheme for video games, digital compasses, interactive browsers or any other application that can be enhanced with inertial-measuring ability, as shown in Fig. 13.3. However, even though inertial sensors are lightweight and cheap, they have to be corrected for drift errors caused by such integration process (Rolland, Baillot, & Goon, 2001).

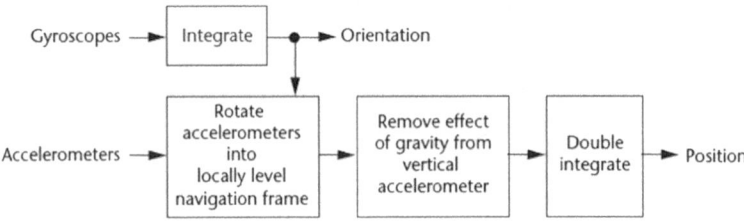

Fig. 13.2 Workflow to obtain position and orientation from the accel-gyro sensor. Image courtesy of (Welch & Foxlin, 2002)

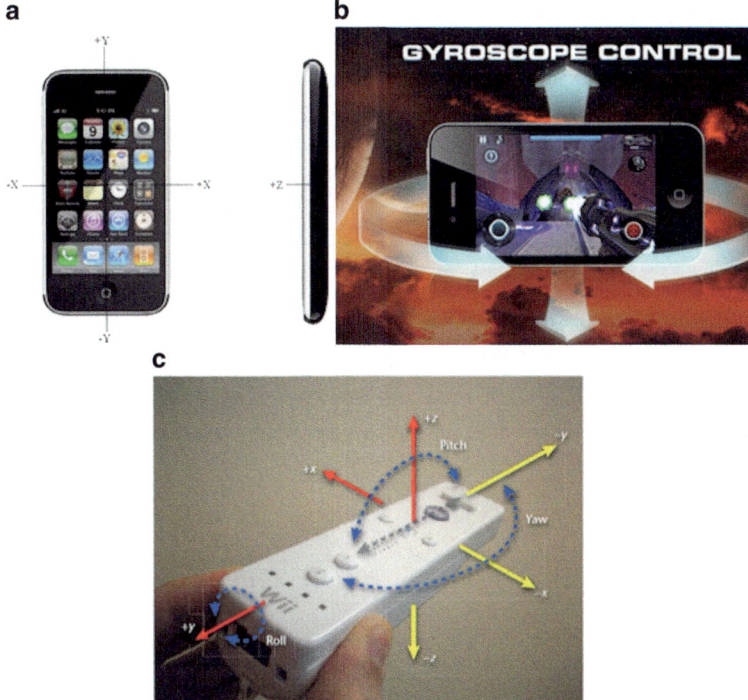

Fig. 13.3 Installed accelerometer (**a**) and gyroscope (**b**) enhance the interactivity of modern smartphone by providing position measurement ability. A Wiimote from Nintendo has a built-in accelerometer inside. Image (**a**) courtesy of Lee (2010), image (**b**) courtesy of Lim (2012), image (**c**) courtesy of Wingrave et al. (2010)

A basic, simplest camera model is a pinhole camera as shown in Fig. 13.3. An image plane lies in the camera's focus f in the z-direction of the Euclidean coordinate system. Pinhole camera model captures a point resides at position $X = (X, Y, Z)^T$ into the image plane. The coordinate center of image plane lies in the principal point p having a coordinate of (p_x, p_y). The point is then projected into the image plane with respect to camera center C as x, which by congruency can be calculated as Eqs. (13.1)–(13.4):

$$x = \left(f\frac{X}{Z} + p_x, f\frac{Y}{Z} + p_y \right)^T \tag{13.1}$$

while ignoring the depth coordinate. A mapping between the 3D world into a 2D plane is achieved by projection from X to x, refer to Fig. 13.4.

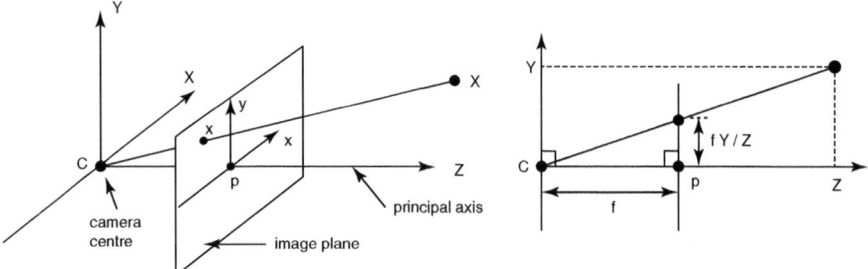

Fig. 13.4 A pinhole camera model. A camera lies in origin C. Image courtesy of Hartley and Zisserman (2003)

Central projection of the camera can be expressed by matrix operation associated with the mapping as:

$$\begin{bmatrix} X \\ Y \\ Z \\ 1 \end{bmatrix} \rightarrow \begin{bmatrix} fX + Zp_x \\ fY + Zp_y \\ z \end{bmatrix} = \begin{bmatrix} f & & p_x & 0 \\ & f & p_y & 0 \\ & & 1 & 0 \end{bmatrix} \begin{bmatrix} X \\ Y \\ Z \\ 1 \end{bmatrix} \tag{13.2}$$

so that the image and real-world coordinate can be written as:

$$x = K \, [I|0] \, X \tag{13.3}$$

where K is defined as camera parameters, or camera calibration matrix, that models the parameter inside one particular camera.

$$K = \begin{bmatrix} f & & p_x \\ & f & p_y \\ & & 1 \end{bmatrix}$$

The position of an object can be described as a coordinate with respect to the world coordinate frame. Likewise, camera pose can be determined by calculating its world coordinate. A relationship between camera's coordinate system and world coordinate system, as illustrated in Fig. 13.5, is described by means of translation and rotation matrix. A translation shifts a coordinate system to a new position whereas rotation changes its orientation.

A camera coordinate system $\tilde{X}$ can be described in the world coordinate system as $\tilde{X}_{CAM}$ by the relationship:

$$\tilde{X}_{CAM} = R\tilde{X} + t \tag{13.4}$$

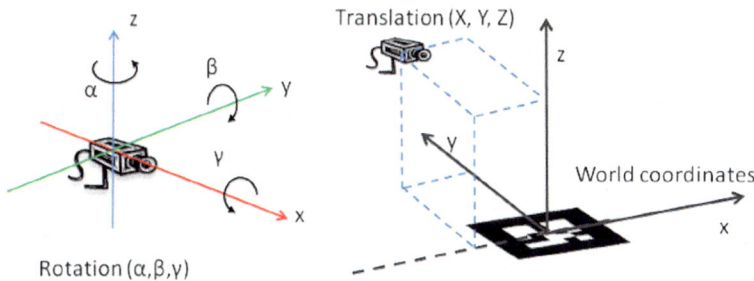

Fig. 13.5 Rotation and translation of the camera coordinate system relative to the world coordinate system. Image courtesy of ShahSani et al. (2017)

where R is a 3-by-3 rotation matrix and t is a 3-by-1 translation matrix. Combining with, an image position in the world coordinate system is determined as:

$$x = K \, [R|t] \, X \tag{13.5}$$

In other words, an image position is determined by nine elements, three from camera parameters(f, p_x, p_y), three from the translation matrix and three from the rotation matrix. If the camera parameters are obtained by means of calibration, the camera pose can be obtained by solving 6-DOF coordinates of rotation and translation.

13.3   Methods

The process is started by gathering the data including GPS locations for POI then stores in a database. The system will use the camera and GPS sensor for calibrations to determine the location. Once the location is detected, it will initiate the encoding process for every POI at that particular location. Finally, the process for POI management such as: update and insert and delete is described in Fig. 13.6. The insert process will be responsible for adding new POI into the database by adding the geolocation, photos or description of the POI. Whereas, update and delete are responsible for the process of changing the information or coordinate of the POI. The sound and haptic activation will be triggered when the stimulation occurred, e.g. Person closed to the destination, the person next to other POI.

Figure 13.7 shows the detailed methodology used for this research, in short ways, the system architecture of the proposed system is described in Fig. 13.9.

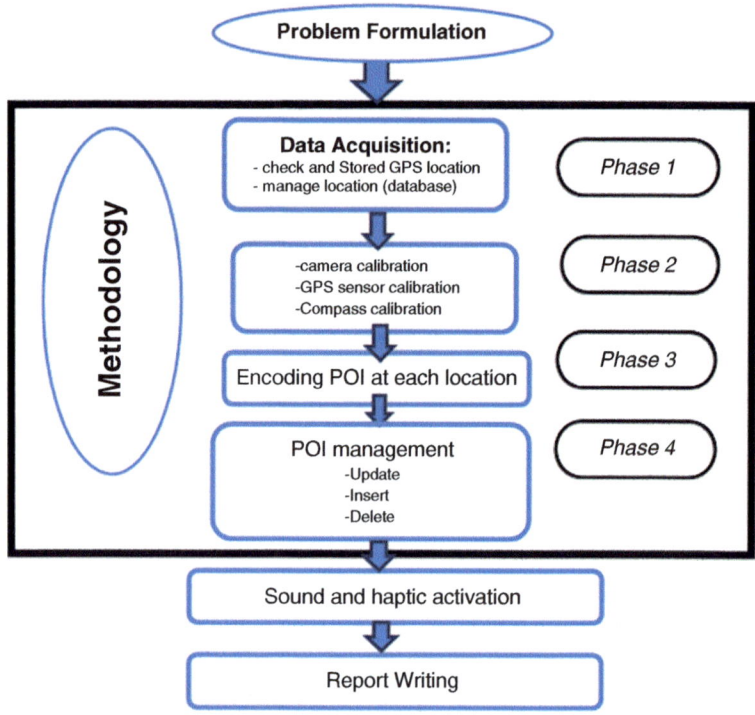

Fig. 13.6 The methodology of the project

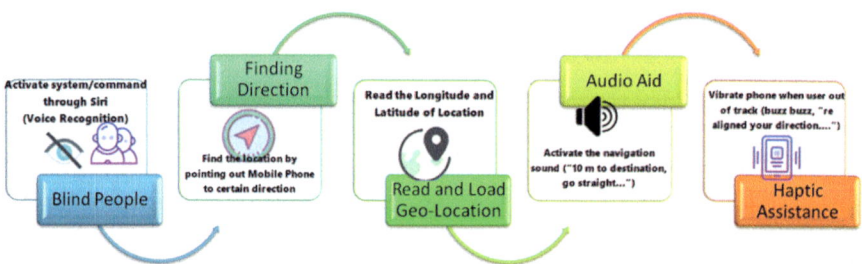

Fig. 13.7 System architecture

The user will activate the system through Siri (voice recognition) then will give the command to find a certain location. It will process the request and find the geolocation. If the location is found then measure the distance between the user and the location. In this case, we used a campus location for initial implementation to give easiness update or tracking for user testing. The sound will aid the user by a certain phrase such as:" 10 m to the destination, keep straight . . . ", while haptic will alert them when they are diverting from the original direction. The haptic approach will keep them on the right track. If somehow their track is diverted a little bit, the system will be asked to realign their path.

13.4 Tests and Evaluation

The new HapAR (Smart KAU) has several features such as the main interface that consist of three sign option for interaction: Google or guest account or directly through Siri. Figure 13.8a shows the main interface of the proposed system, while Fig. 13.8b is Siri features to activate voice command for the smart KAU. Guest account has limited functionality, they are only able to view and use the apps without the capability of updating or deleting the point of interest (POI). However, for visually impaired person user, the aid guidance will be more important rather than update or management of the POI.

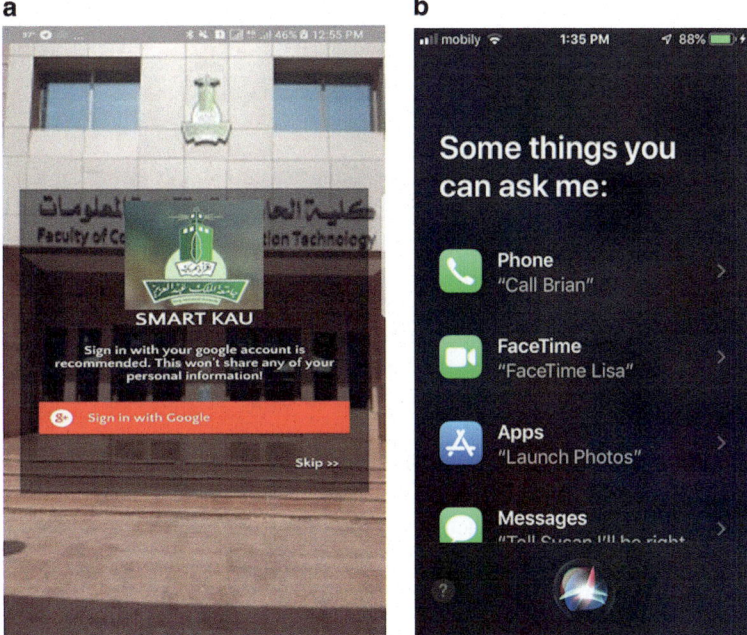

Fig. 13.8 Main interface of HapAR (Smart KAU)

Fig. 13.9 POI of King
Abdulaziz University
Rabigh-branch

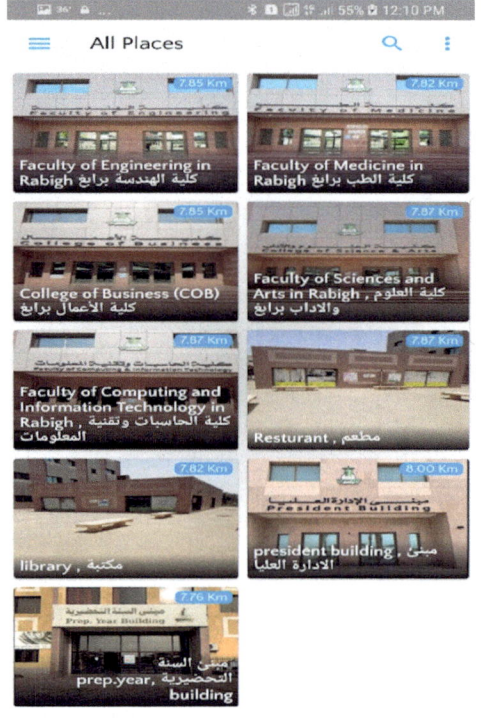

If users want to start the application, they need to choose the way to sign in. After user sign with their account, they will be provided with an interface as shown in Fig. 13.9. It is called all places that illustrate the most important building information in KAU Rabigh, refer to Fig. 13.9.

Figure 13.9 shows the POI of Faculty of Engineering, Faculty of Medicine, College of Business, Faculty of Sciences and Arts, Faculty of Computing and Information Technology, Restaurant, Library, President Building and Preparatory Year building. Each building presentation will have distance and description English and Arabic.

The other features are categorized-based menu that can filter the POI according to certain criteria as shown in Fig. 13.10.

The initial testing was conducted and the POI has been loaded successfully in accordance with the user's command. Figure 13.11 shows Faculty of Engineering location has been loaded with 20 m distance.

Figure 13.12 illustrates an optional menu for Non-Visually Impaired people. They may click the building image to gain additional information such as faculty description, vision and mission, etc.

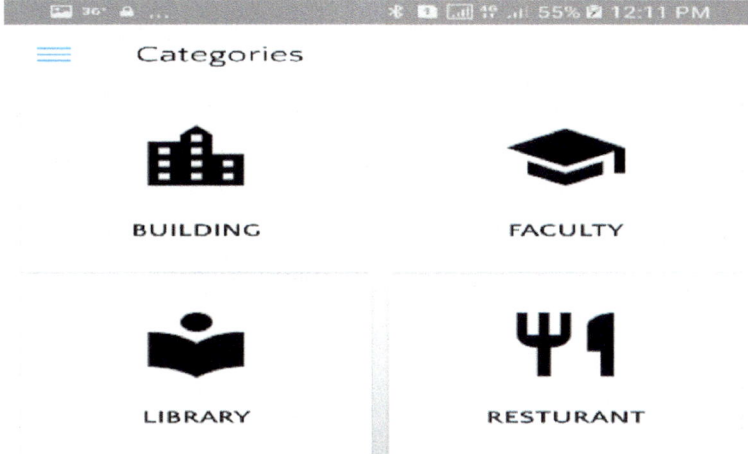

Fig. 13.10 Activity categories

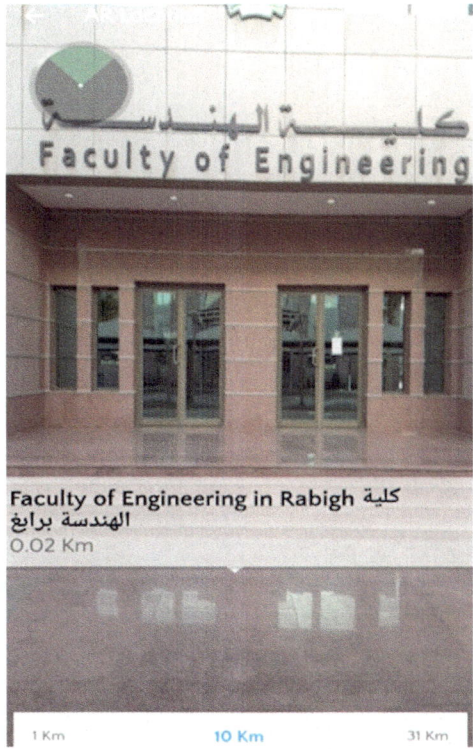

Fig. 13.11 Faculty of engineering POI

Fig. 13.12 Building description

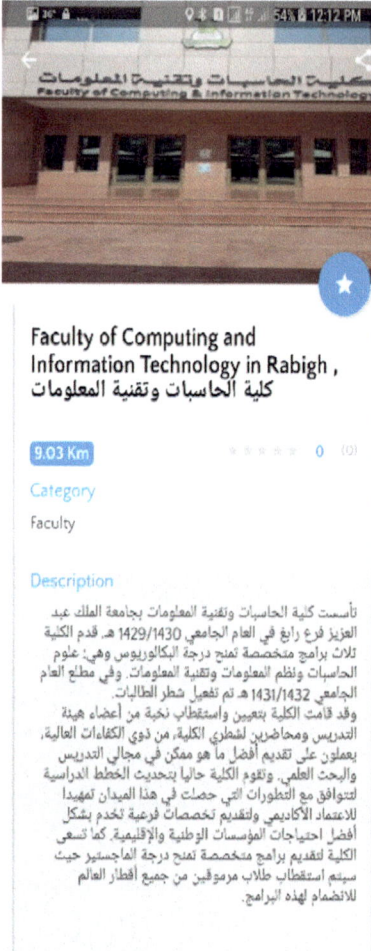

Once building description is loaded, the user can read the description, continued with uploading photos to the apps of detail information regarding the building. Non-visual impaired used may give rates and reviews for evaluating the particular location, refer to Figs. 13.13 and 13.14.

The user can give their feedback for each building toward the rating and review menu, they may give stars and comment based on their experience.

Fig. 13.13 Upload features for non-visually impaired user

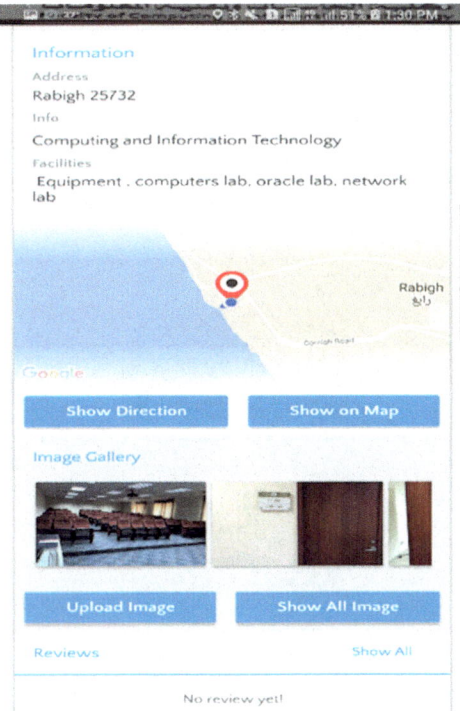

The usability testing was conducted with five respondents that blindfolded purposely to measure the capability of the software on providing a guide toward the visually impaired person. Their response is quite promising as shown in Fig. 13.15.

Figure 13.15 portrays a very promising result for our software, five healthy subjects were blindfolded purposely to measure the four criteria of our proposed apps: software control, haptic feedback, sound feedback and Siri command. The software control overall has a very good rating since the user mostly satisfied with the POI searching just pointing out the handphone. While haptic and sound feedback also receive a positive response even though some respondent gives little bit low feedback. This sound feedback usually disturbed by outdoor environment factors such as wind and people voices, while the haptic feedback depends on the vibration motor for each phone that has different magnitude force. The Siri command is very positive and they like this feature since they only need to activate the application through their voices.

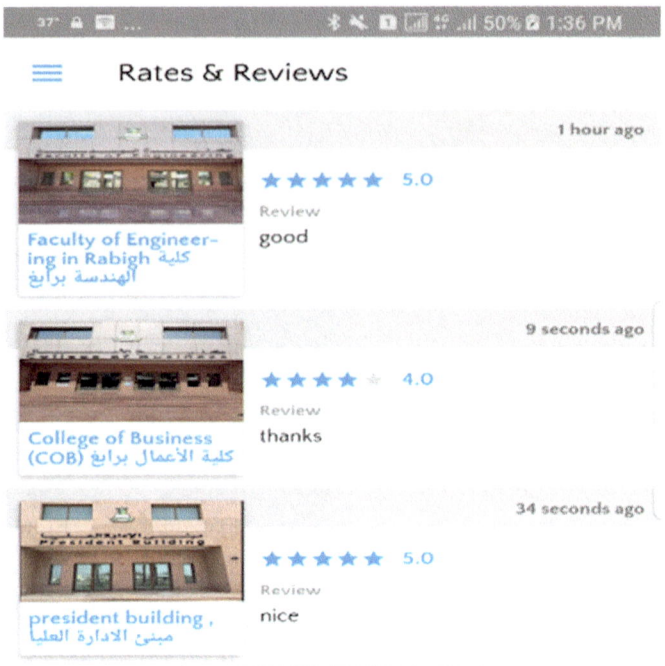

Fig. 13.14 Rating and reviews

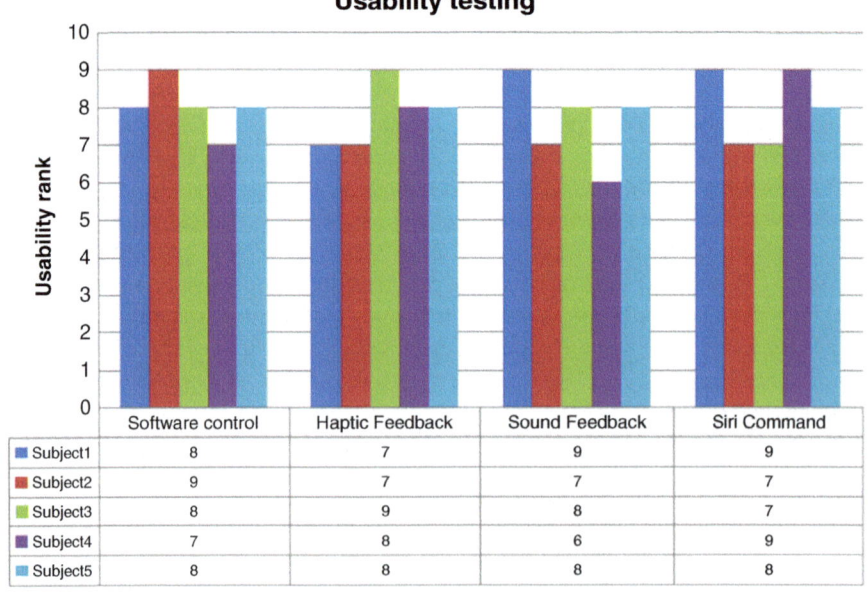

Usability testing

	Software control	Haptic Feedback	Sound Feedback	Siri Command
■ Subject1	8	7	9	9
■ Subject2	9	7	7	7
■ Subject3	8	9	8	7
■ Subject4	7	8	6	9
■ Subject5	8	8	8	8

Fig. 13.15 Usability testing result

13.5   Future Work and Conclusions

HapAR is a mobile augmented reality app with the sternly exclusive role and essence which is transferred efficiently to the user. This system is being introduced to improve the user happiness and simplify the self-touring familiarity within the King Abdulaziz Rabigh branch for the visually impaired user. It uses Siri (Voice Recognition) for command interaction, and then it will find the specific location based on the geo-location reading. The location of the building is predefined and already stored in the database, and it can be compared with the latest location from the user in real time once they run the app.

The user will be guided through audio instruction, which is to provide interactive assistance that reveals how close they are to their destination and the obstacles that exist on the route. In case users get diverted from the track, haptic will alert them and make sure they are on the right track along with audio assistance. The future work that remains challenging for this system is sonar implementation that may give better localization and early warning when the user is approaching an obstacle, so it will increase the safety of the user during their journey toward the destination.

Acknowledgments   This work was supported by the Deanship of Scientific Research (DSR), King Abdulaziz University, Jeddah Saudi Arabia. The authors, therefore, gratefully acknowledge the DSR technical and financial support.

References

Afif, F. N., Basori, A. H., & Saari, N. (2013). Vision based tracking technology for augmented reality: A survey. *International Journal of Interactive Digital Media, 1*(1), 46–49.

Afif, F. N., & Basori, A. H. (2013). Orientation control for indoor virtual landmarks based on hybrid-based markerless augmented reality. *Procedia - Social and Behavioral Sciences, 97*(6), 648–655.

Albaqami, N. N., Allehaibi, K. H., & Basori, A. H. (2018). Augmenting pilgrim experience and safety with geo-location way finding and mobile augmented reality. *International Journal of Computer Science and Network Security, 18*(2), 23–32.

Azuma, R. (1997). A survey of augmented reality. *Presence, 6*(4), 355–385.

Basori, A. H., Afif, F. N., Almazyad, A. S., Abujabal, H. A., Rehman, A., & Alkawaz, M. H. (2015). Fast markerless tracking for augmented reality in planar environment. *3D Resesearch, 6*, 41. https://doi.org/10.1007/s13319-015-0072-5

Bhowmick, A. S., & Hazarika, M. (2017). An insight into assistive technology for the visually impaired and blind people: state-of-the-art and future trends. *Journal of Multimodal User Interfaces, 11*, 149–172. https://doi.org/10.1007/s12193-016-0235

Caudell, T. P., & Mizell, D. W. (1992). *Augmented reality: An application of heads-up display technology to manual manufacturing processes. The 25th Hawaii international conference on system sciences* (pp. 659–669). Honolulu, HI: University of Hawaii at Manoa.

Coughlan, J. M., & Miele, J. (2017). AR4VI: AR as an accessibility tool for people with visual impairments. *International Symposium on Mixed and Augmented Reality, 2017*, 288–292. https://doi.org/10.1109/ISMAR-Adjunct.2017.89

Findlater, L., Stearns, L., Du, R., Oh, U., Ross, D., Chellappa, R., & Froehlich, J. (2015). Supporting everyday activities for persons with visual impairments through computer vision-augmented touch. In *The 17th international ACM SIGACCESS conference on computers & accessibility (ASSETS '15)* (pp. 383–384). New York, NY: ACM. https://doi.org/10.1145/2700648.2811381

Gleason, C., Fiannaca, A. J., Kneisel, M., Cutrell, M., & Morris, M. R. (2018). FootNotes: Georeferenced audio annotations for nonvisual exploration. *Proceedings of the ACM Interactive, Mobile, Wearable Ubiquitous Technology, 2*(3), Article 109. https://doi.org/10.1145/3264919

Hartley, R., & Zisserman, A. (2003). *Multiple view geometry in computer vision* (2nd ed.). Cambridge: Cambridge University Press.

Katz, B. F. G., Kammoun, S., Parseihian, G., Gutierrez, O., Brilhault, A., Auvray, M., . . . Jouffrais, C. (2012). NAVIG: Augmented reality guidance system for the visually impaired. *Virtual Reality, 16*(4), 253–269.

Lee, W.-M. (2010). *Using the accelerometer on the iPhone, iPod touch*. Retrieved 16 April, 2019, from http://www.devx.com/wireless/Article/44799

Lim, P. H. (2012). *Gyroscope in smartphones*. Retrieved 11 October, 2012, from http://www.mobile88.com/news/read.asp?file=/2012/4/21/20120421165938

Milgram, P., Takemura, H., Utsumi, A., & Kishino, F. (1994). Augmented reality: A class of displays on the reality-virtuality continuum. *Telemanipulator and Telepresence Technologies, 2351*, 282–292.

Perrois, J. A., Laviole, J., Briant, C., & Brock, A. (2018). Towards a multisensory augmented reality map for blind and low vision people: A participatory design approach. In *Conference on human factors in computing systems, April 2018*. Montréal, QC: ACM.

Rolland, J. P., Baillot, Y., & Goon, A. A. (2001). A survey of tracking technology for virtual environments. *Fundamentals of Wearable Computers and Augmented Reality, 1*, 67–112.

ShahSani, R. K., Ullah, S., & Rahman, S. U. (2017). Automated marker augmentation and path discovery in indoor navigation for visually impaired. In L. De Paolis, P. Bourdot, & A. Mongelli (Eds.), *Augmented reality, virtual reality, and computer graphics. AVR 2017. Lecture Notes in Computer Science, Vol. 10324*. New York, NY: Springer.

Siltanen, S. (2012). *Theory and applications of marker-based augmented reality*. Espoo: VTT.

Stearns, L., Findlater, L., & Froehlich, J. E. (2018). Design of an augmented reality magnification aid for low vision users. In *The 20th international ACM SIGACCESS conference on computers and accessibility (ASSETS '18)* (pp. 28–39). New York, NY: ACM. https://doi.org/10.1145/3234695.3236361

Tapu, R., Mocanu, B., & Zaharia, T. (2018). Wearable assistive devices for visually impaired: A state of the art survey. *Pattern Recognition Letters*. https://doi.org/10.1016/j.patrec.2018.10.031

Welch, G., & Foxlin, E. (2002). Motion tracking: No silver bullet, but a respectable arsenal. *Computer Graphics and Applications, 22*(6), 24–38.

Wingrave, C. A., Williamson, B., Varcholik, P., Rose, J., Miller, A., Charbonneau, E., . . . LaViola, J. J., Jr. (2010). The wiimote and beyond: Spatially convenient devices for 3D user interfaces. *IEEE Computer Graphics and Applications, 30*(2). https://doi.org/10.1109/MCG.2009.109

Yazdi, N., Ayazi, F., & Najafi, K. (1998). Micromachined inertial sensors. *Proceedings of the IEEE, 86*(8), 1640–1659.

Zhao, Y., Bennett, C. L., Benko, H., Cutrell, E., Holz, C., Morris, M. R., & Sinclair, M. (2018). *Enabling people with visual impairments to navigate virtual reality with a haptic and auditory cane simulation. CHI conference on human factors in computing systems (CHI '18). Paper 116* (p. 14). New York, NY: ACM. https://doi.org/10.1145/3173574.3173690

Zhou, F., Duh, H. B.-L., & Billinghurst, M. (2008). *Trends in augmented reality tracking , interaction and display: A review of ten years of ISMAR. The 7th international symposium on mixed and augmented reality (ISMAR 2008)* (pp. 193–202). New York, NY: ACM & IEEE.

Chapter 14
A Context-Aware Voice Operated Mobile Guidance System for Visually Impaired Persons

Kavi Kumar Khedo, Kishan Yashveer Bhugul, and David Young Ten

14.1 Introduction

In recent years there has been much advancement in technologies that can support visually impaired persons. Indeed, the latest developments in accessible computing technologies have helped millions of visually impaired persons across the world in their daily life (Ehrlich et al., 2017; Pal et al., 2017). Fortunately, all the challenges associated with visual impairments are being addressed at an amazingly rapid pace with stunning modern technologies (Silman, Yaratan, & Karanfiller, 2017). Research on how to improve the everyday life of a visually impaired person is now common and scientists have come up with different solutions to ease the life of those persons. Simple solutions such as text-to-voice output to more complex ones such as the braille impression printer have been proposed. However, as far as navigation solutions are concerned, not so many contributions have been made for the visually impaired persons and this limits their mobility severely.

The most important travelling aid for the visually impaired person is still the white cane. It is after all an excellent example of a good travelling aid as it is multifunctional, cheap and reliable. It also gives an indication to others that the person is visually impaired. In studies about visually impaired person navigation systems (Helal, Moore, & Ramachandran, 2001), it has been noted that even a small amount of extra information about the environment makes a remarkable increase in performance and ease of movement. Therefore, the provision of extra information, through the use of common technologies, that can help the visually impaired people needs to be further investigated.

K. K. Khedo (✉) · K. Y. Bhugul · D. Y. Ten
Department of Digital Technologies, Faculty of Information, Communication and Digital Technologies, University of Mauritius, Reduit, Mauritius
e-mail: k.khedo@uom.ac.mu

© Springer Nature Switzerland AG 2020

335

S. Paiva (ed.), *Technological Trends in Improved Mobility of the Visually Impaired*,
EAI/Springer Innovations in Communication and Computing,
https://doi.org/10.1007/978-3-030-16450-8_14

Nowadays, modern technologies are within the reach of all. It is therefore possible to make use of them and develop a reliable tool to efficiently augment the user's actual navigating techniques. For example, it is now possible to use mobile technologies to make a person with visual impairments more aware of his/her immediate environment. Many researchers like Dey, Abowd, and Wood (1998) have described how contextual information may be used to better understand the situation of users and provide automated customized services accordingly.

In this chapter, a context-aware voice operated mobile guidance system for visually impaired persons named Mobile Vision is proposed and described. The Mobile Vision application is an innovative android application that is used to augment a visually impaired person's pedestrian experience with enough information so as to ease his movement from one location to another. Innovative interaction mechanisms have been developed in Mobile Vision to allow visually impaired persons to use the mobile phone.

14.2 Context Awareness and Navigation Systems for Visually Impaired Persons

The term "context-aware" was brought and defined by Schilit and Theimer (1994) to describe the location, identities of nearby people, objects and changes to the objects. To describe these three factors, four characteristics are used namely: the identity factor that characterizes the object; the location factor that includes the position of the entity and the direction as well as information about regional relations to other entities (e.g. neighbouring entities); the status factor contains properties, which can be perceived by a user.

14.2.1 Types of Context

Any piece of information that is utilized to clarify, specify or determine an event's meaning is called its context. Mobile learning mainly aims at encouraging the user to achieve the maximum level of efficiency in the use of mobile learning solutions. We can broadly categorize context into two types namely intrinsic context and extrinsic context (Thüs et al., 2012).

Intrinsic Context

This category of the context is concerned with the user behaviour. These attributes are his motivational level, his concentration and his knowledge level. Each learner has a different level of knowledge. The application should be able to decide what content to be delivered to the user level of experience and maturity. When registering on a learning system the user is required to answer a few questions that would assess his knowledge on the subject. Based on the assessment, the user is provided with an adapted course content. Then at the end of course he or she is provided a small test to verify if he or she has understood the chapter. The results of this test will decide whether he can proceed to the next level if he needs to spend more time on the same level before taking the test again.

Extrinsic Context

This category contains the information about the current environment of the user. The extrinsic context includes the objects that the user is currently dealing with, the learning time, the position of the user on a map. Peer pressure of a user also forms part of the extrinsic context.

Since the context where a person is located changes rapidly, these changes have to be taken into consideration while designing context-aware systems, especially those that are highly interactive. In context awareness, mobility is an important aspect since the context varies in function of where one is located. With a wide range of possible user scenarios, a mechanism for system services to adapt appropriately and implicitly is needed. For instance, context awareness has to be treated differently at home and at the workplace.

Context awareness can significantly improve navigation systems for visually impaired persons by making them aware of their location and obstacles around them in real-time. This is a crucial aspect while travelling from one place to another as visually impaired persons cannot perceive possible dangers around them. Thus, their other senses such as touch, hearing and smell are heavily used to get an 'image' of their location.

Visually impaired persons generally make use of a white cane or a guide dog, to get more information about their surroundings. However, those two aids do not provide much information that significantly improves context awareness. Visually impaired persons who do not have access to the context-aware technologies, like the GPS, often prefer to rely on repetitive and regular situations that are their past experiences. Unfortunately, visually impaired persons may not be aware of other unexpected hazards. This is where voice recognition and synthesis can help a lot and make them more conscious of the hazards. Any contextual information that may be used to enhance the navigation experience of the visually impaired persons should be fully exploited (Yelamarthi, Haas, Nielsen, & Mothersell, 2010). Modern mobile technologies are equipped with a plethora sensor that can help to detect various contextual information of the user, however these have not been investigated and very limited efforts have been made to develop context-aware navigation systems for visually impaired persons.

14.2.2   Navigation Systems

Navigation systems generally consist of one or several signal emitting devices and a signal receiving device for each user—generally one sender and several receivers. Technologies ranging from the radio frequency identifier description to the global positioning system can be used to provide information like position and environment details. Technologies such as Global Positioning System and Geographic Information System are used for navigation purposes and they can offer contextual information to visually impaired persons (Zöllner, Huber, Jetter, & Reiterer, 2011). Optimized routes can be computed based on the user preference and constraints such as traffic congestion and dynamic obstacles. To get more information about the environment and landmarks of where the person wants to navigate, a spatial database can be queried and output through voice cues.

The main objective of a navigation system is to generate the best path in terms of distance, minimum obstacle and other useful parameters. Some common path determination algorithms (Fallah, Apostolopoulos, Bekris, & Folmer, 2013; Tiwari, 2012) include Dijkstra's algorithm, graph path planning approach and grid path planning approach.

Dijkstra's algorithm can be used to calculate shortest path from a particular point to another. In navigational systems, generally, the shortest path is not the safest one and still the shortest path may not necessarily mean that it will take less time to travel. Furthermore, shortest paths can be complex with many turns and people can get lost if, for instance, they do not turn on at the right place. The best route is the one with the least obstacles or any other hazards that can be a possible danger to the traveller. For example, the path to bypass busy lanes can be longer but safer. The path generated from the graph after applying Dijkstra's algorithm must be translated in directions in order for the person to understand and use it to reach the destination.

In the graph path planning approach, the environment is divided into nodes and edges. Depending on the limitations, each node can represent an object such as an intersection. Then, each edge may be given a weight depending on different criteria such as how dangerous the object can be while navigating. For example, edges with stairs will be of higher weight. Figure 14.1 illustrates the graph approach.

In the grid path planning approach, the environment is divided into cells and each cell contains information about objects at this position. There can be information such as the terrain type for a cell and from the type of terrain, the cell can be classified as traversable or not. For instance, if there is vegetation or snow, the cell is classified as non-traversable. The degree of traversability can be determined from the height of the terrain compared to a reference level which can be determined by the actual location of the user.

There exist some specialized existing navigational systems for visually impaired persons. However, most of these systems are limited in their functionalities and do not fully exploit context-awareness in order to provide better navigation capabilities. For example, Drishti (Helal et al., 2001) is a pedestrian navigation system for visually impaired and disabled persons. It can be used to guide the users to his/her

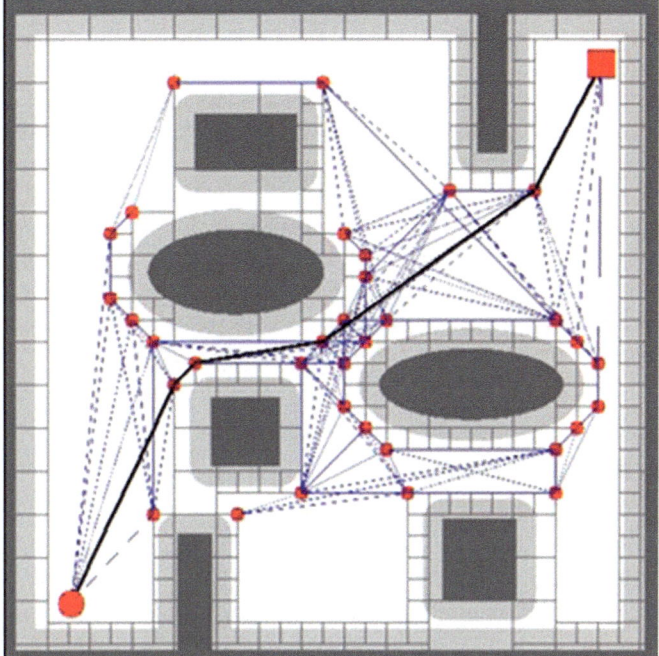

Fig. 14.1 Graph path planning approach

chosen destinations through voice directions feedback. Drishti can also be utilized for tourist guidance. Voice is output from the device on which the system is installed. Along the route towards the users' destinations, warnings of nearby obstacles such as ramps or stairs are given. If other paths are available, the user has the option to choose other routes where he will be more comfortable. Another functionality of the system is that the user can add notes on where he is positioned. For instance, he can add a note about an obstacle that he has discovered on his path for future notices.

Wearable obstacle detection system for visually impaired people (Cardin, Vexo, & Thalmann, 2005) is a system that can be used to caution about neighbouring obstacles while travelling. This is done using a stereoscopic sonar system and then a haptic response is given to the user about the location of the obstacle. Animate obstacles may produce noise and thus non-sighted people can have an idea about the positions of the objects. Yet, static obstacles do not produce sounds and touch has to be used and the person must be nearby the items. Since haptic feedback is used, the hearing sense of the user is not required when interacting with the system. Thus, the user can use his hearing sense for other purposes such as for listening to the surrounding. The sonar sensor has two ultrasonic transducers which are attached together. One emits an ultrasonic wave while the other captures the echo of the ultrasonic wave which had been sent. Using the time at which the signal is emitted and the time at which the echoed signal is received, calculations are done so as to get the distance of the nearest obstacle.

Voice operated outdoor navigation system (Koley & Mishra, 2012) is a transportable system that is useful in congested places. Using a low power GPS, along with voice and the ultrasonic sensor, the user is given necessary information to avoid obstacles along his way. As input, a joystick is used to choose direction and as output, a speaker or headphones are used. For instance, if the East direction is chosen, information about that direction is played via the speaker/headphones. The GPS receiver gets the latitude and longitude of the user's actual position which is then compared in a CSV file on the SD memory card of the device. Place names are stored in the SD card and then are played back to the user from an audio file. If there is an obstacle near the retrieved location, a warning is played back.

14.3 Technological Analysis

In this section, an analysis of technologies available for navigation and interaction systems for the visually impaired is carried out. Latest smartphones are equipped with a wide range of components and sensors such as accelerometer, Wi-Fi and GPS that are useful for navigation systems. Moreover, smartphones have audio capabilities which are very helpful for a visually impaired person. The main mode of communication with the mobile phone is via the in-built microphone and/or speaker for a visually impaired person. Another in-built component is the camera. With the advancements in technologies, image processing can be done with images taken from the camera. On the other hand, if the mobile device does not have enough computing resources, the processing may be done remotely. The different components of mobile devices have made a number of interaction mechanisms possible with visually impaired persons.

Shake input: Shake input is a technology that became popular with the arrival of smartphones in 2007. It generally makes use of an accelerometer sensor; a dynamic sensor capable of a vast range of sensing. Accelerometers that are available can measure acceleration in one, two or three orthogonal axes. Through specific movements of the mobile device different inputs, instructions may be generated. Accelerometers are typically used in one of three modes:

- As an inertial measurement device of velocity and position.
- As a sensor of inclination, tilt, or orientation in two or three dimensions, as referenced from the acceleration of gravity (1 g = 9.8 m/s^2).
- Or as a vibration or impact (shock) sensor.

The shake input method, using the accelerometer sensor, has been mostly used for functionalities like shuffling music in smartphones and MP3 players or gaming like in the Nintendo WII device. The shake method can be used to trigger functionalities for a blind or visually impaired person. For example, one shake voices out the time and two shakes voice out the date.

Voice recognition: With voice recognition software, the right hardware, some time and patience, it is possible to train a device to recognize voice commands issued. Today this technology has become very powerful and the most recent example is the Google Assistant which makes use of natural language for interaction. Voice Recognition technology can be of great help to blind or visually impaired people as they can give voice command such as "Call mum" and the voice is analysed and the action triggered within seconds. However, the use of this technology requires a fast internet connection and works best in a noise free-place.

Text-to-speech output: Text-to-speech tools on mobile devices allow blind or visually impaired users to listen to the text displayed on the screen using a speech synthesizer. A screen reader is the interface between the device's operating system, its applications, and the user. The user may instruct the speech synthesizer to speak automatically when changes occur on the device screen.

Haptic feedback: This technology is used in several ways for the blind and visually impaired. Some applications are using it to relay information about nearby objects back to the user using some vibration motors. The user can feel the distance by the frequency at which the motor pulses; the faster the motors pulse, the closer the object. This kind of feedback can be used whenever it is hard for the user to hear sound alerts. Sound alerts use the same principle, with sound pulses, to relay information to the user but this technique cannot be used in noisy places.

14.4   Mobile Vision: A Context-Aware Voice Operated Mobile Guidance System for Visually Impaired Persons

In this section, the proposed context-aware voice operated mobile guidance system for visually impaired persons, named Mobile Vision is described. The Mobile Vision application aims to augment a visually impaired person's outdoor pedestrian experience with enough information so as to ease his movement from one location to another. Several innovative interaction mechanisms have been developed in Mobile Vision to allow visually impaired persons to interact with a mobile phone.

Due to the highly interactive nature of the system, accurate information is provided to the users in real-time. For example, the user is prompted to turn in a particular direction before passing a junction and not after. In other words, a real-time service should be ensured. Movements of the user are considered in real time and GPS coordinates updated accordingly and properly modelled on the navigation map. New path is determined in case the user takes another direction and the shortest route is still ensured. Different algorithms are considered to ensure the redetermination of routes in case the user takes the wrong direction.

14.4.1 Navigation Map Modelling

The guidance system needs a map to guide the user and notify him about the objects in his immediate surroundings. To model the map, the main objects that should be included are obstacles and places. So as to facilitate the collection of locations, obstacles and places the Google Earth (http://www.google.com/earth/download/ge/) is used. Through site surveys places of interest and other objects are identified and markers are added on the map along with necessary information that will be used by the system. Some places of interest (POI) are already available on Google Earth, thus only the category and other useful information about the places are surveyed. However, to add GPS locations to the map for objects that are not present yet, especially obstacles, a GPS device is used to record the coordinates at the place where the object is found. Furthermore, the information about the obstacles and places are uploaded on a remote server.

The landmark and environment geographic condition are placed on the map during the modelling phase (obstacles, point-of-interest, buildings, opening hours, etc.) and then selected maps are pre-loaded on the mobile device before the start of the journey. It is assumed that routes frequently used by the visually impaired persons will be pre-loaded and synchronized as and when good internet connectivity (minimum 3G) is available. Moreover, a facility is provided so as the mobile device may synchronize with any computer that has the maps through Bluetooth.

14.4.2 Overall System Architecture

The Mobile Vision guidance system for visually impaired persons operates on a mobile device. Sensors are used when required and the system reads and writes files such as maps. Some files have to be downloaded from an online repository. Figure 14.2 gives an overview of the three layers in the Mobile Vision system.

The Mobile Vision system uses different components of the Android OS of the mobile device such as sensors and audio capabilities. The Navigation component is meant to guide the user while the Schedule component gives context information at regular intervals. Figure 14.3 shows the component diagram of the Mobile Vision system.

14.4.3 Path Determination Algorithm

Given a destination, the system gives the safest path to the destination. A combination of a modified version of the Dijkstra's algorithm and a graph-based algorithm is used for this purpose. In order to use the algorithms, a graph must be constructed

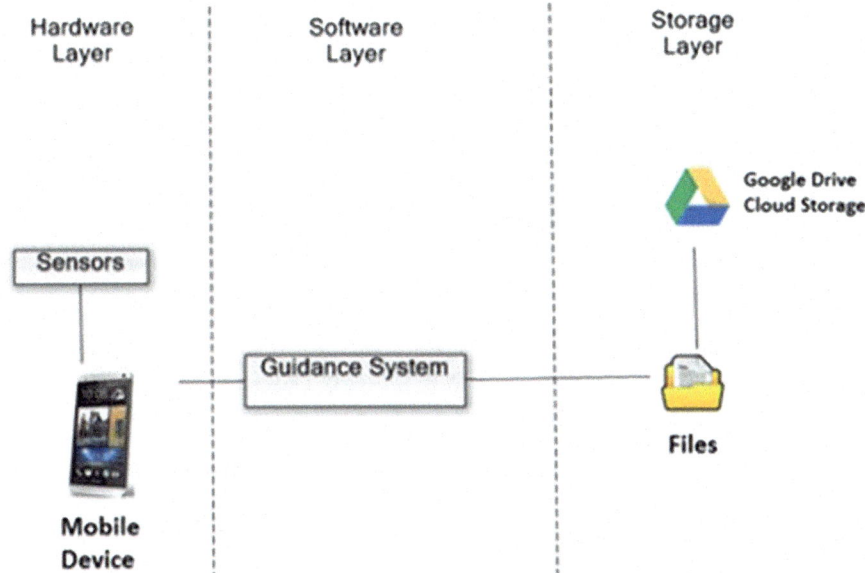

Fig. 14.2 Mobile vision overall system architecture

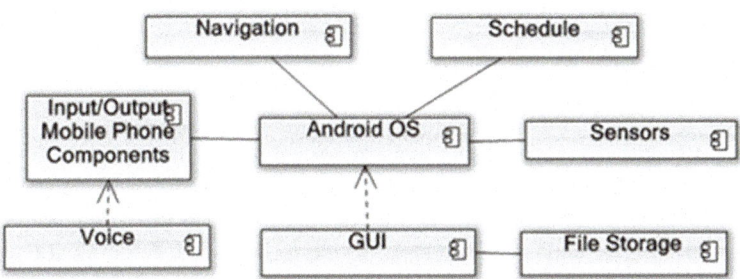

Fig. 14.3 Mobile vision component diagram

which represents the map. An illustration of the construction of a graph based on a customized map is shown in Fig. 14.4.

The following logic is used to construct the graph:

- Each point, whereby there is a change of direction, is taken as a node.
- The path whereby the user can travel between two nodes is taken as edges.
- Each obstacle is given a weightage. The higher the weightage, the more dangerous the obstacle is for the user.
- The weightage of the edges is determined by the sum of the weightages of the obstacles between the two nodes connected by the edge.

As a result, the path which has the lowest weightage is considered as the safest.

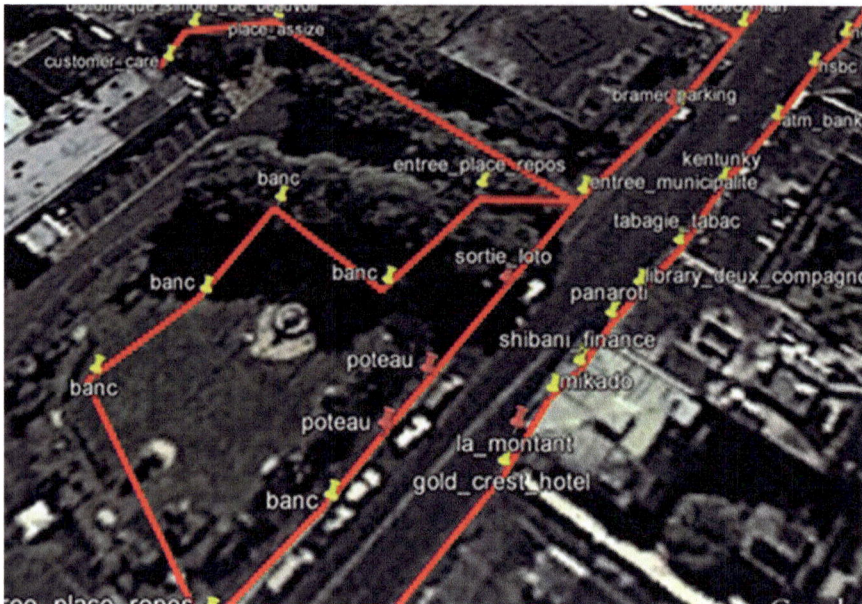

Fig. 14.4 Construction of a graph based on a customized map

14.4.4 Determination of User Orientation

Like for all GPS navigation tools, it is important to get the user heading that is
in which direction the user is walking. To get the user heading, the magnetometer
sensor is usually used, which acts as a compass. The main disadvantage with this
technique is that it requires the mobile device to be in a specific position, either
horizontal or vertical. This is why another technique which consists of flattening the
map and getting the user heading using two GPS coordinates has been derived.

$$\text{Heading Angle} = \text{atan2}\left(\cos\left(\text{lat1}\right) \times \sin\left(\text{lat2}\right) - \sin\left(\text{lat1}\right) \times \cos\left(\text{lat2}\right)\right.$$
$$\left. \times \cos\left(\text{lon2} - \text{lon1}\right), \sin\left(\text{lon2} - \text{lon1}\right) \times \cos\left(\text{lat2}\right)\right)$$

The above equation returns the heading angle in radian from $-\pi$ to π in a four
quadrants fashion. Figure 14.5 shows how to interpret the angle obtained on the
flatten map.

14.4.5 Obstacle Detection Mechanism

The weightage of an edge is determined by the sum of the weightage of obstacles
between two nodes forming the edge. Obstacles that are present between two nodes

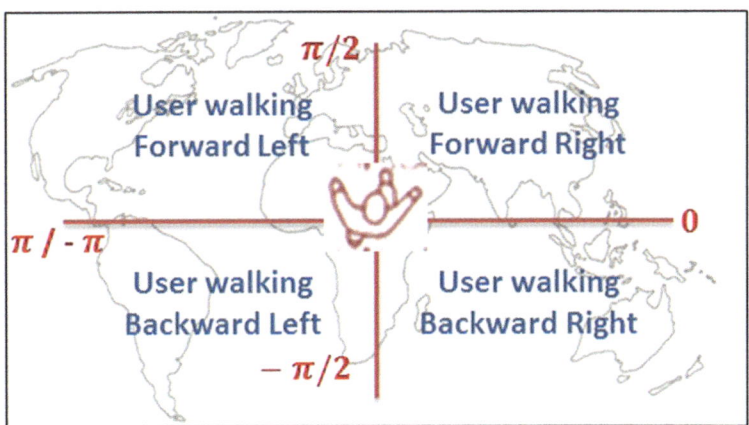

Fig. 14.5 User heading on the flatten map

must be determined. To determine the presence of the obstacles, the heading angle equation from the previous section is used. The system alerts the user about the obstacle when the device is at a distance of three meters from the obstacle and/or a place of interest. This mechanism uses the GPS sensor to get the current location of the device. The current location is then compared to a list of GPS locations of obstacles and places.

14.4.6   Power Consumption Management

The remaining battery level of the mobile device is an important consideration in the Mobile Vision system. The visually impaired person is expected to be very dependent on the system and therefore, its continued operation is vital during a trip. In order to cater for low battery level of the mobile device, two scenarios are considered in Mobile Vision. If the battery level reaches 30%, then user is automatically alerted that the battery is getting low and if the battery life reaches 25% then the system will automatically be switched to an emergency mode. The emergency mode consists of disabling features like haptic feedback and urging the user to set the next destination to a safe place where the mobile device may be powered.

14.4.7   Interaction Mechanisms Used in Mobile Vision

The different interaction modes that are provided in the Mobile Vision system are described in this section. These modes aim to ease the interaction between the visually impaired person and the system.

Voice Feedback Mechanism

To voice out an instruction to the visually impaired persons, the MediaPlayer inbuilt function in Android system is used. It is important that the navigation application gets the audio focus in order to prevent any other applications on the mobile phone to use the sound output function. Other applications on the mobile device should not prevent useful instruction from Mobile Vision being missed by the visually impaired person. To get the audio focus, the audio manager is used.

By default maximum volume is used to voice out an instruction in the Mobile Vision system. A haptic feedback mechanism is used to capture the user's attention before voicing out any instructions. As for any other inbuilt device/sensor in an Android phone, the system service for the vibrator is used. For all voice instructions the user has the option to use a mobile phone headset.

Voice Recording Mechanism

To record a voice, the MediaRecorder inbuilt function in Android system is used. For example, at his current location, a visually impaired person may want to add voice cue of an obstacle/place that is not found in the Keyhole Markup Language (KML) file. Thus an easy interaction mechanism is provided in the Mobile Vision system so as to allow visually impaired persons to record specific voice cues.

Shake-to-Respond Mechanism

The Shake-to-Respond mechanism is extensively used to allow the user to interact with the Mobile Vision system. The accelerometer sensor is used to get shakes by the user. The Android operating system has been investigated in order to be able to catch the shakes of the mobile device and appropriate functions have been implemented to implement the shake-to-respond feature. The sensor listener is first activated and the sensor manager uses the accelerometer sensor. The sensor listener provides a function that executes when there are changes in the accelerometer sensor.

Haptic Feedback Mechanism

The vibrate function is used to capture the user's attention before voicing out any instructions. As for any other inbuilt device/sensor in an Android phone, the system service for the vibrator is required. Once obtained, the vibrator device can be called by specifying the number of times it should vibrate in milliseconds. The haptic feedback is used in several components of the Mobile Vision system wherever the immediate attention of the user is required.

Table 14.1 Context triggered actions

Module	Context aware information used	Action triggered
Safest Path	Obstacles	The safest path is determined
	Current GPS position	
	Destination GPS position	
	Weather information	
	Current time	
User Heading Module	Movement of the user through GPS coordinates	Set the moving direction and angle of the user
Timer Alarm Module	Thirty minutes timer	Voices out the current time, weather information and street name
	Current time	
Navigation	Current GPS position	Voice out surrounding objects like obstacles, interesting places and voice annotation
Shake-to-Respond	A shake action of the user	Select an option based on the number of shakes
Volume Button	A press action of the user	Select an option based on the number of presses
Voice Annotation	Current GPS position	Save the current GPS position to an XML file and start voice recording
Emergency Mode	Battery level information	Urge user to go to initial position, (if user chooses) new path built
	Current GPS location	

14.4.8   Context Triggered Actions

Most of the modules implemented in the Mobile Vision system are dynamic and respond to specific context information. Context-aware information is used by the different modules and an appropriate action is triggered. Table 14.1 shows the module, the context awareness information used and the action being triggered.

14.4.9   Mobile Vision System Components

In this section, the most salient features of the Mobile Vision system are described.

Voice Operated Navigation Support

Given a destination, Mobile Vision automatically determines the best path to be taken by the user. The number of obstacles present, road conditions and weather conditions are all taken into consideration in order to determine the safest path

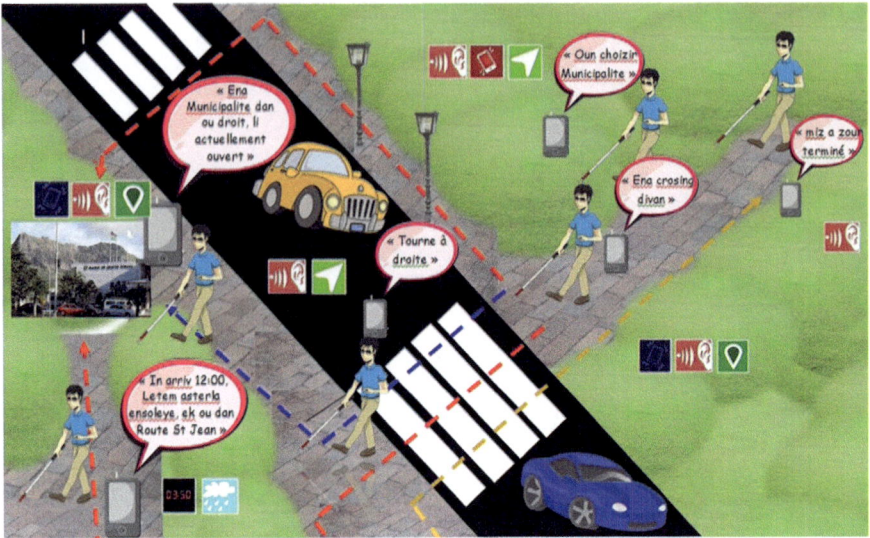

Fig. 14.6 Voice operated navigation support

to the destination. Mobile Vision provides turn-by-turn voice instructions to help the visually impaired persons to move from one place to another. A custom map has been built, which takes into consideration the nearby environment including obstacles, places of interest, actual weather information, the time and day of the week to better guide the user. The application continuously provides feedback to the user about the surroundings. Moreover, Mobile Vision provides a re-routing mechanism that recalculates the best path towards the destination, when the user goes away from the established path. Figure 14.6 shows the best path to the chosen destination of user and the different voice instructions that are given to the user. Only objects relevant to the path are shown on the map.

Innovative Interaction Mechanisms

A Shake-to-Respond mechanism has been developed in Mobile Vision to allow the visually impaired persons to easily interact with the application. Shake-to-Respond allows the visually impaired user to choose from a set of options voiced out by the application by simply shaking the mobile device. Moreover, the Mobile Vision application provides a voice annotation facility which allows the user to easily record a voice description of a particular place of interest. Another mechanism that Mobile Vision application uses to interact with the user is the haptic feedback, which is the vibration facility of the mobile device (Fig. 14.7). The vibrate function is used to capture the user's attention before voicing out any instructions.

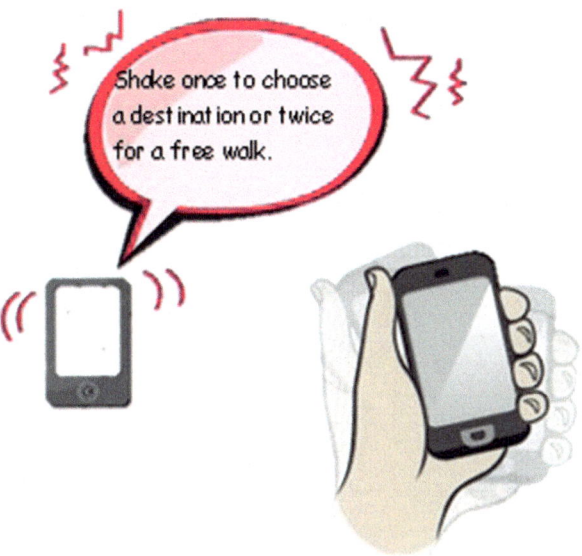

Fig. 14.7 Shake-to-respond interface

Real-Time Environmental Information

Context awareness is any information that can be used to characterize the situation of an entity. Several contextual information are used in Mobile Vision to ease the movement of visually impaired persons. Useful information such as the street name, actual weather information and the time of the day are regularly voiced out to the user (Fig. 14.8). Based on the walking speed of the user, the system automatically calculates the time at which to voice out information about the presence of obstacles.

Back End Cloud Service

A custom map has been built where the objects/places of interest and obstacles are plotted at the appropriate location. Special marking design is provided to add different objects on the map. The map has been implemented using the Google Drive cloud storage to ease maps update process in the mobile device. When Mobile Vision application is started on the mobile device the latest map is loaded from the Google Drive. The map provided is generic and can be built independently for different regions by adding objects such as obstacles and places of interests along with their descriptions (Table 14.2).

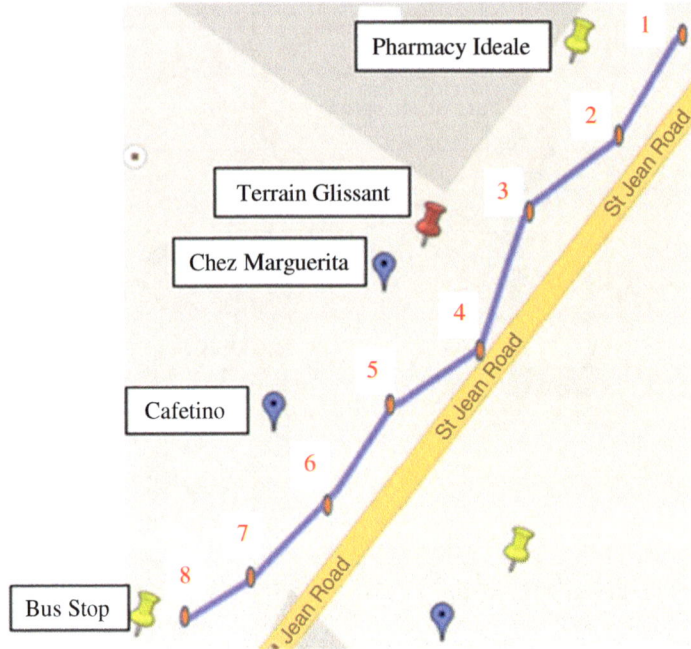

Fig. 14.8 Real-time environmental information

Table 14.2 Salient features of mobile vision system

Features	Description	Features	Description
	Mobile Vision automatically determines the best path to be taken by the user		The voice annotation facility allows the user to easily record a voice description of a particular place of interest
	Frequent weather forecasts are voiced out regularly		The Shake-to-Respond feature allows the user to interact with the application by simply shaking the mobile device
	Real-time information such as nearby interesting places, rest places and obstacles are voiced out		The haptic feedback (vibrate function) is used to capture the user's attention before voicing out any instructions
	All turn-by-turn instructions, options, time, places are voiced out in Creole language		The current time is voiced out to the user every 30 min

14.5   Evaluation of Mobile Vision System and Future Works

Each of the components implemented in the Mobile Vision system has been tested individually. After integration of the different components overall system testing was carried out including accuracy test and performance test. Around 200,000 of places and obstacles were able to be loaded in the system's memory before the application crashes. It is to be noted that the system has been designed in such a way that the minimum number of items are loaded in memory at any particular given instant. The two different options to trigger tasks on the Mobile Vision system were tested. The first one is using shaking, the number of shakes corresponds to the task number and the other option is by using the volume button, again the number of press on the volume button corresponds to the task number.

A thorough user acceptance test was carried out with five volunteer visually impaired persons. To assess the shake sensitivity, the tests were based on hundred attempts. The maximum number of continuous shakes was set to four. The test scenario for the shake-to-respond was as follows:

- The tester had to choose the operation he/she wanted to execute.
- The tester had to shake the mobile device the number of times needed to execute the particular operation.
- For each tester, the number of successful attempts was recorded.

The shake-to-respond feature has been tested for different situations including: while walking; while sitting; while standing; and using different hands. It is to be noted that this module is sensitive enough to detect users' shakes with a success rate of around 96%. Likewise, the other features of the Mobile Vision were systematically tested by the five visually impaired persons and the results were recorded accordingly. It was observed that users were able to recognize an obstacle on average 92% of the time and they were able to understand 94% of the voice instructions given to them during a journey. It was noted that only 75% of the trials for the voice annotation facility were completed successfully by the users. The voice annotation feature requires a number of steps and some users were not able to understand all of them, therefore the usability of this feature should be improved. It was also observed that users were able to capture the haptic feedback 98% of the time and they found this feature to be very useful. The local Creole language has been used to record instructions and information. This is because the Creole language was the preferred language among visually impaired persons who tested the system.

A number of live testing of the Mobile Vision system was carried out with the visually impaired persons after a short training session. It was observed that, after the safest path had been established, precise voice instructions were given to the user. As the testers were navigating, all the required instructions were given depending on the current GPS location. Special care had to be taken in the algorithm to adapt to the user's way of navigating. If ever the user decided to change the path for some reason, the system automatically adapted to the change and regenerated another path from the current location.

The main limitation of the Mobile Vision system was the accuracy of the GPS device of smartphones. Most smartphones have quite inaccurate GPS devices and are not proper for high precision navigation system. This is because GPS devices on smartphones connect only to a limited number of GPS satellites which are generally not precise enough to get the user's exact current location. Through a number of live testing of the Mobile Vision system carried out, it is noted that there is an average deviation of 1.2 m between the predefined location and the location obtained on the fly. The accuracy of the localization service can further be improved by using better GPS receivers.

Moreover, it is observed that as the number of obstacles increases at a particular location, the number of nodes increases and thus the resources required to calculate the path also rises. It should be noted that smartphones have a limited amount of memory and cannot allocate more than a defined amount to a particular application. To overcome this, a device with a larger amount of memory should be used or a more efficient algorithm that can cater for a large number of obstacles at a particular location should be used.

14.5.1 Future Works

The Mobile Vision system provides a solid foundation for an effective and easy to use navigation system for the visually impaired. Further works are required so as to improve the accuracy of the location detection measurements. Moreover, more contextual information can be explored in order to improve the experience of the users of Mobile Vision. The Mobile Vision system can be implemented using better devices such as the Google Glass. The latter has a very accurate GPS device which research has been optimized for walk navigation. Devices like the Google Glass are also equipped with a high-resolution camera at the eye level which can allow identification of objects based on their position and location. Image processing techniques can be used to perform the identification of objects and names of objects can then be voiced out objects in real time instead of fully depending on a custom map.

The path determination algorithm may be improved using machine learning techniques. Based on how the user navigates, on which days, at what time, the places of interest, how obstacles are tackled and which path is used, the system may learn the characteristics of the navigation environment. The paths from starting point A to destination B can be determined based on the user's previous personal experiences. More research should be carried out on the way the safest path is determined. The main algorithm that has been adapted for the Mobile Vision System is the Dijkstra's algorithm. More efficient algorithms should be investigated that will consume less memory and less processing power and that give better paths. Moreover, in the Mobile Vision application only static obstacles have been considered. Mobile obstacles require a different set of algorithms for detection and will be considered in the future.

14.6   Conclusion

In this chapter, the implementation of a context-aware voice operated mobile guidance system for visually impaired persons is presented. A number of innovative mobile user interfaces such as shake-to-respond and haptic feedback have been used in the Mobile Vision system. The Mobile Vision application aims to augment a visually impaired person's outdoor pedestrian experience with enough information so as to ease his movement from one location to another. Several innovative interaction mechanisms have been developed in Mobile Vision to allow visually impaired persons to interact with the mobile phone. Environmental conditions and landmark information along their route are provided on the fly through simple explanatory voice cues. The application can advise the user where he/she is currently located, and provide spoken directions to travel to a particular destination. Optimized routes are computed based on the user preference and constraints such as traffic congestion and dynamic obstacles. To get more information about the environment and landmarks of where the person wants to navigate, a spatial database is queried and the information is output through voice cues.

Live testing was carried out to test the accuracy and performance of the Mobile Vision system. All the components and algorithms developed in the systems were thoroughly tested. It was observed that visually impaired persons were effectively using the system just after a short training of one hour. Moreover, the different interaction mechanisms developed greatly ease the interaction between the users and the system in order to execute the different navigational tasks. The system greatly helps the visually impaired by improving their navigation experience. A number of possible avenues for extending and improving the Mobile Vision system have been identified.

References

Cardin, S., Vexo, F., & Thalmann, D. (2005). Wearable obstacle detection system for visually impaired people. In *VR workshop on haptic and tactile perception of deformable objects* (No. VRLAB-CONF-2005-019, p. 50).

Dey, A. K., Abowd, G. D., & Wood, A. (1998). CyberDesk: A framework for providing self-integrating context-aware services. *Knowledge-Based Systems, 11*(1), 3–13.

Ehrlich, J. R., Ojeda, L. V., Wicker, D., Day, S., Howson, A., Lakshminarayanan, V., & Moroi, S. E. (2017). Head-mounted display technology for low-vision rehabilitation and vision enhancement. *American Journal of Ophthalmology, 176,* 26–32.

Fallah, N., Apostolopoulos, I., Bekris, K., & Folmer, E. (2013). Indoor human navigation systems: A survey. *Interacting with Computers, 25*(1), 21–33.

Helal, A., Moore, S. E., & Ramachandran, B. (2001). Drishti: An integrated navigation system for visually impaired and disabled. In *Proceedings of the Fifth International Symposium on Wearable Computers, 2001* (pp. 149–156). Piscataway, NJ: IEEE.

Koley, S., & Mishra, R. (2012). Voice operated outdoor navigation system for visually impaired persons. *International Journal of Engineering Trends and Technology, 3*(2), 153–157.

Pal, J., Viswanathan, A., Chandra, P., Nazareth, A., Kameswaran, V., Subramonyam, H., ... O'Modhrain, S. (2017). Agency in assistive technology adoption: Visual impairment and smartphone use in Bangalore. In G. Mark, S. Fussell, C. Lampe, M. C. Schraefel, J. P. Hourcade, C. Appert, & D. Wigdor (Eds.), *Proceedings of the 2017 CHI Conference on Human Factors in Computing Systems* (pp. 5929–5940). New York, NY: ACM.

Schilit, B. N., & Theimer, M. M. (1994). Disseminating active map information to mobile hosts. *IEEE Network, 8*(5), 22–32.

Silman, F., Yaratan, H., & Karanfiller, T. (2017). Use of assistive technology for teaching-learning and administrative processes for the visually impaired people. *Eurasia Journal of Mathematics, Science & Technology Education, 13*(8), 4805–4813.

Thüs, H., Chatti, M. A., Yalcin, E., Pallasch, C., Kyryliuk, B., Mageramov, T., & Schroeder, U. (2012). Mobile learning in context. *International Journal of Technology Enhanced Learning, 4*(5-6), 332–344.

Tiwari, R. (Ed.). (2012). *Intelligent planning for mobile robotics: algorithmic approaches: algorithmic approaches*. Hershey, PA: IGI Global.

Yelamarthi, K., Haas, D., Nielsen, D., & Mothersell, S. (2010, August). RFID and GPS integrated navigation system for the visually impaired. In *2010 53rd IEEE International Midwest Symposium on Circuits and Systems (MWSCAS)* (pp. 1149–1152). Piscataway, NJ: IEEE.

Zöllner, M., Huber, S., Jetter, H. C., & Reiterer, H. (2011, September). NAVI–a proof-of-concept of a mobile navigational aid for visually impaired based on the microsoft kinect. In *IFIP Conference on Human-Computer Interaction* (pp. 584–587). Berlin: Springer.

Chapter 15
Modelling the Creation of Verbal Indoor Route Descriptions for Visually Impaired Travellers

Johannes Tröger, Sarah Schnebelt, and Jan Alexandersson

15.1 Introduction

For navigating the environment, humans build upon orientation and mobility skills. These skills are required both in familiar environments and in unfamiliar environments. In familiar environments people often navigate using non-spatial strategies (Iaria, Petrides, Dagher, Pike, & Bohbot 2003), the so-called path-integration strategies which are based upon a single point of reference (Loomis, Klatzky, & Golledge 2001), which is typically the destination point. Relying solely on one single point of reference, like using the starting point alongside path-integration strategies, also might be applied for exploring unfamiliar environments, or sight-seeing. Nevertheless, when navigating unfamiliar environments, humans tend to spontaneously use a landmark-based strategy (Iaria et al. 2003) supported by either cognitive or external maps and by localising themselves through perceptual cues. This highlights two key factors for effective human navigation in unfamiliar environments: (1) landmark-based navigation strategies and (2) the use of cognitive or external maps as support. Visually impaired users (VIs) typically experience great difficulties navigating in unfamiliar environments, as vision is ideal for fast mapping of large environmental layouts (Kalia, Legge, & Giudice 2008; Michon & Denis 2001), reducing the necessary amount of physical exploration, as well as recognising landmarks at distance (Tsuji, Lindgaard, & Parush 2005; Ungar 2000) and most analog support systems like classic signs and maps are restricted to visual perception which makes this support inaccessible for VIs. Large-scale mapping services like *Google Maps* or *OpenStreetMap* model environments digitally and help VIs to overcome the *print barrier* of classic maps and signs. In combination with

J. Tröger (✉) · S. Schnebelt · J. Alexandersson
German Research Center for Artificial Intelligence (DFKI), Saarbrücken, Germany
e-mail: johannes.troger@dfki.de; sarah.schnebelt@dfki.de; jan.alexandersson@dfki.de

© Springer Nature Switzerland AG 2020   355
S. Paiva (ed.), *Technological Trends in Improved Mobility of the Visually Impaired*,
EAI/Springer Innovations in Communication and Computing,
https://doi.org/10.1007/978-3-030-16450-8_15

accessible interfaces like *BlindSquare* these services have significantly reduced the disadvantages VIs encounter when navigating unfamiliar outdoor environments. In indoor navigation such ubiquitous services do not exist yet. Additionally, navigating indoors holds a higher chance of losing orientation (Radoczky 2003).

In line with the fast developing domain of technology-supported outdoor navigation, considerable progress has been made in the field of supporting indoor navigation. This includes localisation of the user, language-based user interfaces, hybrid modelling of the environment in a machine-readable way and adaptive routing algorithms—for an overview see Fallah, Apostolopoulos, Bekris, and Folmer (2013). But still there is a big gap concerning

- the identification of semantic landmarks geared towards the needs of VIs,
- the way of connecting them in order to generate reliable routes and
- the generation of verbal route descriptions (VRDs) communicating this to the traveller via speech driven interfaces.

This paper contributes to fill this gap by introducing and validating a formalised way of building landmark-based indoor VRDs for VIs. In order to reach this goal, this contribution starts with a short note on VIs' mobility and orientation skills which are often disregarded by sighted people, especially when it comes to sighted people trying to help or design supportive solutions for VIs (Williams, Galbraith, Kane, & Hurst 2014).

15.2 Orientation and Mobility (O&M) Skills

Sighted people often underestimate the navigation skills of blind persons (Gomez, Langdon, & Clarkson 2016). The perception of VIs, having "great difficulties in (a) generating efficient mental maps of spaces, and therefore (b) navigating efficiently within these spaces" (Lahav & Mioduser 2003, p. 172), is based upon the outdated assumption that *spatial cognition*[1] is highly depending on vision. Early theories state that VIs "suffer" from (1) deficient (Von Senden 1960) or (2) inefficient spatial cognition (Fletcher 1980) restraining the generation of cognitive maps and thereby navigational performance.

Assuming that spatial cognition is highly dependent on visual input and VIs lack this input over their lifetime, it would result in **deficient spatial cognition**. Regardless it has been proven that both sighted travellers and VIs use perceptual cues from multiple sensory systems (Tsuji et al. 2005), highlighting that spatial cognition is not exclusively built from visual but multimodal sensory input. Moreover, reviewing this theory, one has to keep in mind that visual impairment ranges from blindness to full sight and some VIs rely significantly on visual input

---

[1]Spatial cognition is concerned with the acquisition, organisation, utilisation and revision of knowledge about spatial environments (Center 2016).

while navigating (Kulyukin, Nicholson, & Coster 2008) for determining windows or even discriminating different levels of brightness on surfaces. More recent theories assume that visual impairment is not classified as a total absence of spatial understanding but rather an **inefficient spatial cognition**. The inefficiency theory is mainly supported by empirical studies conducted in small artificial laboratory set-ups, differing significantly from the sensory variation of a realistic indoor navigation environment (Kitchin, Blades, & Golledge 1997). Building cognitive maps in those environments is heavily biased towards the use of *global frames of reference*[2] for spatial coding. Tasks, determining spatial cognition, typically involve pointing at indirectly connected landmarks along a route (Dodds, Howarth, & Carter 1982) or indicating locations after exploration on two-dimensional maps (Fletcher 1980). Both named tasks suggest the use of global frames of reference, which in turn favours sighted people as "vision provides very reliable information about external frames of reference (i.e. the relationship between external surfaces)[but], touch, hearing and movement do not" (Ungar 2000, p. 232). In other words: sighted people have learned to mainly rely on global frames of reference for spatial coding, which is a strategy they also employ in laboratory experiments being blindfolded, which gives them an advantage in the successive measurements, resulting in higher scores and eventually undermining the view of a more efficient spatial cognition. In real-world navigation tasks—including the whole spectrum of sensory input, as well as allowing for body-centric frames of reference—results have shown that VIs perform just as well as blindfolded sighted people which provides strong evidence for a very efficient spatial cognition, as long as the tasks support VIs' strategies (Loomis, Klatzky, Golledge, Cicinelli, Pellegrino, & Fry 1993; Klatzky, Golledge, Loomis, Cicinelli, & Pellegrino 1995).

Therefore, both the deficiency and inefficiency theory have been revised, and current research argues in favour of a third model—the difference theory—which says being visually impaired may result in qualitatively different spatial cognition, but functionally equivalent to those of sighted people (Ungar 2000). This paves the way for a new understanding of VIs cognitive as well as external maps, which are different than those of sighted persons. The general mechanism of organising maps around landmarks is the same for VIs and sighted travellers though (Iaria et al. 2003; Loomis et al. 2001; Ungar 2000; Kitchin et al. 1997; Kitchin 1994; Passini & Proulx 1988).

Michon and Denis (2001) highlight the role of landmarks in building cognitive maps of environments and classify their navigational functions as follows: (1) form cognitive maps, (2) reference actions/decisions, (3) re-orient/approve after decisions. Emphasising their importance as reference for navigational decisions and orientation, they also serve as emotional confirmation for being on the right route. Landmarks "have features that make them stand out to be recognisable from the environment" (Saarela 2015, p. 3). But as mentioned earlier, features that stand out

---

[2]Global frames of reference allow to locate other places within the same frame of reference, as for example, using latitude/longitude values (Kitchin et al. 1997, p. 233).

are somehow different for VIs than for sighted people. Studies have shown that there is a significant difference in the subset of landmarks VIs choose compared to sighted travellers (Passini & Proulx 1988; Golledge, Loomis, Klatzky, Flury, & Yang 1991). It is the way today's world supports landmark-based navigation—based upon vision and visual signage—that imposes an enormous challenge on VIs. Given the print barrier, VIs need significantly more time for creating and learning new landmarks and building cognitive maps than sighted travellers (Qin et al. 2015). Tackling this challenge, verbal or even verbo-tactile, descriptions of the environment can be used as an effective means for supporting non-visual learning in familiar, as well as unfamiliar indoor layouts (Giudice, Bakdash, & Legge 2007; Papadopoulos, Barouti, & Koustriava 2016). The verbal description of geometric concepts (e.g. flight of stairs) is thereby mentally transformed into abstract spatial form enabling the formation of cognitive maps.

To sum up, VIs have, according to the difference theory, no functional limitations due to spatial cognition when it comes to navigation, but rely heavily on alternative sensory inputs. Relying on auditory or tactile sensory input takes typically more time and negatively affects, but in general does not restrict, VIs' navigation ability. The lack of adequate support geared towards VI-specific cognitive mapping forces them to rely on little but robust techniques with long establishment periods and imposing high dependencies. Therefore, innovative approaches are needed that leverage VIs' existing navigation skills to provide the key-elements of personal empowerment.

15.3 Related Work

The key-elements to empower VIs while navigating indoors are (1) underlying hybrid—geometrical and semantic—models, (2) adaptive routing algorithms which work on top of them and provide VIs adequate routes and (3) the provision of VRDs accordingly. As localisation is one of the key enablers for emergency and fall-back functionalities, this paper regards it as one of the prerequisite elements but not a key-element. Considerable technological progress has been made regarding these key-elements—for a comprehensive overview see Fallah et al. (2013). This section will briefly overview these advancements and critical review of them.

15.3.1 Localisation

According to Fallah and colleagues "all navigation systems must include a basic form of localisation" (Fallah et al. 2013, p. 22). This is naturally true when the goal of a navigation system is set to encompass the complete navigation of an individual, including determining a user's location and orientation.

On the contrary, there are scenarios where travellers (1) simply like to localise themselves, (2) do not want to convey their position for localisation or (3) do not meet the technical prerequisites to be properly localised. For instance, many travellers rely on self-localisation with navigational aids, such as the classic, analog map. More strikingly, as path-integration is the best way of exploring unfamiliar areas and building efficient cognitive maps, there is evidence that relying heavily on location-empowered navigation services can negatively affect one's orientation and mobility skills (Aporta & Higgs 2005). In addition, privacy concerns are among the major hurdles for solutions with built-in localisation functionality (Kaasinen 2003). Of course, many users, when navigating foreign environments, accept these drawbacks for the convenience of using navigation services based on fine-grained localisation.

Affordable, GPS-capable mobile devices equipped with global coverage significantly changed the way both VIs and sighted people navigate outdoors. Applications like *BlindSquare* draw upon this effect and are widely used by VIs with smartphones. However, an equivalent service for indoor navigation has yet to be made widely and feasibly available. The latest version of BlindSquare allows for indoor localisation but has major drawbacks. The application, built upon Apple's proprietary *iBeacon* protocol which allows positioning via direct sensing based on bluetooth (Ruffa, Stevens, Woodward, & Zonfrelli 2015; Saarela 2015), is vulnerable to security threats and the accuracy of the localisation—using triangulation instead of proximity—is highly dependent on the number of external beacons distributed (ibid.) in the setting. Relying on and maintaining a large number of technical devices makes this approach prone to error and less than desirable.

Other technical solutions, which accomplish localisation based on alternative technical sensors, include visual pattern matching, users' confirmatory input combined with dead-reckoning or lean approaches that use direct sensing. These are also error-prone as they rely solely on wireless communication fingerprints of preinstalled devices (Schwartz, Stahl, Müller, Dimitrov, & Ji 2010).

15.3.2 Hybrid Models of Environments

One major reason why VIs face less problems with outdoor navigation is the sheer amount of semantic data within a comprehensively charted environment. Google's navigation service, including Google Maps, is primarily based on the enormous potential of modelling the environment with a hybrid of 3D geometric data, information on infrastructure, traffic, points of interest or even visual patterns. It is clear that the depth of this data supports the travellers' cognitive maps at the highest possible degree. Efforts to provide comparable modelling indoors is still in its infancy, although there are OSM-based services like *OpenLevelUp* which also models indoor environments and allows for navigation built upon volunteers' data (Goetz & Zipf 2013). As previously mentioned, landmarks chosen by VIs differ to those chosen by sighted travellers (Passini & Proulx 1988; Golledge et al. 1991), which needs to be reflected in the semantic models of indoor environments. Existing approaches draw upon hybrid models which combine geometrical information with an ontology based on semantic information (Nicholson, Kulyukin, & Coster 2009). This enables *semantic location-based services* (sLBS) or even human-centred LBS, to react dynamically to changes of the spatial semantics or user semantics—e.g. users in wheelchairs asking for navigation vs. VIs asking for navigation (Tsetsos, Anagnostopoulos, Kikiras, & Hadjiefthymiades 2006). The major challenge of this approach lies in the generation of the semantic layer. This can be extracted automatically, requiring significant computation power and engineering effort, or manually created. Manual semantic descriptions of indoor environments by VIs for other VIs ensure a certain validity of the semantic description (Gaunet & Briffault 2005). Community driven semantic data-collection and modelling exploits exactly this effect (Kulyukin et al. 2008; Qin et al. 2015) and raises "the Accessibility Floor by Crowd-sourcing Applications" (Zeng & Weber 2015, p. 348). Although the validity of the constructed semantic information is good, the ontologies of routes have to be carefully harmonised with an individual's O&M training. For example, verbs of movement are part of this training, and if a VI uses a white cane for guidance, this brings four new and different concepts of movement/exploration (Kulyukin et al. 2008).

Leveraging the organic nature of crowd-based ontologies, hybrid models might also include temporary barriers, which are reported as a user encounters them (Chen, Lin, Liu, Zhang, & Yue 2015). This feature enables a connected routing algorithm to produce dynamically personalised routes, although the availability of real-time data limits this functionality.

15.3.3 Adaptive Routing Algorithms

Adaptive or personalised routing algorithms build upon the principle that different users have different preferences when navigating buildings. As there are indeed significant differences in the movement profile of VIs depending on whether they use a cane or a dog (Gaunet & Briffault 2005, p. 282) or whether they have residual vision left or not, different strategies are employed. Research on indoor navigation for VIs tends to marginalise these issues under the homogeneity assumption of the VI target group (Gaunet & Briffault 2005; Giudice et al. 2007), resulting in significant oversimplification. Taking this into account, there are approaches which use sLBS alongside user profiles, modelling preferences according to the use of certain route sections (Tsetsos et al. 2006; Karimi & Ghafourian 2010; Koide & Kato 2005; Swobodzinski & Raubal 2009). In this case navigation turns also into a personalised path-finding problem, which requires more sophisticated algorithms than just the minimisation of the Euclidian distance between start and end points. This can be implemented by a rule-based selection of suitable paths and some quality assessment, eventually proposing the path with the highest score to the user. Other systems use the inverse approach by using a cost-function-based algorithm on top of links between landmarks, tagging, for example, open hallways for some VI with higher costs than corridors (Chen et al. 2015; Koide & Kato 2005). Only three of the reported approaches have been applied to indoor navigation (Tsetsos et al. 2006; Karimi & Ghafourian 2010; Swobodzinski & Raubal 2009), which of course comes with a different set of rules to be implemented. Although technically very promising, two of them do not report any evaluation with actual users (Karimi & Ghafourian 2010; Swobodzinski & Raubal 2009) and one of them reports a preliminary evaluation with a single user (Tsetsos et al. 2006). Nevertheless, a follow-up publication—implementing results from 2006 into a system called *MINISIKLIS* (Kikiras, Tsetsos, Papataxiarhis, Katsikas, & Hadjiefthymiades 2009)—states that "a number of trials with real users are underway" (Papataxiarhis et al. 2009, p. 275), but have until today, writing this text, not been published. Supporting indoor navigation for VIs through personalised routing is thus a very specific case which has not been addressed in depth and more importantly not been evaluated sufficiently. This might also be due to the fact that the actual generation of VRDs is very difficult per se, as VIs need not only suitable routes but also richer information than just a list of left/right turns (Brunner-Friedrich & Radoczky 2006).

15.3.4   *Verbal Route Descriptions (VRDs)*

VIs typically receive comprehensive O&M training resulting in the ability to effectively describe familiar routes to other VIs in a way they can then effectively enact them (Gaunet & Briffault 2005). Although there is broad evidence that VRDs for VIs work both indoors and outdoors there is very limited information on how these descriptions were actually produced and their underlying rules.

Multiple researchers report effective indoor VRDs which are either displayed as recorded audio messages (Koustriava & Papadopoulos 2016) triggered by iBeacon-based localisation (Havik, Kooijman, & Steyvers 2011) or RFID tags (Ivanov 2011). All three papers do not report a formalised method to generate these descriptions. One way to deal with this is by learning how to generate VRDs from existing ones produced by VIs on familiar routes. This method exploits the fact that VIs are able to generate effective VRDs. In 1999, Denis and colleagues used a corpus of routes to identify a skeleton for VRDs which were used for generating descriptions of new routes (Denis, Pazzaglia, Cornoldi, & Bertolo 1999). The results are nevertheless restricted to outdoor navigation and sighted travellers. Implementing a similar approach, Nicholson, Kulyukin and Marston report a solution for automatic landmark extraction from natural language VRDs (Nicholson, Kulyukin, & Marston 2009). Their *route analysis engine* (RAE) uses auto-tagging based on a set of linguistic and grammatical patterns which infer landmarks from spatial prepositions like across, about, away, to the right of, etc. Training data is based on a survey with VIs, resulting in a corpus of 104 VRDs (Kulyukin et al. 2008). The automatically generated landmarks are used in a *Collaborative Route Information Sharing System*

(CRISS), synthesising new routes from existing landmarks. The performance of RAE was evaluated and yielded positive results, but unfortunately it was "not possible, for example, to actually test someone attempting to follow one of the routes described" (Nicholson 2010, p. 149). This of course drastically reduces the validity of the reported approach. An evaluation with actual VIs on unfamiliar routes, following the newly generated VRDs, would be crucial for understanding the feasibility of this approach. Moreover, this approach is based on the comprehensive training data of a precise area, relying on a critical size of VIs providing valid VRDs, as all corpuses do. The danger of circular reasoning is obvious: VIs need VRDs to travel in unfamiliar areas but therefore VRDs generated from other VIs, having already travelled this areas, are needed. This fact represents a major limitation in terms of feasibility.

Taking this into account, explicit formalised rules, that allow for the creation of VRDs in indoor layouts, merit investigation, for VIs as well as sighted persons. To solve this, Gaunet and Brifault propose an experimental set-up for outdoor navigation which includes three steps: (1) VIs travel familiar outdoor environments and explain the route like they would do for another VI, (2) rules to build VRDs are extracted and applied to build new descriptions for unfamiliar routes and (3) the new paths are evaluated again through VIs (Gaunet & Briffault 2005).

Regarding the state of the art, one major drawback is the lack of standardised, sufficient evaluation of personalised routing (Swobodzinski & Raubal 2009; Chen et al. 2015; Tsetsos et al. 2006; Papataxiarhis et al. 2009; Karimi & Ghafourian 2010) with actual VIs. Building upon the insights Gaunet and Brifault regarding the generation of outdoor VRD routes (Gaunet & Briffault 2005), this contribution addresses the following challenges:

- the **identification of suitable landmarks** geared towards the needs of VIs,
- the way of connecting them in order to generate **valid routes** and
- the **generation of VRDs** communicating this to the traveller via speech driven interfaces.

15.4   Iterative User-Centred Approach

In resolution to the aforementioned gap of sufficient evaluation in personalised routing, user-centred design methodologies have been successfully applied in the area of human–computer interaction (Lowdermilk 2013; Gulliksen et al. 2005; Tröger et al. 2016). This user-centric design emphasises VIs in all stages of development, and ensures focus on the intended demographic, a necessity for evaluating and reporting results. In general, the user-centred approach in this study can be described in four phases: (1) acquisition and analysis of data, (2) synthesising formal models, (3) generating VRDs with unknowing sighted persons and (4) evaluating these descriptions with VIs; the four-step sequence was iterated again after the first cycle—compare also Fig. 15.1.

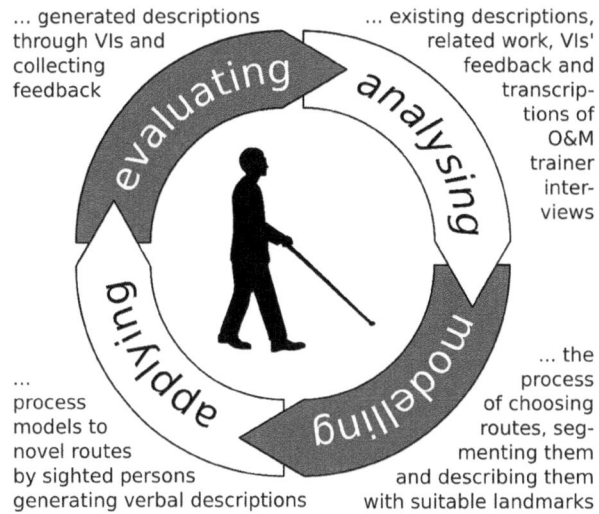

... generated descriptions through VIs and collecting feedback

... existing descriptions, related work, VIs' feedback and transcriptions of O&M trainer interviews

... the process of choosing routes, segmenting them and describing them with suitable landmarks

... process models to novel routes by sighted persons generating verbal descriptions

Fig. 15.1 The applied user-centred design cycle

Both evaluation phases and the second data acquisition phase involved VIs. The eleven participating VIs were between 24 and 63 years old: eight were born without sight and three have been blind since 22, 26 and 37 years of age. All have been skilled cane users for 18–40 years and would, for initially visiting unknown buildings, arrange sighted company, ask an employee to pick them up at the entrance of the building or ask random bystanders to describe directions to a specific spot. One of the test persons stated that they occasionally carry a dictaphone to record verbalised descriptions while travelling in order to find the same routes again. All mentioned VIs participated in the data acquisition phase and three congenitally completely blind persons visited the campus of Saarland University to test and assess the navigation instructions in, for them, an unknown environment.

15.4.1 Acquisition and Analysis

In the first cycle, VRDs for three routes in the authors' office building were analysed. These descriptions had already been evaluated with two VIs and proven to be feasible. The data was linguistically analysed, based on existing state-of-the-art ontologies for route descriptions (Allen 1997; Kulyukin et al. 2008). For the second cycle, comments for improvements of the newly generated VRDs were collected and additionally, several interviews with VIs and O&M instructors were carried out. The comments were recorded on audio while the VIs followed the novel VRDs and also afterwards answering the debriefing questionnaire. The interviews with O&M trainers were based on a 37 items survey, comprising open questions on strategies, as well as the use of concrete possible landmarks.

Linguistic Structure of Verbal Route Descriptions

The analysis revealed that VRDs consist of two components: (1) directions (Where am I going?) and (2) context (Where am I?). This mirrors related work (Havik et al. 2011; Allen 1997) which typically classifies two types of communicative statements for VRDs: Route Information and Environment Information or Directives and Descriptives. The latter describes the environment of the building or room, and its features, as well as declaring important *fixed objects* (FOs) and their position. Directions, however, comprise the actual orientation and mobility instructions. Both types of elements were classified according to four categories: *environmental features* (sound, smell, touch, sense, named FOs), *delimiters* (countable, descriptive, localisation, spatial, distance), *verbs of movement* and *state-of-being verbs* (egocentric, exocentric). Directions include references to the relevant *FOs* which are introduced in the context of the previously described categories. After evaluating the generated VRDs, additional insight was gained in the use of context in descriptions. To best support the creation of cognitive models, context descriptions should immediately refer to floor numbers and the label of the part of the building. VIs mentioned that as soon as buildings' labels are absent, this causes confusion and a break in continuity.

Sequence of Directions

Descriptions are compiled from smaller sections which are typically based on architectural layouts. A section might only be a large room with a complex layout, or a sequence of directions guiding through an entire part of the building with a simpler structure. The algorithm for constructing analysed descriptions is modelled as follows:

- A VRD always starts with an environmental description (context)
- One or more directions are attached which lead to the next section
- In the new section a context specification follows[3]
- A VRD ends with the notification that the user has reached the goal

A pilot study with one VI and interviews with O&M trainers confirmed the structural analysis of existing VRDs: blind people prefer having knowledge about the environment, in advance, which conveys an additional sense of safety and autonomy; therefore the context is of high importance. The context information also helps to build cognitive maps of the surroundings, therefore it has to be given for each section introducing architectural features, as well as FOs and their positions to be referred to within the directions.

---

[3]Steps 2 and 3 are repeated until the target destination is reached.

Fixed Objects as Landmarks

The analysed routes typically used FOs as landmarks (e.g. handrails or stairs; architectural features like walls, windows or pillars). After the pilot evaluation, the VI mentioned concern about the use of elevators due to the lack of a standard interfaces and being possibly unable to react in an emergency situation. Another verbalised concern was the use of countable delimiters in directions, especially in the case of counting doors: according to the general sound scenery, VIs have to bypass doors very closely to notice them through the echo of their footsteps, which causes them discomfort, as they don't want to give the impression of entering some stranger's office.

Careful analysis of basic building blocks of VRDs gives an idea of their linguistic structure, how they can be modelled as a sequence of directions and contexts, and the use of FOs as suitable landmarks. However, the analysis in combination with the architectural layout on site reveals that the sequence of directions following landmarks is typically just one possible strategy out of multiple to navigate to the respective destination. This raises the following question: what strategy allows for choosing from multiple existing landmarks and connecting them through directions in order to build effective VRDs? Such a strategy or model would be essential to enable a third unexperienced instance, like any sighted person or software, to create effective VRDs for VIs.

15.4.2   Synthesising a Formal Model

Solving this part of the equation for VIs is more difficult than for other travellers with special preferences. Visual impairment does not physically restrict VIs in a direct way, like in the case of moving in a wheelchair (Tsetsos et al. 2006). Therefore, routing strategies were deduced from existing VRDs and interviews with O&M trainers, resulting in the following skeleton: (1) definition of starting point and destination, (2) choice of navigable route, (3) segmentation of the route into handy subsections and (4) development of strategies for each section (Fig. 15.2).

The definition of starting point and destination is typically given by task and therefore not subject to the formal model. Still, it was mentioned by VIs after the first cycle that the information on how to enter/access the starting point should be included—the description should, for example, not start in the main hall but standing outside the building.

Choice of Suitable Route

In most cases several routes lead to a destination and the shortest might not necessarily be the most suitable one. If more structural possibilities are available, such as stairs and elevators, the indoor navigation system should either take the

Fig. 15.2 The final flowchart
for generating VRDs

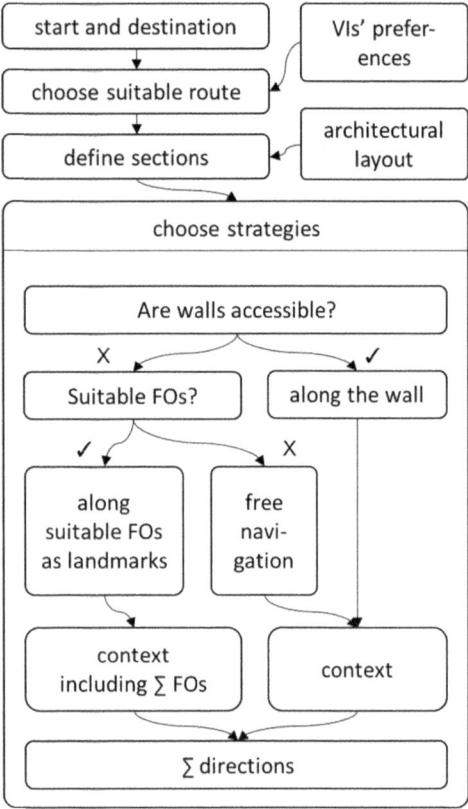

user's preferences into consideration or introduce the various alternatives (using elevator vs. climbing stairs). Thereby, a certain degree of independence and the opportunity to make own decisions can be given by an indoor navigation systems.

Segmentation of the Route

The segmentation of a route into convenient subsections serves two goals: reducing the mental load of the traveller and fostering the generation of modular cognitive maps. The pilot test clearly demonstrated that by the segmentation of VRDs, the VI was able to give more valid VRDs than when trying to describe the whole route at once. The boundaries of the sections are in most cases given by the architectural layout on site and follow the boundaries of rooms or corridors, although in some cases it makes sense to subsegment large rooms or long corridors. This makes sense especially when the environmental features change significantly enough for VIs to recognise—for example, concrete walls which are succeeded by a glass facade in a corridor.

Development of Strategies for Segments

Within each section the VI is guided according to, in the context introduced, suitable FOs serving as landmarks.

Suitable FOs Both evaluation phases showed that direction strategies need to carefully avoid harm-causing objects. This was also underlined by the professional O&M trainers: objects at stomach or head level cannot be detected with the most important navigation aid of VIs, the white cane and therefore, have to be widely avoided and are categorised as non-suitable FOs. Otherwise, descriptions are built in relation to suitable FOs, elements that do not move, which fulfil the criteria of landmarks and are in most cases recognisable through tactile or even auditive senses, described by environmental features. After the two evaluations with VIs new insights were gained and the strategies were updated concerning three issues: (1) although fixed objects that are frequently in use by people were first instructed to be avoided, VIs claimed that they are used in crowded areas and have no problems with that. (2) Moving objects like umbrellas, blocking the entrance, were also classified as familiar and easily managed issues. (3) FOs that are narrow, small or low and located in the middle of route sections/rooms are typically easy to miss and should not be used as landmarks. One example which occurred multiple times during the evaluation was the pillar in the middle of the hall, which fulfils exactly these characteristics—see Fig. 15.3.

Navigating Along Walls Each landmark connects to other landmarks via directions. VIs feel the safest when they are guided along vertical walls using rectangular turns. However, occasionally buildings' architectural layout is more complex so that either paths along walls are not available, and/or turns are not rectangular. If that is the case, VIs can also walk rather close to walls and still recognise the presence of a wall.

Navigating Freely Given the case that walls are rather inaccessible, VIs have to navigate freely in the room. This can also include walking in a diagonal direction to cross the room. Therefore, interviews with O&M trainers yielded the following: in order to specify the range of rotation/degree of turning, the clock system and relations of the body to FOs can be used, e.g. with the wall in your back or walk facing eleven o'clock.

These insights, concerning the choice of suitable routes, the segmentation of routes and the development of strategies were synthesised in the next step and resulted in two instructive documents, a flowchart, including explanations for all steps and a dictionary, which serve as objective tools for third persons to generate new VRDs even if they are unfamiliar with the way VIs move indoors.

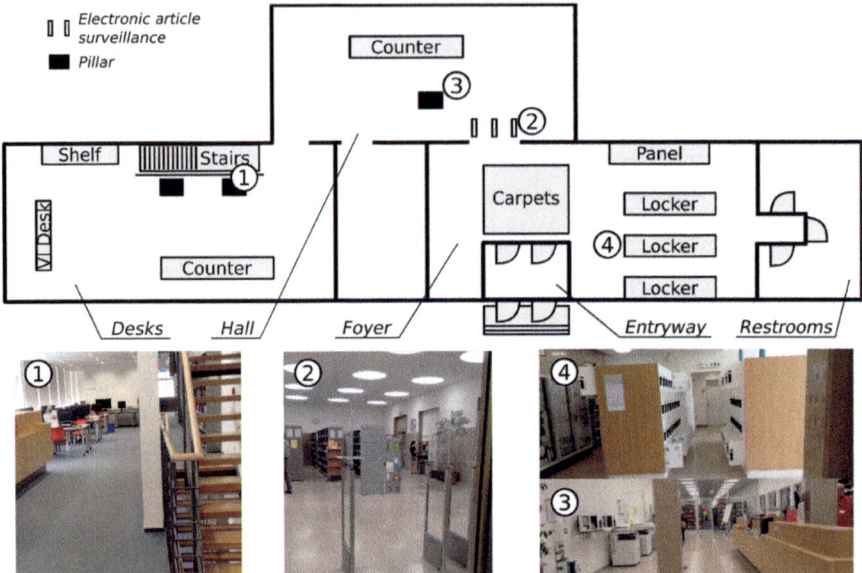

Fig. 15.3 The general architectural layout of the SULB, displaying the test-route from the entrance to the VI desk and from the entrance to the restrooms

15.4.3   Generating Verbal Route Descriptions

In order to evaluate the formal model for generating VRDs, an environment was chosen that was unfamiliar for all participating VIs. Sighted subjects who had no former experience with VIs were using the instructions to generate new VRDs while being on site. Four sighted subjects (20–46 years old) generated descriptions—two each cycle. The environment that was chosen for the new descriptions was the university library of the University of Saarland (SULB) which comprises a dedicated workplace for people with visual impairment. Therefore, the routes to be described were covering the path from the entrance to these workplaces and from the entrance to the restrooms and vice versa—compare Fig. 15.3.

The participating sighted subjects were met on site and given the task, as well as time to acquaint themselves with the foreseen routes. They were then provided with the two instructive documents, a notepad and pencils. An experimenter was always near by to answer questions on the method but did not answer questions on the content of the task at hand. After all sighted participants completed their descriptions their results were compared and if possible synthesised into a single VRD. If that was not possible, all options were juxtaposed to present them to the VIs during the adjacent evaluation phase. The descriptions were compared, regarding the categories discussed in the previous section–synthesising formal models: (2) choice of navigable route, (3) segmentation of the route into handy subsections and (4) development of strategies for each section. In general, all four subjects implemented

Table 15.1 Directions used to describe route 1—entrance to the VI workplaces and route 2— entrance to the restrooms—with the maximum, minimum and mean number of directions over all four subjects, as well as the number of directions which yielded a total accordance over all four subjects and the number of directions which yielded at least an accordance of two over all four subjects

	N directions			Accordance	
Route	Max	Min	$\bar{x}$	4/4	$\geq$2/4
1	19	15	17.25	7	17
2	7	3	5.75	2	4

the foreseen routes by the same route, but with different amounts of segmentation of the route into sections. Three of four subjects described the route (1) from the entrance to the visually impaired's workplaces by five sections and one subject described it by six sections; the route (2) from the entrance to the restrooms was described by two sections, over all four subjects. Within the two addressed routes the sighted subjects generated VRDs with up to 24 (1) and seven (2) possible different directions, which yielded an accordance of all four subjects for seven (1) and two directions (2) and a partial accordance of at least two subjects for 17 (1) and four directions (2), respectively—compare Table 15.1.

In order to analyse the used landmarks, the contexts and the directions were analysed according to the used FOs. Hereby, FOs that were used by only one sighted subject to support a direction, but not by the other sighted subject were classified as mismatch, whereas FOs that were described by both subjects in the context but not used in the directions were classified as matches, as well as FOs that were used by both subjects in their contexts and their directions accordingly. In order to assess the reliability of the instructive material for generating VRDs, the inter-rater reliability can be used, for which Cohen's kappa coefficient is an approved statistical indicator (Bortz 2005). In both cycles the two sighted subjects yielded κ coefficients around 0.40 which is typically regarded as moderate or fair agreement between raters (Landis & Koch 1977)—compare also Table 15.2.

After completing the VRD descriptions each participant filled out a meta-survey gathering feedback on the instructive materials and the process of generating VRDs for VIs. In both the first and second cycle the subjects classified the instructive materials as intelligible. However, in the first cycle, they stated that the instruction was too extensive and therefore hard to apply in such a short amount of time; accordingly, the instructions were adapted with this feedback for the second cycle.

15.4.4 Evaluation of Verbal Route Descriptions

The evaluation of the generated VRDs represents the fourth phase within the user-centred methodology. This evaluation serves as an assessment of the validity of the generated VRDs within a special group of subjects, VIs. Validity, in this context,

Table 15.2 Inter-rater
reliability for the generated
VRDs by sighted subjects in
cycle 1, upper panel, and
cycle 2, lower panel

		S1				
		Used	Not used	$\sum$		
S2	Used	11	5	16	p_0	0.72
	Not used	2	7	9	p_e	0.51
	$\sum$	13	12	25	κ	0.43
		S3				
		Used	Not used	$\sum$		
S4	Used	13	5	18	p_0	0.74
	Not used	1	4	5	p_e	0.56
	$\sum$	14	9	23	κ	0.41

Comparing fixed objects used as landmarks and these mentioned in the description though not used as landmarks in the directives, whereby the relative observed agreement among both raters p_0 and the hypothetical probability of chance agreement p_e result in the coefficient κ

is defined as the degree to which VIs efficiently and safely arrive at the foreseen destination of a route or route sections, indicated by VIs behaviour and comments while following the VRDs. The three VIs that followed the VRDs were asked to comment on the feasibility of the encountered descriptions while following them. This included comments in free format and also dedicated comments on the used strategy composing these sections. The situation was observed by the experimenter who took notes and rated the sections' validity. A section's validity was rated as *poor* when a subject could not succeed to the next section in a reasonable time, intentionally stopped to follow the directions, the experimenter had to intervene to protect the subject from harm, or the next section was reached unintentionally, meaning the subject didn't follow the VRD but reached the next section by chance. In this case the experimenter intervened and asked for feedback and suggestions for improvement according to the invalid section. A section's validity was rated as *medium*, when a subject succeeded to the next section but claimed that the VRD should be significantly improved and suggested a possible alternative for a chosen strategy. A section's validity was rated as *high*, when a subject uttered no negative feedback, succeeded to the next section and had no or insignificant suggestions on improvements. After completing the navigation tasks all VIs answered questions from a debriefing survey.

Technical Setup

ELENA (ELEvator Navigation App) is an indoor navigation App prototype which runs on Android devices which was developed in the DFKI in former projects. It already includes some VRDs in Saarbrücken's DFKI office building. In order to synchronise ELENA's VRDs with the physical localisation, the user can either use preinstalled near field communication (NFC) tags on site, or the built-in UbiSpot system, which requires trained wireless communication fingerprints on the route to enable a more effective localisation (Schwartz et al. 2010). Building on this framework ELENA implements an interface for location-based services especially for operating the elevator via the smartphone interface, depending on the momentary position within the building. The VRDs follow the aforementioned structure of *descriptives* and *directives* and are verbalised by the built-in Android text-to-speech engine. The user can repeat descriptions through the interface and also confirm progress on route manually. For the evaluation, the generated descriptions were transcribed into digital text and then included in the existing ELENA application to be read out by the text-to-speech engine. For the evaluation within this study ELENA was additionally equipped with bone conductance headphones, in order to deliver the VRDs without interfering with the subjects' primary sensory system.

Results

According to the mentioned two types of assessed feedback, the results will be divided into results from the formal feasibility evaluation and results from the free comments.

Formal Feasibility The sighted persons VRDs of the two addressed routes—(1) entrance to the VI workplaces and (2) entrance to the restrooms—were evaluated by three VIs which resulted in four directions having poor validity and three directions having medium validity—compare Fig. 15.4 and Table 15.1. Poor direction's validity was due to the following reasons:

- Undetectable small FOs like the electronic article surveillance detectors in the hall—see Fig. 15.3
- Problems with straight free walking in large rooms

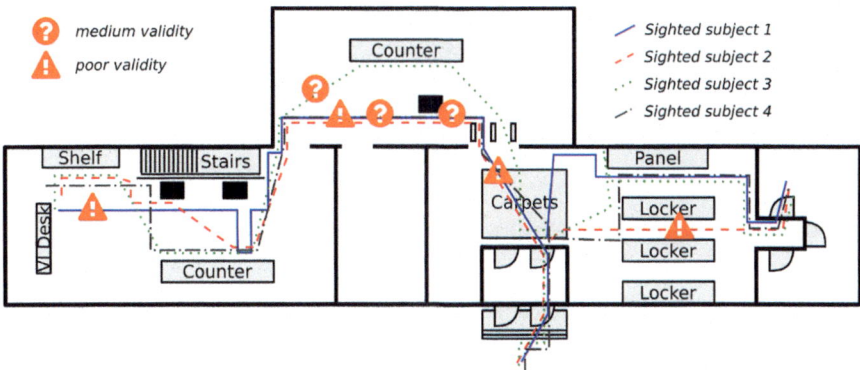

Fig. 15.4 The generated route descriptions—generated by subject one and two within the first cycle and subject three and four within the second cycle—and their validity evaluated by VIs

- Navigating along harm-causing objects like open locker doors at height of the head which might be detected to late and might cause accidents

  Medium direction's validity was due to the following reasons:

- Unexpected movable objects like umbrellas or other visitors blocking the described direction
- Problems with diagonal free walking in large rooms
- Undetectable thin FOs like the pillar in the hall—see Fig. 15.3

In order to gain more insights in trouble-causing directions, comments of the VIs were collected and VIs completed the debriefing questionnaire after navigating through both test-routes. These comments and answers were analysed as free comments.

Free Comments As indicated above, FOs which were potentially harm-causing haven't been classified as harm-causing or have been overseen by the sighted subjects, which indicated that the instructions on harm-causing objects were not accurate enough. Therefore, the strategy flowchart was revised and suitable FOs are better described in the final model. Comparing the reactions on chosen landmarks, VIs did not always agree on the suitability of FOs as landmarks. For example, carpets were both accepted as suitable FOs and as movable objects and therefore classified as unsuitable. FOs which are not necessarily perceivable such as the pillar and the detectors were treated differently. For sighted persons the pillar and detectors are large enough to not be overseen, but their total volume is relatively small and therefore hard to locate through auditive echo from VIs' steps. Accordingly, these FOs were also explicitly categorised as unsuitable. The third and fourth VRD from the second cycle did not include the electronic article surveillance, but VIs stated afterwards that they preferred to know about the detectors although they are hard to find. Asking for preferences between different strategies, VIs' preferences were only partly overlapping. One VI preferred to navigate free in the room whereas another VI preferred directions along FOs and architectural components. According to the debriefing questionnaire, one subject felt more confident when travelling in unknown areas than the others. This subject also preferred the strategy, navigating free in the room. Finally, all three VIs agreed that noises or odours should not be included as landmarks in VRDs.

15.5   Discussion and Conclusion

This study set out to provide a formal model for the creation of VRDs and evaluate it with VIs. The model was evaluated in two consecutive cycles yielding positive results among the evaluating VIs.

Emphasising that novice sighted subjects with no prior experience with VIs, or their travelling methods, were able to generate VRDs which yielded valid ratings proves that the presented model answers the need for a formalised step-by-step manual for the generation of indoor VRDs. This result is remarkable, as former studies have shown, in that especially sighted persons have difficulties understanding how VIs navigate though VRDs (Williams et al. 2014). The reliability of the used instructive material was assessed in both cycles and showed a fair inter-rater reliability which is acceptable. This serves as evidence for the applicability of the model which is also supported by the general positive feedback on the feasibility of the model. Still some subjects created invalid directions which did not serve to help VIs efficiently and safely arrive at the determined destination of the route. In some case, a correct application of the model could have prevented invalid directions. In other cases, the model had to be adapted for special cases like hardly perceivable FOs or harm-causing FOs. In contrast to former ontologies of suitable landmarks for VIs (Kulyukin et al. 2008), noises and odours were found to be unsuitable and VIs stated that such environmental features should not be included as landmarks. The final model is in line with the respective analysis of outdoor VRDs (Gaunet & Briffault 2005; Allen 1997) and fills the gap of how to generate valid indoor VRDs for VIs.

Although preliminary findings are reported, a comprehensive evaluation of the model's reliability and validity, as a step-by-step tool, is beyond the scope of this study, representing one major limitation. In order to systematically evaluate this approach's reliability and validity the instructive materials and generated VRDs need to be treated separately. A larger pool of subjects is needed to generate a sufficiently large number of VRD instances of the same route, to calculate advanced reliability measures for the generated VRDs, like consistency. Advanced evaluations of the generated VRDs should also consider the psycho-linguistic processes of VIs, including the understanding and coding of VRDs as well as translation into locomotion making use of O&M skills. The interaction with or new generation of cognitive maps should also be evaluated, connecting to results from aforementioned work in this field (Iaria et al. 2003; Loomis et al. 2001; Ungar 2000; Denis et al. 1999; Kitchin et al. 1997; Kitchin 1994; Passini & Proulx 1988). Hereby, one should carefully decide on which level of granularity VRDs should be evaluated—route level, sections level or even directions and context level. This study reports first results on the level of directions, as the pool or roots were not large enough to create a representative body of data for generalisable statements about the models' validity on a route level.

The gathered qualitative data resulting from VIs free comments and answers to the debriefing questionnaire revealed an, in the literature mainly unattended, angle on the topic of indoor navigation for VIs: although VRDs for VIs represent a niche in the field of research on pedestrian navigation, preferences regarding the choice of landmarks or routing strategies vary enormously upon VIs. This study especially revealed different preferences for routing strategies which should be, as indicated by qualitative data, in relation to VIs' confidence for travelling in unfamiliar environments and VIs' self-efficacy. This hypothesis could be subject to further investigations in this field, clarifying whether greater self-confidence in VIs correlates with preferences towards shorter and more direct strategies navigating free in rooms and if less self-confidence correlates with preferring longer routes, along fixed objects and architectural structure components. The relationship between such preferences and the received O&M training could also be within the scope of such a research activity. This promising angle should be taken into consideration in future activities in this field of research.

Acknowledgements The authors would like to thank Hali Lindsay and Alarith Uhde for helpful feedback and proofreading on an earlier version of the manuscript.

References

Allen, G. L. (1997). From knowledge to words to wayfinding: Issues in the production and comprehension of route directions. In *International Conference on Spatial Information Theory* (pp. 363–372).

Aporta, C., & Higgs, E. (2005). Satellite culture: Global positioning systems, inuit wayfinding, and the need for a new account of technology. *Current Anthropology, 46*(5), 729–753. https://doi.org/10.1086/432651

Bortz, J. (2005). *Statistik für human- und sozialwissenschaftler* (6th ed.). Berlin: Springer. https://doi.org/10.1007/b137571

Brunner-Friedrich, B., & Radoczky, V. (2006). Active landmarks in indoor environments. In S. Bres & R. Laurini (Eds.), *Visual information and information systems* (pp. 203–215). Berlin: Springer.

Center, B. B. S. C. (2016). *Spatial cognition.* Retrieved August 14, 2016 from http://bscc.spatial-cognition.de/node/12

Chen, M., Lin, H., Liu, D., Zhang, H., & Yue, S. (2015). An objectoriented data model built for blind navigation in outdoor space. *Applied Geography, 60,* 8494. https://doi.org/10.1016/j.apgeog.2015.03.004

Denis, M., Pazzaglia, F., Cornoldi, C., & Bertolo, L. (1999). Spatial discourse and navigation: An analysis of route directions in the city of Venice. *Applied Cognitive Psychology, 13*(2), 145–174. https://doi.org/10.1002/(SICI)1099-0720(199904)13:2h145::AID-ACP550i3.0.CO;2-4

Dodds, A. G., Howarth, C. I., & Carter, D. C. (1982). The mental maps of the blind: The role of previous visual experience. *Journal of Visual Impairment & Blindness, 76*(1), 5–12.

Fallah, N., Apostolopoulos, I., Bekris, K., & Folmer, E. (2013). *Indoor human navigation systems: A survey* (vol. 25, no. 1). Oxford: Oxford University Press. https://doi.org/10.1093/iwc/iws010

Fletcher, J. F. (1980). Spatial representation in blind children. 1: Development compared to sighted children. *Journal of Visual Impairment and Blindness, 74*(10), 381–385.

Gaunet, F., & Briffault, X. (2005). Exploring the functional specifications of a localized wayfinding verbal aid for blind pedestrians: Simple and structured urban areas. *Human–Computer Interaction, 20,* 267–314.

Giudice, N. A., Bakdash, J. Z., & Legge, G. E. (2007). *Wayfinding with words: Spatial learning and navigation using dynamically updated verbal descriptions* (vol. 71, no. 3). https://doi.org/10.1007/s00426-006-0089-8

Goetz, M., & Zipf, A. (2013). Indoor route planning with volunteered geographic information on a (mobile) web-based platform. In *Progress in location-based services* (pp. 211–231). Berlin: Springer.

Golledge, R. G., Loomis, J. M., Klatzky, R. L., Flury, A., & Yang, X. L. (1991). Designing a personal guidance system to aid navigation without sight: Progress on the GIS component. *International Journal of Geographical Information System, 5*(4), 373–395.

Gomez, J., Langdon, P. M., & Clarkson, P. J. (2016). Navigating the workplace environment as a visually impaired person. In M. Antona & C. Stephanidis (Eds.), *Universal access in human-computer interaction. Users and context diversity* (pp. 566–576). Cham: Springer.

Gulliksen, J., Göransson, B., Boivie, I., Persson, J., Blomkvist, S., & Cajander, Å. (2005). Key principles for user-centred systems design. In *Human-centered software engineering—integrating usability in the software development lifecycle* (pp. 17–36). Berlin: Springer.

Havik, E. M., Kooijman, A. C., & Steyvers, F. J. (2011). The effectiveness of verbal information provided by electronic travel aids for visually impaired persons. *Journal of Visual Impairment & Blindness, 105*(10), 624.

Iaria, G., Petrides, M., Dagher, A., Pike, B., & Bohbot, V. D. (2003). Cognitive strategies dependent on the hippocampus and caudate nucleus in human navigation: Variability and change with practice. *The Journal of Neuroscience: The Official Journal of the Society for Neuroscience, 23*(13), 5945–5952.

Ivanov, R. S. (2011). A low-cost indoor navigation system for visually impaired and blind. *Communication and Cognition, 44*(3), 129.

Kaasinen, E. (2003). User needs for location-aware mobile services. *Personal and Ubiquitous Computing, 7*(1), 70–79.

Kalia, A. A., Legge, G. E., & Giudice, N. A. (2008). Learning building layouts with non-geometric visual information: The effects of visual impairment and age. *Perception, 37*(11), 1677–1699. https://doi.org/10.1068/p5915

Karimi, H. A., & Ghafourian, M. (2010). Indoor routing for individuals with special needs and preferences. *Transactions in GIS, 14*(3), 299–329.

Kikiras, P., Tsetsos, V., Papataxiarhis, V., Katsikas, T., & Hadjiefthymiades, S. (2009). User modeling for pedestrian navigation services. In *Advances in ubiquitous user modelling* (pp. 111–133). Berlin: Springer.

Kitchin, R. M. (1994). Cognitive maps: What are they and why study them? *Journal of Environmental Psychology, 14*, 1–19.

Kitchin, R. M., Blades, M., & Golledge, R. G. (1997). Understanding spatial concepts at the geographic scale without the use of vision. *Progress in Human Geography, 21*(2), 225–242. https://doi.org/10.1191/030913297668904166

Klatzky, R. L., Golledge, R. G., Loomis, J. M., Cicinelli, J. G., & Pellegrino, J. (1995). Performance of blind and sighted persons on spatial tasks. *Journal of Visual Impairment and Blindness, 89*(1), 70–82.

Koide, S., & Kato, M. (2005). 3-D human navigation system considering various transition preferences. In *2005 IEEE International Conference on Systems, Man and Cybernetics* (vol.1, pp. 859–864). https://doi.org/10.1109/ICSMC.2005.1571254

Koustriava, E., & Papadopoulos, K. (2016). The impact of orientation and mobility aids on wayfinding of individuals with blindness: Verbal description vs. audio-tactile map. In *International conference on universal access in human-computer interaction* (pp. 577–585). https://doi.org/10.1007/978-3-319-40250-5

Kulyukin, V., Nicholson, J., & Coster, D. (2008). Shoptalk: Toward independent shopping by people with visual impairments. In *Proceedings of the 10th International ACM SIGACCESS Conference on Computers and Accessibility* (pp. 241–242). https://doi.org/10.1145/1414471.1414518

Lahav, O., & Mioduser, D. (2003). A blind person's cognitive mapping of new spaces using a haptic virtual environment. *Journal of Research in Special Educational Needs, 3*(3), 172–177. https://doi.org/10.1111/1471-3802.00012

Landis, J. R., & Koch, G. G. (1977). The measurement of observer agreement for categorical data. *Biometrics, 33*(1), 159–174.

Loomis, J. M., Klatzky, R. L., & Golledge, R. G. (2001). Navigating without vision: Basic and applied research. *Optometry and Vision Science: Official Publication of the American Academy of Optometry, 78*(5), 282–289. https://doi.org/10.1097/00006324-200105000-00011

Loomis, J. M., Klatzky, R. L., Golledge, R. G., Cicinelli, J. G., Pellegrino, J. W., & Fry, P. A. (1993). Nonvisual navigation by blind and sighted: Assessment of path integration ability. *Journal of Experimental Psychology: General, 122*(1), 73.

Lowdermilk, T. (2013). *User-centered design: A developer's guide to building user-friendly applications*. Sebastopol: O'Reilly Media.

Michon, P.-E., & Denis, M. (2001). When and why are visual landmarks used in giving directions? In D. R. Montello (Ed.), *Spatial information theory* (pp. 292–305). Berlin: Springer.

Nicholson, J. (2010). Generation and analysis of verbal route directions for blind navigation. All graduate theses and dissertations. 672. https://digitalcommons.usu.edu/etd/672

Nicholson, J., Kulyukin, V., & Coster, D. (2009). ShopTalk: Independent blind shopping through verbal route directions and barcode scans. *The Open Rehabilitation Journal, 2*(1), 11–23. https://doi.org/10.2174/1874943700902010011

Nicholson, J., Kulyukin, V., & Marston, J. (2009). Building route based maps for the visually impaired from natural language route descriptions. In *Proceedings of the 24th International Cartographic Conference (ICC 2009)* (pp. 15–21).

Papadopoulos, K., Barouti, M., & Koustriava, E. (2016). The improvement of cognitive maps of individuals with blindness through the use of an audio-tactile map. In M. Antona & C. Stephanidis (Eds.), *Universal access in human-computer interaction. Interaction techniques and environments* (pp. 72–80). Cham: Springer.

Papataxiarhis, V., Riga, V., Nomikos, V., Sekkas, O., Kolomvatsos, K., Tsetsos, V., et al. (2009). Mnisiklis: Indoor location based services for all. In *Location based services and telecartography ii* (pp. 263–282). Berlin: Springer.

Passini, R., & Proulx, G. (1988). Wayfinding without vision an experiment with congenitally totally blind people. *Environment and Behavior, 20*(2), 227–252. https://doi.org/10.1177/0013916588202006

Qin, H., Rice, R. M., Fuhrmann, S., Rice, M. T., Curtin, K. M., & Ong, E. (2015). Geocrowdsourcing and accessibility for dynamic environments. *GeoJournal, 81*(5), 699–716. https://doi.org/10.1007/s10708-015-9659-x

Radoczky, V. (2003). *Kartographische unterstützungsmöglichkeiten zur routenbeschreibung von fußgängernavigationssystemen im in-und outdoorbereich.* (Unpublished doctoral dissertation), WienInstitut für Kartographie und Geo-Medientechnik, Wien.

Ruffa, A. J., Stevens, A., Woodward, N., & Zonfrelli, T. (2015). Assessing iBeacons as an assistive tool for blind people in Denmark. Worcest. Polytech. Inst. Interact. Qualif. Proj. E-Proj.-050115–131140.

Saarela, M. (2015). Solving way-finding challenges of a visually impaired person in a shopping mall by strengthening landmarks recognisability with iBeacons. Technical report. Häme University of Applied Sciences, Finland. http://www.hamk.fi/english/collaboration-and-research/smart-services/matec/Documents/solving-way.pdf

Schwartz, T., Stahl, C., Müller, C., Dimitrov, V., & Ji, H. (2010). UbiSpot - A user trained always best positioned engine for mobile phones. In *2010 ubiquitous positioning indoor navigation and location based service, UPINLBS 2010* (vol. 11). https://doi.org/10.1109/UPINLBS.2010.5654313

Swobodzinski, M., & Raubal, M. (2009). An indoor routing algorithm for the blind: Development and comparison to a routing algorithm for the sighted. *International Journal of Geographical Information Science, 23*(10), 1315–1343. https://doi.org/10.1080/13658810802421115

Tröger, J., Alexandersson, J., Britz, J., Rekrut, M., Bieber, D., & Schwarz, K. (2016). Board games and regulars' tables—extending user centred design in the mobia project. In *International Conference on Human Aspects of it for the Aged Population* (pp. 129–140).

Tsetsos, V., Anagnostopoulos, C., Kikiras, P., & Hadjiefthymiades, S. (2006). Semantically enriched navigation for indoor environments. *International Journal of Web and Grid Services, 2*(4), 453. https://doi.org/10.1504/IJWGS.2006.011714

Tsuji, B., Lindgaard, G., & Parush, A. (2005). Landmarks for navigators who are visually impaired. In *Proceedings of XXII International Cartographic Conference a Coruña 2005 Proceedings, CD*.

Ungar, S. (2000). Cognitive mapping: Past, present and future. In *11 New Fetter Lane, London EC4P 4EE* (1st edn., pp. 221–248). London: Routledge.

von Senden, M. (1960). Space and sight: The perception of space and shape in the congenitally blind before and after operation. Oxford, England: Free Press of Glencoe. https://psycnet.apa.org/record/1960-35029-000

Williams, M. A., Galbraith, C., Kane, S. K., & Hurst, A. (2014). Just let the cane hit it: How the blind and sighted see navigation differently. In *Proceedings of the 16th International ACM Sigaccess Conference on Computers & Accessibility* (pp. 217–224). https://doi.org/10.1145/2661334.2661380

Zeng, L., & Weber, G. (2015). A pilot study of collaborative accessibility: How blind people find an entrance. In *Proceedings of the 17th International Conference on Human-Computer Interaction with Mobile Devices and Services*.

Chapter 16
An Aid System for Autonomous Mobility of Visually Impaired People on the Historical City Walls in Lucca, Italy

Massimiliano Donati, Fabrizio Iacopetti, Alessio Celli, Roberto Roncella, and Luca Fanucci

16.1 Introduction

According to the Italian Institute of Statistics (ISTAT) (Istituto Poligrafico e Zecca dello Stato, 2007), the number of visually impaired people in Italy is 350,000 and, among them, the number of blind people is 60,000. In Europe, visually impaired people are about 30 million (European Blind Union, 2008).

For many people with visual impairments, autonomous mobility is often limited to the well-known home environment or to the surroundings, due to the dangerousness of moving alone: from obstacles encountered on the path (e.g. stairs, holes, etc.) to the danger represented by motor vehicles, subways, etc. However, having some possibility of autonomous mobility beyond a limited context may improve the overall quality of life of these people, favoring relationships and increasing self-esteem.

People with visual impairments, and in particular blind people, need to acquire some specific skills before moving autonomously outside a well-known context. Moreover, the use of mobility aid devices to recognize the current position on a route and to detect and avoid obstacles and dangers is often required. Before walking alone on a route, it is generally needed to have built a mental map of the route, enriched with reference points such as trees, building corners, lamps, sidewalks, stairs, etc., which can help the person to recognize his/her position.

Because of the difficulties and dangers involved in autonomous mobility, many people with visual impairments have often to give up moving alone.

M. Donati (✉) · F. Iacopetti · A. Celli · R. Roncella · L. Fanucci
Department of Information Engineering, University of Pisa, Pisa, Italy
e-mail: massimiliano.donati@unipi.it; fabrizio.iacopetti@unipi.it; alessio.celli@unipi.it; roberto.roncella@unipi.it; luca.fanucci@unipi.it

© Springer Nature Switzerland AG 2020   379
S. Paiva (ed.), *Technological Trends in Improved Mobility of the Visually Impaired*,
EAI/Springer Innovations in Communication and Computing,
https://doi.org/10.1007/978-3-030-16450-8_16

The present work describes the continuation of the research project "The Walls for All" (in Italian "Le Mura Per Tutti") (Fanucci, Roncella, Iacopetti, Donati, & Giannelli, 2014) and its current outcomes. The goal of the project is the realization of a mobility aid system for visually impaired people in a public outdoor place of free time, tourist and cultural interest. The project aims at promoting autonomous mobility on a predefined safe path installed on the historical walls of Lucca City, Tuscany, Italy. The developed solution provides the user with guidance and context information by means of a modified traditional white cane equipped with embedded electronics (Smart Cane), buried cables identifying the safe path (virtual path), and a specific Android application running on a mobile device. The project is being carried out at the Department of Information Engineering, University of Pisa, Italy.

Hereafter, Sect. 16.2 reports the state-of-the-art analysis of mobility aid systems. The proposed mobility solution and the installation site are respectively described in Sects. 16.3 and 16.4. Finally, conclusions are drawn in Sect. 16.5.

16.2   State of the Art in the Field of Mobility Aids for Visually Impaired People

In the field of mobility aids for visually impaired users, different solutions have been proposed until now. The most recent solutions rely on modern ICT technologies and different working principles, while some others are traditional and well-known (e.g. white cane, dog guides, etc.).

Each proposed solution typically addresses some specific aspects and requirements of autonomous mobility. For example, the detection of obstacles in front of the user, the provision of navigation information to reach the desired destination, the tactile feedback as a mean of guidance on a route, etc. The different proposed solutions have their own advantages and drawbacks.

The current section illustrates the main categories of mobility aid systems for people with visual impairments, providing some examples of ICT-based solutions that have reached the commercial or pre-commercial stage, and citing also some in progress or finished research projects (Elmannai & Elleithy, 2017).

16.2.1   GPS-Based Geo-Localization and Guidance

This category of mobility aid systems relies on geo-localization and guidance information based on the current user's position and on a map. Such systems exploit the GPS (Global Positioning System) signal and in some cases also terrestrial enhancement signals aiming at improving positioning accuracy (Easy Walk, n.d.; Elmannai & Elleithy, 2017; The Cittabile Project, n.d.; The MAPPED Project, n.d.).

Guidance information provided to the user are usually vocal messages and/or vibration feedback.

GPS-only based solutions rely on GPS positioning accuracy. In outdoor scenarios, the minimum accuracy is in the order of one/few meters, but near buildings, trees, etc., accuracy can raise up to 10 m or more. Such accuracy is therefore not completely suitable for mobility of visually impaired pedestrians, especially in an urban scenario, where routes are complex and present several obstacles (e.g. sidewalks, traffic lamps, etc.) and dangers (e.g. vehicles, stairs, etc.). Moreover, GPS-based systems cannot be used inside buildings due to the lack of the GPS signal coverage.

Two main sub-categories of GPS-based systems exist: (1) applications for mobile devices and (2) stand-alone dedicated devices.

Among applications for mobile devices, an example is represented by the Android app Corsair (n.d.). Similar apps are available for different operating systems, as an example the application BlindSquare for iOS (n.d.). Other examples are available in literature (GPS for the Visually Impaired, n.d.).

Corsair is a GPS-based Android app for pedestrian navigation. The application provides the user with information about navigation, Points of Interest (POI) in the surroundings, ordered by category, and can also provide information about public transports (if available). The user is guided by means of vocal messages, or via the vibration of the mobile device that helps the user follow the right direction. The application offers other features that are particularly suitable for people with visual impairments, for example the repetition of the last played messages by pressing the earbud push-button, the provision of messages about the current position, etc. A screenshot of the Corsair application is shown in Fig. 16.1.

The application uses the same maps of other consumer services, but provides an ad-hoc realized user interface. The application exploits the mobile and/or WiFi data communication infrastructure to download the needed maps. No other infrastructure delimiting or identifying the path is needed. The application is freely available to users and is Open Source.

Within the sub-category of GPS stand-alone dedicated devices, Trekker Breeze Plus (n.d.), shown in Fig. 16.2, is a commercial device for pedestrian navigation of visually impaired people. Along the route, the device provides vocal messages concerning street names, the presence of crosses and information on nearby POIs such as public buildings and shops. The device also provides step-by-step instructions on how to use it.

On the producer's website it is not explicitly mentioned whether the terminal exploits data communication networks to retrieve the needed maps, or if maps are pre-loaded or have to be uploaded to the device in other ways (as an example via a personal computer and an Internet connection). The system does not need any infrastructure delimiting or identifying the path.

Other similar commercial devices exist (GPS for the Visually Impaired, n.d.), some of them providing also very specific user interfaces like Braille Note GPS that features a Braille interface (Braille to Note GPS Website, n.d.).

Fig. 16.1 A screenshot of the
Corsair application for
Android mobile devices

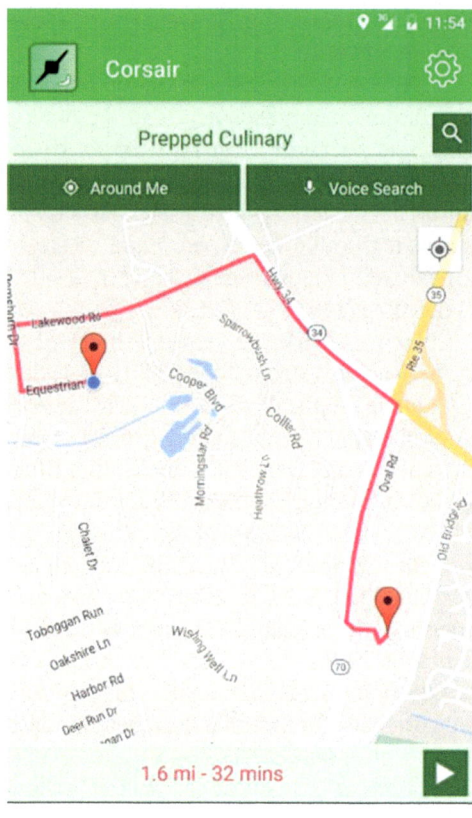

Finally, there are several research projects that led to the development of prototypical GPS-based systems (Malavasi et al., 2009; Xiao, Ramdath, Losilevish, Sigh, & Tsakas, 2013).

16.2.2   Obstacle Detection

Other mobility aid systems for visually impaired people aim at detecting obstacles in front of the user and warning him/her accordingly. Those systems are known as Local Obstacle Detection (LOD) systems and are designed to inform the user about the presence and possibly the position of obstacles.

Such systems are typically implemented by means of electronic devices that are mounted on a traditional white cane or integrated with it, or they are carried by users in their hands. The devices are equipped with detection sensors and provide a human–machine interface. The most used sensing technologies are ultrasounds, infrared and LASER (Elmannai & Elleithy, 2017; Farcy & Damaschini, n.d.).

Fig. 16.2 The stand alone
GPS-based navigation device
Trekker Breeze Plus

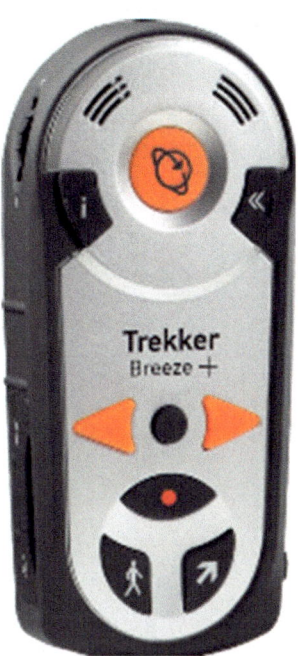

Anyway, currently available devices are not able to detect all obstacles in front of the user, mainly because of the very different geometrical and physical properties of obstacles (e.g. shape, composition, height from the ground, etc.).

Some research projects concerning obstacle detection and classification are focused on RADAR-based systems, as an example (Kwiatkowski et al., 2017). Until now, LOD systems based on RADAR technologies have not reached the commercial stage because the performance of such systems is still not adequate, mainly due to technical difficulties related to their design and miniaturization.

Among commercial LOD systems, Ultracane from BEL (Ultracane System Website, n.d.) is a white cane whose handle embeds ultrasound ranging sensors. The device emits ultrasound beam in different directions and processes the received echoes to obtain information about the presence and the distance of obstacles in front of the cane. Two push-buttons/vibration actuators on the cane handle provide the user with information about obstacles by means of a vibration that is modulated according to the position of the obstacle. The device is able to detect obstacles on the ground and up to a height of about 1.5 m. The device and the detection areas are shown in Fig. 16.3.

Ultracane does not require neither data communication networks nor the installation of any infrastructure on the path. The producer's website underlines the importance of a training phase of at least some days with an instructor to learn how to use the device properly.

Safewalk (n.d.) is another example of LOD cane providing the user with information about the presence of obstacles in front of him/her via vibration

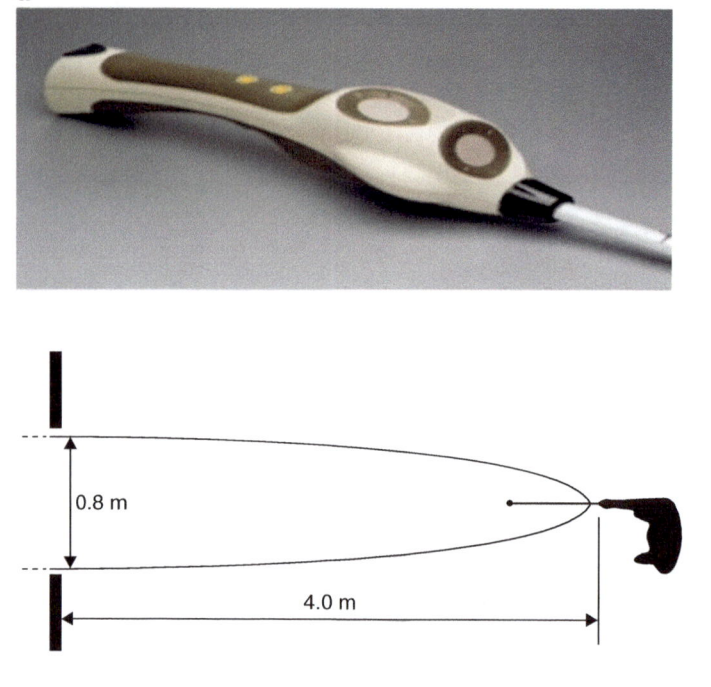

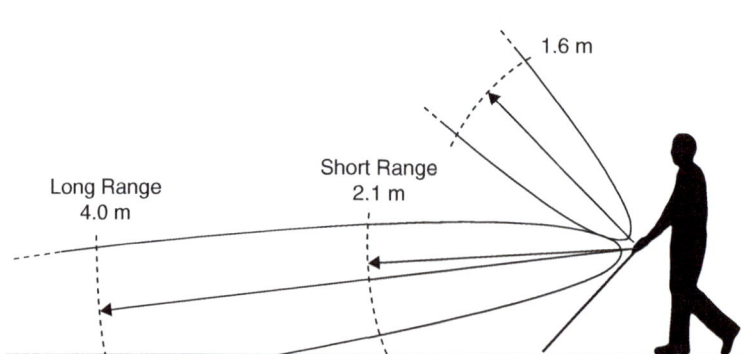

Fig. 16.3 The Ultracane handle (**a**) and the illustration of the detection areas (**b**)

feedback and audio messages. In particular, the user is warned about the danger of falling or stumbling due to changes of the ground level, both uphill and downhill, due to obstacles in front him/her and due to suspended obstacles: lamps, poles, stairs, cars, sidewalks, open blinds, etc. The system, shown in Fig. 16.4, is suitable for both outdoor and indoor environments.

The lower-end of the cane is provided with a double wheel that allows the user to perceive the characteristics and roughness of the ground and to reduce the effort in keeping the cane. The system is made from aluminum in order to be light and

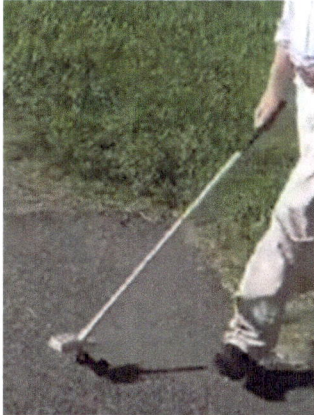

Fig. 16.4 The prototypical version of Safewalk system

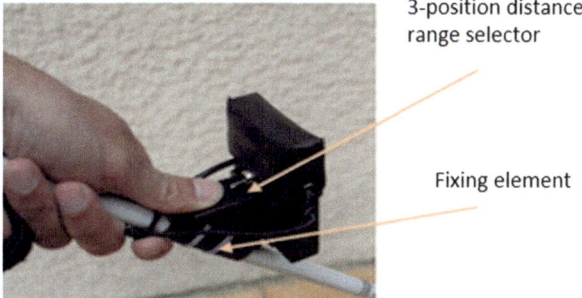

3-position distance
range selector

Fixing element

Fig. 16.5 Tom Pouce II system installed on a traditional white cane

sturdy. It is powered by a rechargeable battery that allows for about 7 days of a typical usage without the need of recharging. Different settings are available, for example the minimum obstacle detection distance.

Safewalk does not use data communication networks and does not require the installation of infrastructures on the path. At the time of writing (July 2018), it is in pre-commercial stage, and the producer offers the possibility of booking the product.

Tom Pouce II (Pollicino), produced by BEL (Tom Pouce II System Website, n.d.), is an example of LOD device to be mounted on the traditional white cane (see Fig. 16.5). The detection approach used in the first version of the device (2011) is based on infrared technology. The detection distance range is selectable by the user by means of a 3-position slide switch. The device provides the user with information about the presence of obstacles via three different types of vibration: continuous vibration, 8 and 15 Hz-modulated vibration, as schematically illustrated in Fig. 16.6.

The modulation of the vibration informs the user about the distance and position of the obstacle: continuous vibration for far obstacles on the ground, 15 Hz-modulated vibration for near obstacles on the ground, 8 Hz-modulated vibration

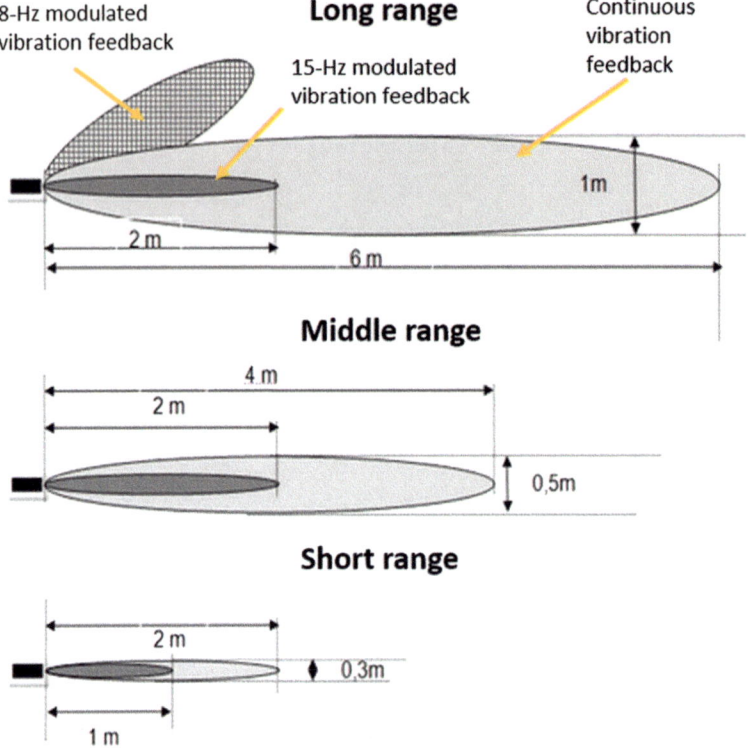

Fig. 16.6 Tom Pouce II system: different types of vibration signaling obstacles in different areas

for near suspended obstacles. The terms "far" and "near" refer to the range of the sensing area selected by means of the slide switch.

On the website, the producer asserts that the complexity for the user in selecting the sensing distance and interpreting the vibration modulations, results in an improvement of the system usability providing a better obstacle awareness.

Tom Pouce II does not use the traditional data communication networks and does not require the installation of any infrastructure on the path. As it occurs with other similar devices, a training course of some days with an instructor is recommended to allow the user to learn using it.

An infrared obstacle detection device to be hold in the user's hand is Pollicino Light (n.d.), produced by BEL and shown in Fig. 16.7. The device is particularly suitable for indoor environments and in case the environment ground structure is known it may avoid the use of the white cane. The detection distance is selectable by means of a 2-way switch and the orientation of one side of the device in the hand with respect to ground (orienting the top or bottom side of the device towards the ground represents a 2-way selection). Four different ranging distances may be selected: 8 m, 4 m, 2 m, and 30 cm.

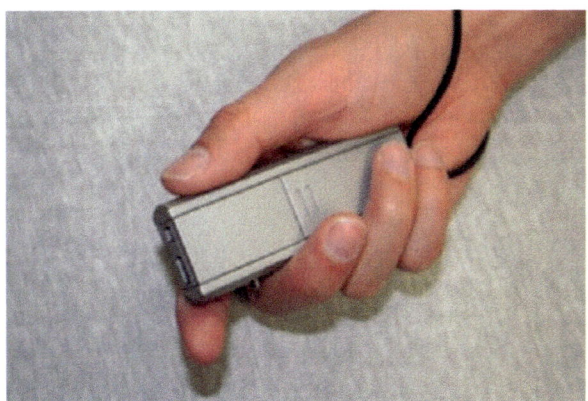

Fig. 16.7   Pollicino Light system

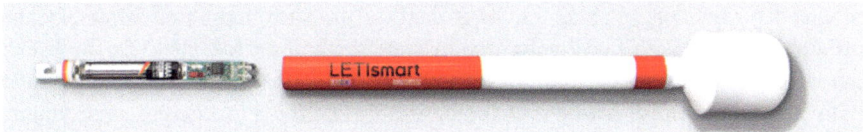

Fig. 16.8   LetiSmart Luce device

Pollicino Light does not use data communication networks and does not require the installation of infrastructures on the path. The device was a commercial product sold in 2014, but at the time of writing (July 2018) it was not possible to know its availability on the market. As with other similar systems, a training course was recommended to allow the user to use it effectively.

Regarding research projects, the results of several activities in the field of LOD systems have been published in literature. For example, the system described in Vítek, Klima, Husnik, and Spirk (2011) is based on ultrasound obstacle detection, but there are many others exploiting different sensing technologies and working principles (Elmannai & Elleithy, 2017).

16.2.3   Enhancement of the User's Visibility

Among mobility aid systems, some solutions aim at making users more visible to other pedestrians or to vehicle drivers, in order to improve safety in autonomous mobility.

An example of such systems is LetiSmart Luce (n.d.), shown in Fig. 16.8. It consists of a kit to be mounted on the bottom end of the white cane to allow for a high visibility in low lighting conditions.

LetiSmart Luce is essentially a battery-powered lighting device, emitting light according to environmental lighting conditions. It is a commercial product and does not require neither data communication networks not the installation of an infrastructure on the path.

In the future, it is foreseen the evolution of LetiSmart Luce into a new device integrated with the city public transport system and/or other city services that will provide users with the vocal information needed to move autonomously in the urban environment in the city of Trieste, Italy.

16.2.4   Obstacle Detection and Environment Recognition by Means of Vision Systems

A different category of mobility aid systems includes devices based on cameras mounted on helmets, glasses, etc. that analyze the surrounding environment and provide the user with vocal information and/or vibration feedback. Such system output aims at helping users to avoid obstacles on the path and at providing them with localization information and the perception of the surrounding environment and of nearby objects.

It is possible to find some vision systems at the prototypical or pre-commercial stage. Horus (n.d.) is an example of vision system for objects and environment recognition that provides the user with vocal information. It consists of cameras mounted on a headset and of a portable processing unit, as shown in Fig. 16.9.

The system learns objects and faces during an initial training phase, then it is able to detect and recognize some objects and the face of known people. Once an

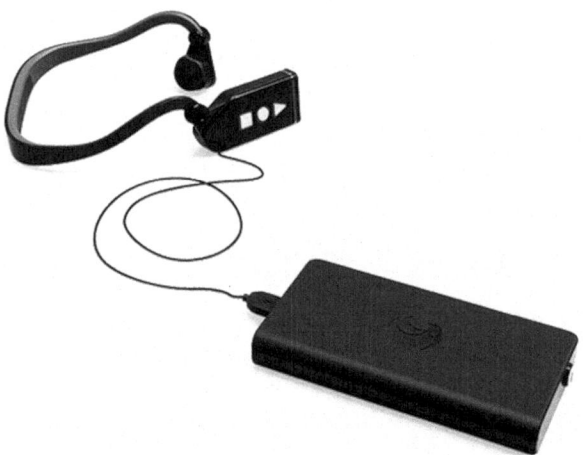

Fig. 16.9 Horus system: cameras mounted on the headset and the portable processing unit

object is recognized, Horus can help the user reach and grab the object via vocal information. Additionally, it can read the text on a book page, on a road sign, on a timetable, etc.

The user interacts with the system by means of some push-buttons on the headset and on the portable unit, which are easily identifiable by their different shapes. Using these push-buttons, the user can navigate the audio menu entries and activate the different device features. In some circumstances, Horus provides some vocal information automatically.

Horus is produced by Horus Technology. At the time of writing (July 2018), the system is in pre-commercial stage, and the producer offers the possibility of booking the product. From the information available on the producer's website, Horus seems not to require any data communication network (e.g. mobile and WiFi networks). The system does not require any specific infrastructure installed in the environment.

There are currently some other obstacle detection and environment recognition systems based on cameras and/or different kind of sensors (Elmannai & Elleithy, 2017). For example, the device described in (Brilhault, Kammoun, Gutierrez, Truillet, & Jouffrais, 2011) exploits the fusion of Artificial Vision and GPS positioning while the one reported in (Fontanesi, Frigerio, Fanucci, & Li, 2015) uses 3D Multisense technology for pedestrian crossing identification.

16.2.5   User Localization via Signal Reception and Processing

In this category of mobility aid systems, the user's position is determined by a portable unit that processes one or more types of signals received from transmitters placed in the environment and possibly also processing data read from kinematic sensors, as in Indoor Positioning Systems (IPS). Typical signals used are WiFi, Ultra Wide Band (UWB), Bluetooth, Infrared (IR), and Light-Fidelity (LiFi). Once determined the position of the user, the localization information are typically provided via vocal messages or vibration feedback, often by means of a smartphone/tablet and a dedicated app.

Such systems are suitable for both outdoor and indoor environment. Indeed, the installation and management of a transmitter network is not always feasible in an outdoor environment.

These systems are usually the prototypical result of research activities, and only seldom they reached the state of commercial product.

An example of a commercial solution for indoor navigation exploiting signals from transmitters in the environment is the StepInside mobile app developed by Senion (n.d.). The application targets the general public, but could be of some use for visually impaired people.

The StepInside app, elaborating the signals received from WiFi transmitters and from Bluetooth beacons and the kinematic data provided by the smartphone sensors, localizes the user on a map of the building with one or even several floors. The working scheme of the user mobile terminal is shown in Fig. 16.10.

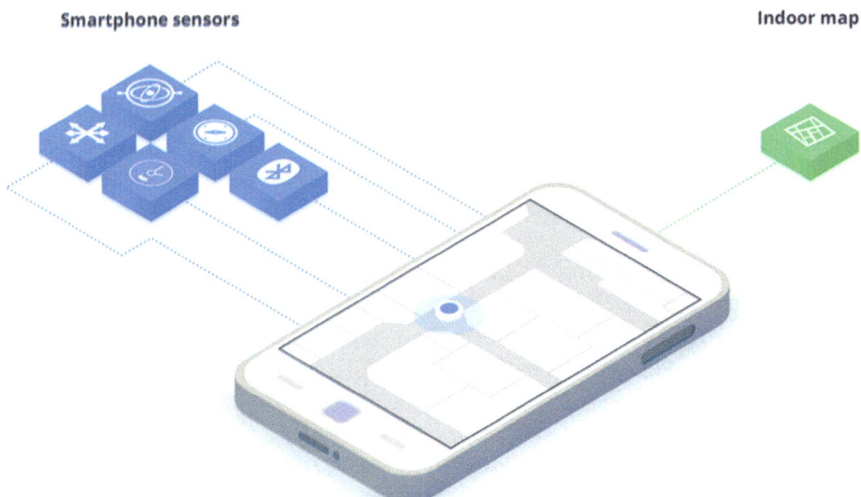

Smartphone sensors   **Indoor map**

Fig. 16.10 Representation of the working scheme of the user terminal in the IPS by Senion

The app is designed for indoor navigation in shopping centers, airports, etc., providing users with information on their position and location-based services.

The local communication/localization infrastructure can be partially exploited to provide other services (e.g. Internet access, etc.). The cost of the system (e.g. management system, map realization, etc.) is customer-specific and is therefore unknown.

There are currently some other guidance systems based on the reception and processing of different kinds of signals (Elmannai & Elleithy, 2017). For example, the system developed in (Li-fi Based Blind Indoor Navigation System for Visually Impaired People, n.d.) exploits the modulation of the light emitted by LED bulbs to transmit LiFi data to a portable device that processes them and determines the position of the user inside mapped buildings. The system described in (Dhruv, 2014) is instead based on a white cane, Bluetooth and IR modules installed in the environment and a user device that receives IR signals, communicates with Bluetooth modules and provides location information to the user.

16.2.6   RFID-Based Guidance Systems

In recent years, guidance systems based on RFID technology were proposed. For example, the system defined in Biader Ceipidor, Medaglia, Rizzo, and Serbanati (2006) uses a predefined safe path identified by means of buried RFID tags that are detected by a RFID reader mounted on a white cane. A mobile user terminal, connected to the reader, provides the user with location and navigation vocal information according to the RFID code read and a predefined online map. At the time of writing (July 2018), no updated information about the system may be found on the Internet, except for some news dated 2016 reporting some work in progress for the improvement of a previous prototypical system.

Another example is represented by Radio Frequency Identification Walking Stick (RFIWS) that was developed to help blind people navigate on the sidewalk (Saaid, Ismail, & Noor, 2009). The system helps the user in detecting and calculating the distance to the sidewalk border.

16.2.7   Guidance Systems Based on Guide Tiles

Predefined paths based on guide tiles (Loges system, n.d.; Apice System, n.d.) are often installed in many public places and buildings (e.g. railway stations, subways, squares, etc.). Guide tiles have different kinds of surface pattern that can be recognized and followed by the user using the tip of the white cane and/or with the feet. The different patterns signal the user the presence of a straight track, a curved one, the proximity to a sidewalk, etc. Figure 16.11 shows some examples of tiles with grooves and reliefs patterns.

The installed paths allow the user to follow a safe route in an indoor and/or outdoor scenario (see Fig. 16.12). However, such guidance system requires the user to obtain a preliminary knowledge of the route.

This guidance system may have a huge impact on existing buildings and places and has high installation costs.

16.2.8   White Cane

The white cane is one of the most traditional mobility aid for visually impaired people. However, its use is not easy at all and specific training courses must be

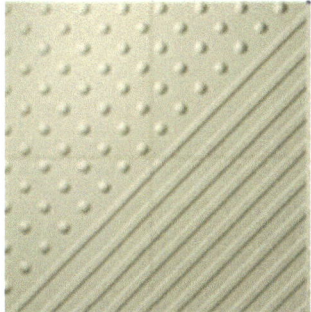
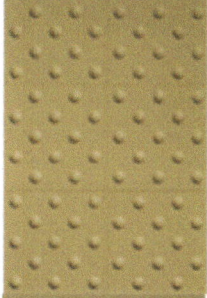

Fig. 16.11 Some different patterns in Loges-Apice guide tiles

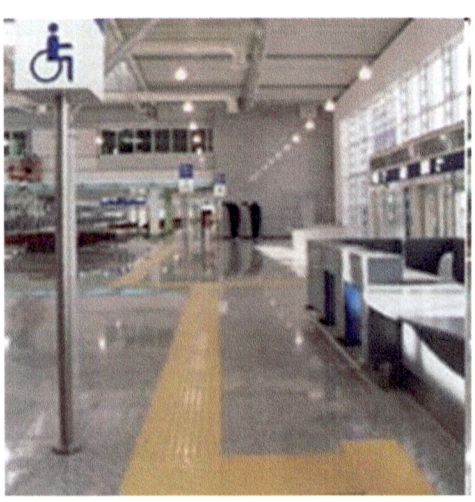

Fig. 16.12 Loges-Apice path installed in a public building

attended in order to learn how to use it for moving alone and for recognizing reference points, obstacles, etc. Moreover, the white cane is not effective in all situations. For example, it does not allow to detect obstacles that are not lying on the ground (e.g. an open blind, etc.).

16.2.9   Dog Guides

The well-known mobility aid represented by the dog guide is effective in many situations, but the interaction between the user and the dog poses some requirements that are not very easy to be managed. The user must in fact establish and maintain a strict, engaging and continuous relationship with the dog (Guide Dogs for Visually Impaired and Blind People, n.d.).

16.3   The Proposed System

The developed aid system addresses an outdoor urban mobility scenario, and in particular living an outdoor public place of tourist/cultural interest. In detail, the proposed system is focused on the provision of GPS-based guidance and context information on a predefined path and not on the obstacle detection approach on a whatever path. The advantage is that the selected path is quite safe, except for the still existing possibility of unforeseen obstacles (e.g. a bicycle that has been parked where it should not be, etc.). However, obstacle detection can be carried out by users via the developed Smart Cane just as if they were using a traditional white cane on their route.

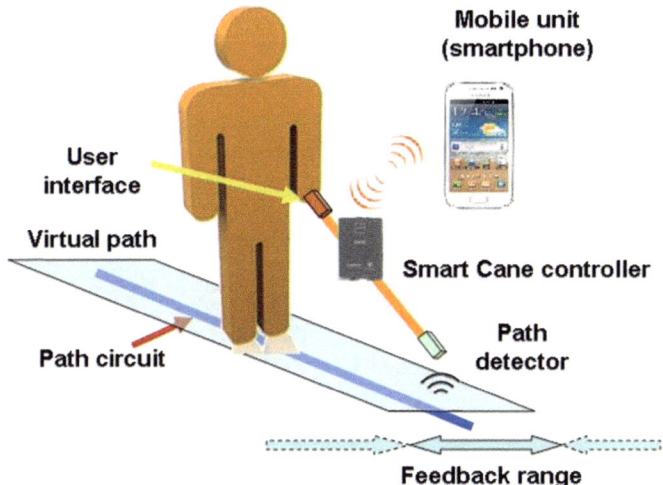

Fig. 16.13 The wall for all system architecture

Since the initial phase of the project, end-users' associations were actively involved in order to better fulfill user requirements. The collaboration started during the requirements definition and continued until prototype testing, carried out directly by some end-users.

The main user requirements in the autonomous outdoor mobility scenario were defined in relation to the control of an electronic device and the kind and amount of information needed for an effective navigation.

The system, further described in the following sections, is schematically illustrated in Fig. 16.13. The system architecture consists of three main elements:

- The virtual path.
- The Smart Cane.
- The mobile device with an ad-hoc Android application.

The guidance feature is realized combining two kinds of information. The first is the tactile vibration feedback produced by the Smart Cane when used on the predefined safe path (virtual path). The second one, provided by an Android app running on a mobile device, consists of vocal messages with navigation information and other information concerning the surrounding environment. Such vocal information is based on the GPS position of the user and on a predefined map for the specific installation site.

Tactile vibration feedback was chosen as the most suitable feedback type to signal the presence of the virtual path and, at the same time, to leave the hearing channel free. The hearing channel is very important for visually impaired people to locate themselves in the environment and to navigate, which is accomplished by detecting and analyzing the traffic noise, recognizing open spaces, etc. For the same reason, the system provides vocal messages mainly on user's request. The content and the detail level of vocal messages were chosen addressing users' needs. In particular, vocal messages were aimed at helping the user build and follow a mental map of the path, providing information about reference points that can be identified along the route and that help the user have awareness of the current position.

The Smart Cane is connected to the mobile device through a Bluetooth link. The user can interact with the system via an 8-switch user interface mounted on the Smart Cane handle. The whole route is shortly described via a vocal help message that can be listened to before facing the route. While walking, the user can repeatedly query the system in order to obtain vocal information about nearby relevant points and the distance from them. In this way it is possible for him/her to locate himself/herself on the mental map of the environment he/she has built.

Vocal information may be listened to via earphone (Bluetooth or wired) or via device speakerphone, allowing for the use of the system with only one hand, as normally no interaction with the mobile device is required.

The mobile device with the Android application is not strictly needed for path detection. In such a case, the only information available is the vibration feedback that signals the presence and position of the virtual path.

The selected installation site was the pedestrian/bicycle lane of about 4 km on top of the historical walls of Lucca city, Tuscany, Italy. This route is very popular among people from Lucca and the surroundings, but also among tourists from other parts of Tuscany. From the lane it is possible to access green areas along the Walls, named "Bastioni" (bastions) or "Baluardi".

16.3.1 The Virtual Path

The virtual path implements the predefined path that the user can walk and explore by means of the Smart Cane. The elements composing the virtual path are the following:

- Tracks.
- Branch points, where three or more tracks join together.
- Points of interest along the path (e.g. benches, etc.).

Another kind of element mapped in the proposed mobility aid system is represented by points of interest far from the path (e.g. historical buildings, etc.). A schematic representation of the above-mentioned elements is shown in Fig. 16.14.

The tracks of the virtual path are realized by means of a couple of parallel electrical wires in which a modulated current, injected by a signal generator, generates a variable magnetic field that is detected by the path detector mounted near the Smart Cane tip. When the smart cane tip is within a range of about 0.25–0.5 m from the center of the track, the Smart Cane handle vibrates with an intensity roughly inversely proportional to the distance of the tip from the center of the track.

The joining of three or more tracks represents a branch point. For a length of about 1 m starting from the joining point, the two cables of each track are replaced

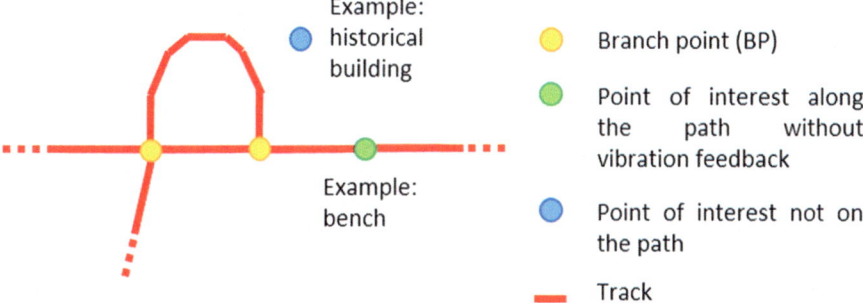

Fig. 16.14 Elements mapped in the proposed mobility aid application

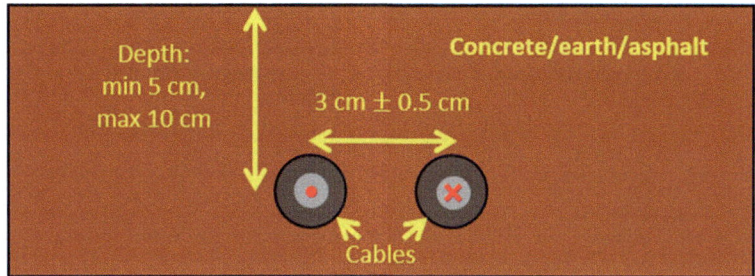

Fig. 16.15 Schematic view of the cable placement

by a unique twisted cable, so that the magnetic field is heavily shielded and is not detected by the Smart Cane. In branch point areas, having therefore a diameter of about 2 m, the Smart Cane provides no tactile vibration feedback.

Points of interest along the path are identified by the cancellation of the magnetic field for a length of about 1 m, which is accomplished using a twisted cable in replacement of the two parallel cables.

Points of interest that are not along the path are not directly reached by the cable infrastructure. They are mapped simply by the GPS coordinates in the Android application and represent relevant cultural/outdoor points outside the walked route.

The placement of cables must occur at a mutual distance of about 3 cm (this value is anyway not critical). In case of a permanent installation of the virtual path infrastructure, as is the case for the walls of Lucca city, the cables can be buried under quite any kind of material up to a depth of about 5–10 cm, as illustrated in Fig. 16.15. At the frequency used (10 kHz), the magnetic field is not shielded by concrete/asphalt/ground soil, both wet and dry.

Another possible type of installation, not realized within the current project, is a surface installation on existing floors (e.g. below a carpet, etc.). In such a case, with minimal installation costs, the system may provide a guidance function (also without exploiting the GPS signal) also inside or around a public building, an exhibition, etc.

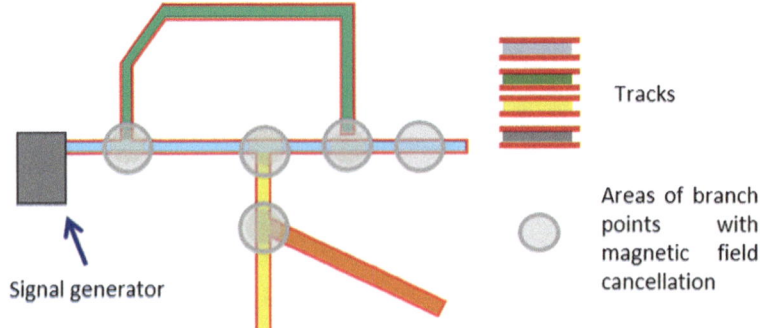

Fig. 16.16 Virtual path circuit architecture

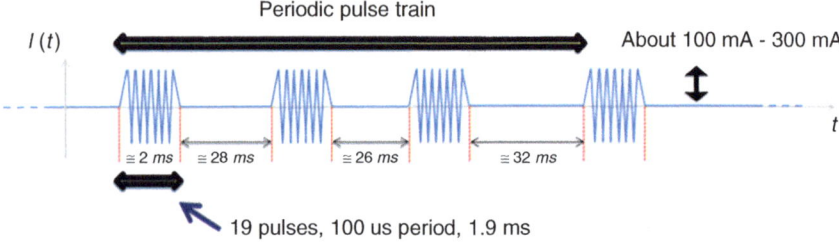

Fig. 16.17 Schematic view of the current waveform in the loop circuit

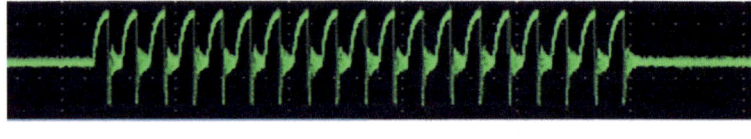

400 us/div, 200 mA/div

Fig. 16.18 Scope view of the current waveform within the cables

The electrical circuit identifying the virtual path must be a closed loop (see Fig. 16.16). A single signal generator is able to drive a path up to about 400 m. For longer paths, it is necessary to use several circuits implementing sub-paths. Two or more loop circuits, driven by different signal generators, usually converge in branch points, where the magnetic field is strongly attenuated and therefore not detected; otherwise, detection issues may arise from the overlap of magnetic fields produced by currents from different generators that have unrelated phases and possibly slightly different frequencies.

Figure 16.17 shows the schematic view of the waveform of the current flowing within the cables; Fig. 16.18 reports the scope view.

Enabling or excluding existing path segments is quite easy and only requires a modification of cable connections within junction boxes. As long as a loop circuit

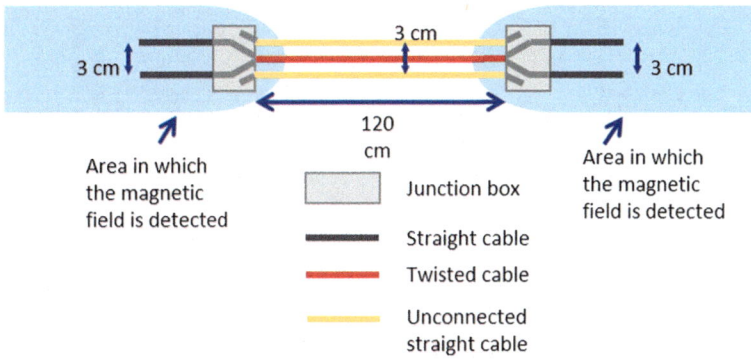

Fig. 16.19 Installation details for a point of interest with magnetic field cancellation

does not exceed the maximum allowed length, the addition of new tracks is possible without the need to add new signal generators. It simply requires to make, in a junction box, the proper connection of the newly installed cables and the already existing circuit. In a similar way, for many of the points of interest with magnetic field cancellation and for some branch points it is possible to enable/disable the magnetic field by simply reconnecting in a different way the cables in some junction boxes (see Fig. 16.19). In fact, in many points the two straight cables and the twisted cable were buried together in order to face possible modifications of the loop circuit, if required in the future.

The user can realize to have approached a relevant point with magnetic field cancellation, expected if he/she queries the system while walking on the route, when the vibration feedback stops.

In case of branch point, the joining tracks can be discovered by moving the Smart Cane in a circular area with a diameter of about 2 m around the point. The detailed information about joining tracks and where they lead to, provided by the application, can help the user to select the desired route.

Concerning points of interest on the path, they are typically related to benches placed within few meters aside from the track. Once the user has detected the short signal interruption, he/she can locate the bench using the smart cane as a traditional white cane, helped by the information provided by the application about on which side and how far it is located from the track.

Due to the relatively low GPS accuracy/precision, which is generally at least some meters or more in the installation site, branch points and points of interest with magnetic field cancellation are placed far from each other at a distance greater than about 15–20 m, so that with the proposed system the GPS accuracy and precision do not represent a fundamental concern.

Fig. 16.20 The Smart Cane

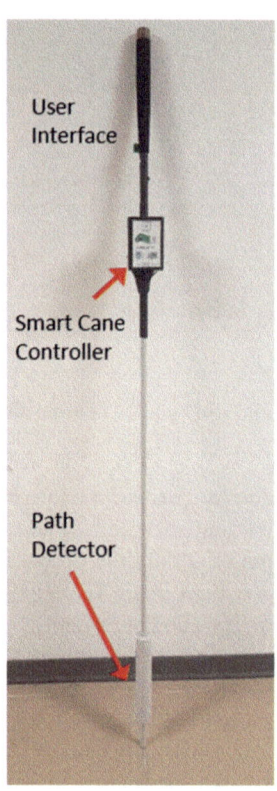

16.3.2   *The Smart Cane*

The Smart Cane is a fiberglass white cane equipped with some interconnected electronic devices and components developed within the project. In particular:

- The Smart Cane Controller (SCC).
- The Path Detector (PD).
- The input/output User Interface (UI).

The Smart Cane, further described hereafter, is shown in Fig. 16.20 and its architecture is illustrated in Fig. 16.21.

The input/output UI was designed and tested by final users during the first project phases. In Fig. 16.22 some details of the user interface are illustrated. The input interface consists of a 5-switch mini-joystick, with Forward, Backward, Left, Right and Central controls, and of a 3-position slide switch, with Forward, Backward and Central controls. The mini joystick can be operated by means of the thumb finger and the slide switch by means of the index finger, without the need to lose the grip on the handle. The output UI includes a vibration motor installed in the cane handle and a buzzer.

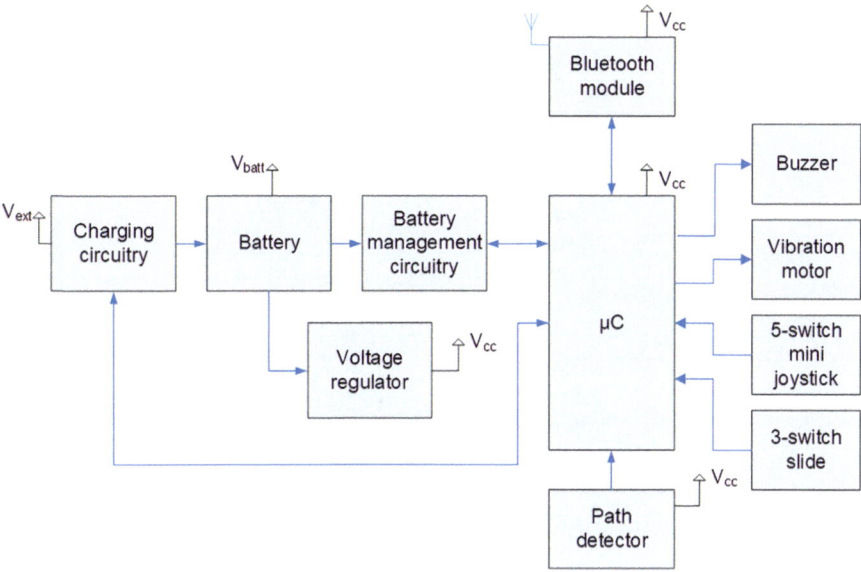

Fig. 16.21 The Smart Cane architecture

The Smart Cane Controller contains the main electronic subsystem of the Smart Cane. Its main components are an ATMega32L 8 bit microcontroller, which executes an embedded C compiled application with a code footprint of about 30 kB, a circuit for battery charging and monitoring, a Bluetooth module, a buzzer and a driver for the vibration motor.

The SCC is connected to the input UI. Each button press/release events is sent to the mobile device via the Bluetooth link and allows the user to control most of the navigation and information functions of the Android application. For user convenience, the buzzer provides audio feedback about press and release events. Moreover, it also warns the user about the low battery condition.

The Path Detector is an electronic circuit (see Fig. 16.23) mounted in proximity of the Smart Cane tip and enclosed in a cylindrical case.

The PD is connected to the microcontroller inside the SCC via a flat cable inside the cane. Within a range of about 25–50 cm from the center of the virtual path cables, the output signal of the PD contains some pulses that are recognized by the SCC microcontroller as belonging to a valid pattern generated by the path magnetic field. Most spikes and other signals due to environmental electrical noise are rejected by the hardware and/or the firmware. Figure 16.24 reports the scope view of the current within the cables and the corresponding path detector output for a given distance from them. When the output signal of the PD is compliant with the expected parameters, the microcontroller activates a vibration motor in the cane handle, with an intensity roughly proportional to the path signal intensity and therefore inversely proportional to the distance from the center of the virtual path.

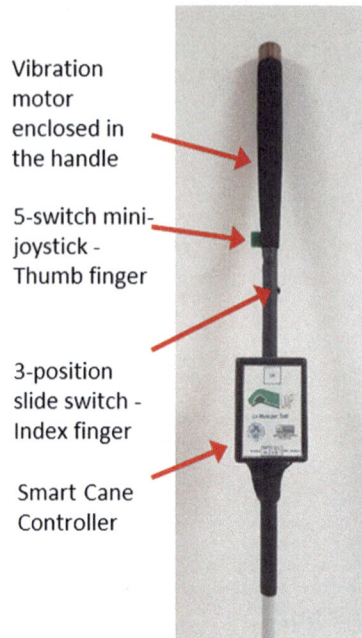

Fig. 16.22 The Smart Cane User Interface (UI) and the Smart Cane Controller (SCC)

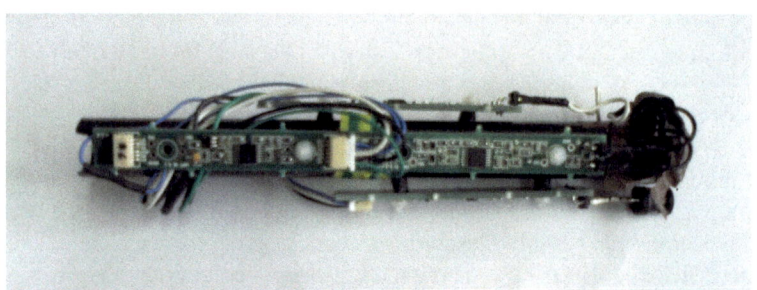

Fig. 16.23 The path detector (PD)

By moving and/or sweeping the cane, the user can locate the side borders of the path and, approximately, its center.

The average overall current draw of the different Smart Cane components is less than 100 mA, and battery life is some hours in a typical scenario. Battery recharging may be performed via a common 6 V to 500 mA mains power supply connected to a dedicated socket on the SCC.

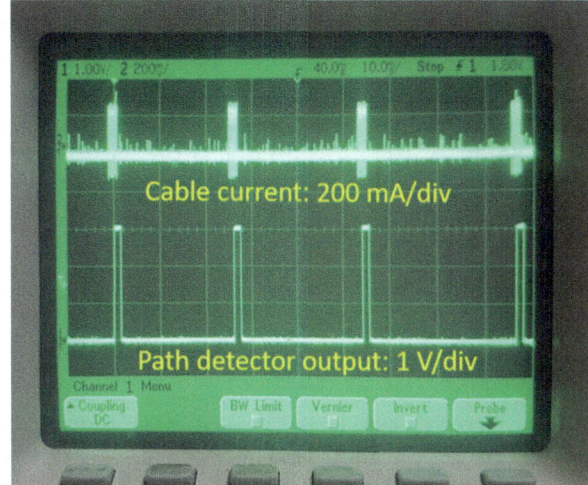

Horizontal division: 10 ms/div

Fig. 16.24 Scope view of the current within the cables vs. the path detector output signal

16.3.3   The Mobile Device and the Android Application

The third element of the system is a mobile device that runs an ad-hoc Android application. Its main task is to track the route of the user and to provide him/her synthesized audio messages when requested by means of the Smart Cane input UI.

The mobile device is required to be equipped with Android OS ≥ 4.0 and ear piece with a mic. Also it has to feature an internal GPS receiver and a Bluetooth interface. No restriction are present on the device screen size and form factor (i.e. smartphones, tablet), nor constraint on memory and processing capabilities.

Considering the middle-range segment of Android devices, the built-in Bluetooth interface is able to manage multiple connections (i.e. to the smart cane and optionally to the earpiece) as required. The internal GPS receivers do not critically suffer from GPS shielding caused by user's body; therefore the mobile device could also be kept leaning to the body or in a pocket. Moreover, the precision of the GPS signal resulted to be generally sufficient in the test and installation site without particular filtering or corrections. In light of these considerations, common commercial devices are suitable for this kind of employment.

The application requires the privileges to operate with the GPS receiver and the Bluetooth interface of the device, as well as to access the phone manager in order to make call or sending SMSs in case of emergency. Additionally, online or preloaded offline text-to-speech voice database is required to play the messages.

Once the application has been launched, generally no interaction with the on-device controls is needed because it is entirely controllable by means of the Smart Cane UI, and the device can be also locked.

Different kinds of guidance/touristic message are available during the walk:

- Overall description of the path, useful to build the mental map of the entire environment.
- Name and distance of recently approached and nearby branch points and tracks joining in them, where they take to and which is the direction to be taken (e.g. left/right).
- Name and distance of next points of interest on the path (e.g. benches, etc.).
- Information about points of interest not on the path (e.g. the description of nearby historical buildings, etc.).

Even if not strictly required to use the system, the application features a graphical user interface, mainly developed for debug/demonstration purposes. Figure 16.25 shows the application running on a Samsung A3 smartphone.

The upper section reports the status of the connections with the Smart Cane and the GPS signal, the presence or absence of the virtual path signal and the Smart

Fig. 16.25 The main window of the Android application

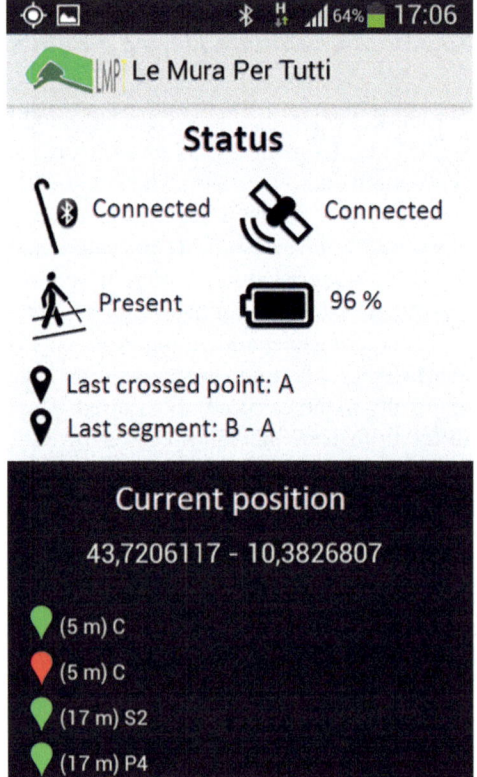

Table 16.1 Configuration and preference parameters of the App

Parameter	Description
Smart Cane Bluetooth address	Selector of the Smart Cane Bluetooth among the list of bonded devices
Detection radius	Distance in meters that makes the relevant point to be considered as crossed in the application
Emergency Phone Number	Phone number to be called or to send to SMSs in case of emergency during the walking
Path log	Storage of the entire path walked by the user using Keyhole Markup Language (KML)
Guidance Message Autoplay	Autoplay of messages when the user reaches an intersection point

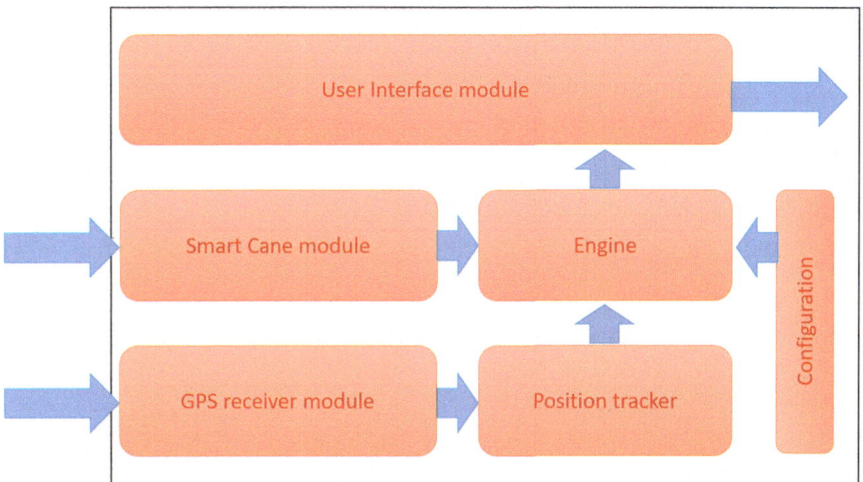

Fig. 16.26 Android Application software architecture

Cane battery level. The information about the last point and segment (couple of the last two points) visited by the user are also available. The lower section provides the coordinates of the current position of the user and the list of relevant points in increasing order of distance from such a point.

The application provides also a configuration window to allow the customization of the list of parameters reported in Table 16.1.

The software architecture is shown in Fig. 16.26. It consists of a series of cooperating modules that implement the desired functionalities: localize the user during the walk and provide information based on the current position and the a priori knowing of the relevant points position in the path.

The Smart Cane module runs in a dedicated thread. It manages the Bluetooth connection with the SCC in order to receive the commands given by the user and the updates of the virtual path detection status in every second.

Also the GPS Receiver module runs in a thread. It reads in every second an updated position of the device from the GPS to localize the user in the space.

The Position Tracker module maintains the information about the current position *CurrPos* of the user (i.e. GPS coordinates) and implements a circular queue *Queue[10]* for the automatic tracking of the last relevant points approached by the user during the walk.

The Engine module is the decision-maker module of the application. It uses the commands coming from the user and the position tracking information to select the messages to be played. Moreover, it monitors the status of the connections with the Smart Cane and the GPS receiver, providing service messages in case of faults, and finally it handles the refreshing of the user interface.

The user interface module is in charge of making available to the user the synthesized messages via built-in or externally connected audio output interfaces. Moreover, this module is responsible for the update of the information that appear on the main window when the device screen is unlocked.

The configuration contains the value of the parameters described in Table 16.1, that affects the behavior of the application, and the map of the entire path, loaded from an XML file, that represents the a-priori knowing of the installation environment. In particular, the map is organized into three sections:

- An array *Arr_path[N]* containing the name and the GPS coordinates of all the relevant point along the virtual path (i.e. branch points and points of interest with signal cancellation);
- An array *Arr_poi[M]* containing the name, the detailed description and the GPS coordinates of all the relevant points in the installation environment of interest outside the virtual path;
- A matrix *Mat[N][N]*, in which both columns and rows represent the relevant points along the virtual path and the elements are defined as follows:

  – *Mat[i][i]* contains the detailed description message for the i-th point.
  – *Mat[i][j]* contains the guidance message for the user that approaches the i-th point coming from the j-th point, if and only if a track between the two relevant points exists.

At the start-up of the application, the Engine loads the configuration and generates the SmartCane and the GPS receiver threads. After few seconds, when the Bluetooth connection with the Smart Cane Controller has been established and the GPS signal locked, a service message informs the user that the system is ready.

From this point on, the Position Tracker updates the *CurrPos* and the *Queue* variables using the coordinates provided by the GPS Receiver while the SmartCane module forwards the virtual path detection status to the Engine. In particular, a new relevant point P is marked as crossed, and put in the head position of the queue, if the distance between P and the *CurrPos* is less than the detection radius parameter:

Queue[head] = *P*, iff *distance(P,CurrPos)* ≤ *detection radius*.

When the user queries the system by means of the Smart Cane joystick, the Engine provides the proper message to the output user interface based on (1) the current position, (2) the virtual path detection status, (3) the queue of the last crossed relevant points and (4) the map of the path in the configuration.

In particular, the Engine firstly orders the arrays of relevant points by distance from the user's position and calculates the target relevant point assuming no inversion of direction:

Ordered_Arr_path = order(Arr_path, CurrPos);
Ordered_Arr_poi = order(Arr_poi, CurrPos);
Target_point = target(Ordered_Arr_path, Queue[head]);

Then, depending on the activated control button, the requested message is played:

- Joystick—Right button: the short names and distances of the two closest relevant points along the virtual path (*Ordered_Arr_path[0].name; Ordered_Arr_path[1].name*).
- Joystick—Left button: the short names and distances of the two closest points of interest outside the virtual path (*Ordered_Arr_poi[0].name; Ordered_Arr_poi[1].name*).
- Joystick—Up button: the information about the current position of the user. In particular:
  - If the user is on the virtual path, the app provides the short name of the closest target branch/interest point the user is moving to (*Ordered_Arr_path[target]. name*);
  - If the virtual path is not detected and the user is within a branch/interest point area, the app provides the name of this relevant point (*Queue[head].name*);
  - Otherwise an "out of path" service message is provided.

- Joystick—Down button: the detailed information on nearby or recently approached branch and interest points. In particular:
  - If the virtual path is detected, the app provides the detailed information (short name and description) of the nearest target branch/interest point the user is moving to (*Mat[target][Queue[head]].message*);
  - If the virtual path is not detected and the user is within a branch/interest point area, the app provides information about joining branches, where they take to and about the direction to be taken (e.g. left/right) with respect to the last walked segment of the track (*Mat[Queue[head]][Queue[head-1]].message*).

- Joystick—Press button stops the current message if a message is being played or provides the overall description of the track otherwise;
- Slide switch—Up button sends an emergency SMS containing also the current GPS coordinates;
- Slide switch—Down button makes an emergency call.

The application can be applied also in different installation sites or scenarios by simply downloading the specific maps configuration file on the mobile device.

16.3.4 The Software for the Service Management

In order to effectively provide a service for the end-user based on the proposed system, a dedicated software application to manage the pick-up/hand-back of Smart Canes and pre-configured mobile devices was developed. The application is web-based and supports multiple concurrent accesses, via login procedure, to allow the service provider to offer different management offices along the route, where the user can pick-up or hand-back the equipment.

Management offices are usually located in a few points along the path, inside tourist information offices or ticket offices in public buildings (e.g. museums, etc.). The availability of multiple management offices allows visually impaired users to pick-up the equipment in a point of the route, after being registered by a logged in operator, and return them also in a different point of the entire path.

16.4 Installation of the System on the Historical Walls of Lucca City

During the development period, a short segment of the virtual path was installed for preliminary on-field tests with some final users recruited in collaboration with the Italian Association for the Blind and Visually Impaired—Section of Lucca. The selected site was the pedestrian lane inside the "Baluardo San Donato", on the walls of Lucca city (see Fig. 16.27).

The installation phase on the walls of Lucca city started in summer 2013, concurrently with some major paving works on a segment of the pedestrian and bike lane. At the present (July 2018), after two further steps of works, the virtual path has been completely installed on the entire ring on top of the Walls and inside two green areas along the Walls (bastions). The total length is about 4 km.

Figure 16.28 shows the map of the final installation, highlighting the tracks of the entire path and the location of branch points and points of interest with and without magnetic field cancellation. Additional service points for development purposes are also shown. Figure 16.29 shows some details of a specific section of the route.

Points of interest with magnetic field cancellation, along the main route, are mainly benches aside the path. Points of interest without field cancellation are not along the virtual path and are represented by some buildings of cultural and historical value. Such points may be changed/extended at any time by just modifying the configuration used by the Android application.

Two starting/ending points of the path are foreseen, where the user can pick-up or hand-back the system equipment (i.e. Smart Cane and pre-configured mobile device). They will be located within tourist offices and/or a museum, not far from the lane on top of the Walls. A candidate point is in proximity of the Baluardo San Salvatore; it just faces the main ring on the Walls and is connected to it by a virtual track. Another pick-up/hand-back point is foreseen on the opposite side of the walls,

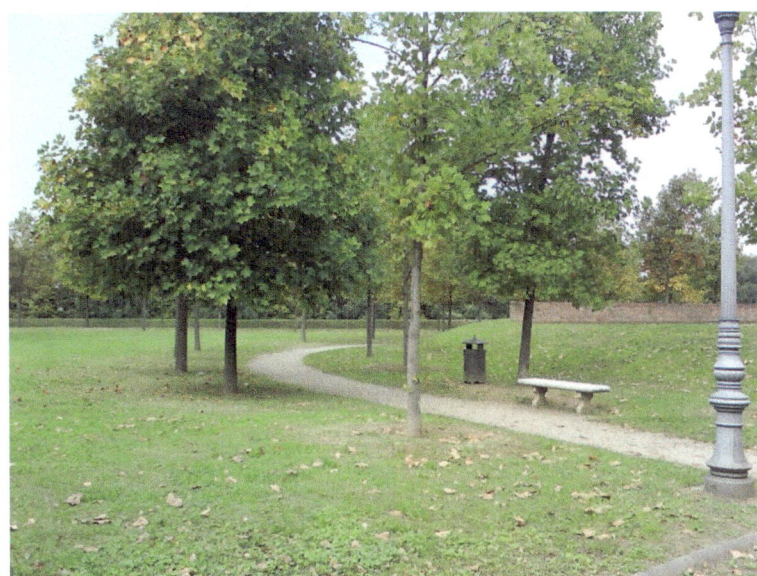

Fig. 16.27 Internal lane on "Baluardo San Donato" used during the preliminary test phase

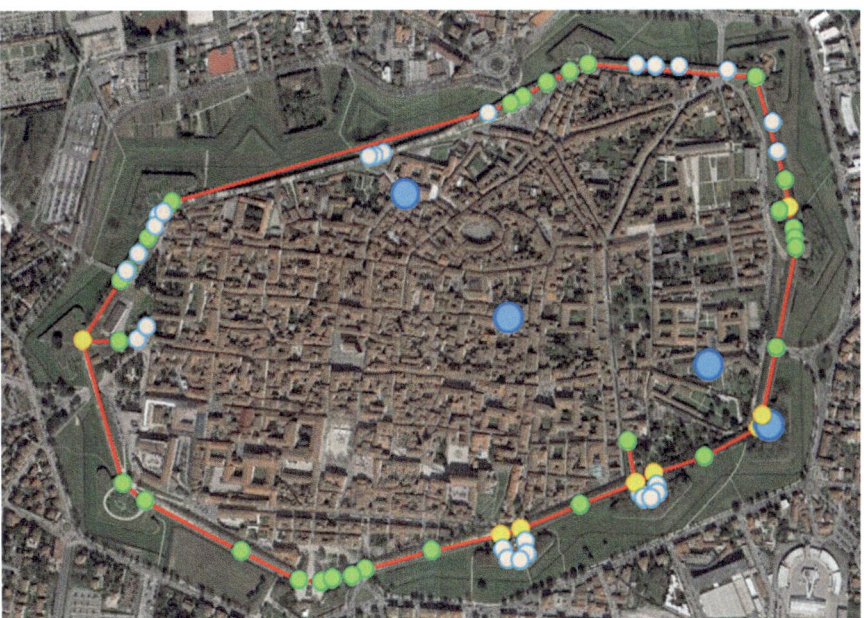

Fig. 16.28 Map of the virtual path installed on the wall of Lucca city. Colored circles represent point of interest, branch points and service points used for development purposes

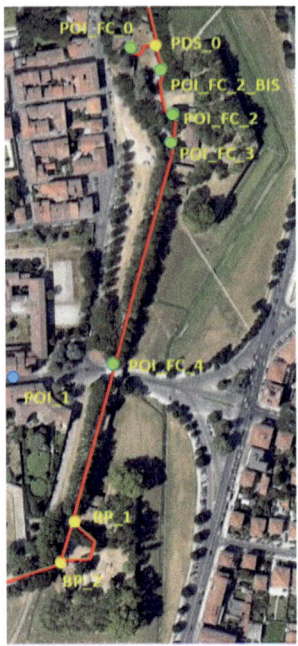

Virtual path (installed cables)

POI_FC – Point of interest along the route with magnetic field cancellation

BP – Branch point with magnetic field cancellation

POI – Point of Interest not along the route

Fig. 16.29 Detailed view of a section of the entire route

not far from Baluardo San Donato; tracks joining it to the main walking path on the walls are under installation.

Before the installation of the virtual path cables, tests were carried out in order to detect possible path detection problems caused by disturbance signals from other sources. Some sectors of the route showed to suffer from noise coming from the mains supply of the public lighting system, some others from sporadic electrical interference due to for example water pumps near the path or to other unidentified noise sources. This electrical noise picked up by the Path Detector in some points of the walking route is rejected by the SCC microcontroller algorithms that generally avoid false positives (recognition of the presence of the virtual path).

Moreover, before the final installation, GPS logs were taken along the route in order to verify possible critical areas concerning GPS accuracy/availability. GPS reception showed to suffer slightly inside Bastioni and in some areas under trees on the main ring, but it does not represent a major issue for the system.

Finally, Fig. 16.30 shows a schematic view of a virtual path segment installed on the Walls while an example illustrating the user asking the system for information about the surrounding environments is shown in Fig. 16.31.

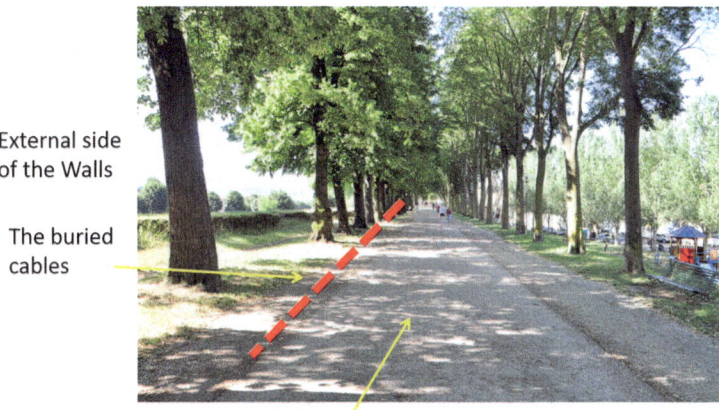

Fig. 16.30   A schematic overview of the path installation on the main route on the walls

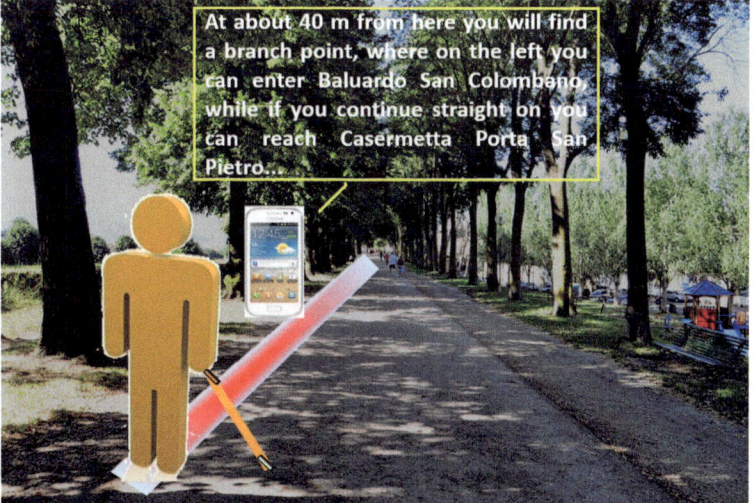

Fig. 16.31   Example of audio message provided by the system during the walk

16.5   Conclusion

The proposed mobility aid system for visually impaired people is particularly suited for historical places such as the medieval Walls of the city of Lucca, since it is completely hidden under the terrain. Indeed, the opportunity was provided by a major paving re-work on the pedestrian and bike asphalt road on the walls which was planned in three steps.

The mobility aid system has been already installed and successfully tested with end-users in the first two path segments.

The installation of the last path segment, from a possible pick-up/handback point to the main route, is currently in progress, and is foreseen to be completed by 2018. Afterward the facility will be opened to the public. End-users will be able to pick up or hand back the smart-cane and the associated smartphone from one of the starting/ending points of the path. Updated information will be available on the following website: http://www.luccaaccessibile.it/le-mura-per-tutti.

Acknowledgments The project "Le Mura per Tutti" has been partially supported by Fondazione Banca Del Monte di Lucca and Fondazione Cassa di Risparmio di Lucca for the design and development of the hardware/software systems and the installation of the infrastructure on the historical walls.

The authors would like to thank Massimo Diodati (President) and all the friends of the Lucca section of the Italian Association of the Blind and the Visually Impaired for their valuable support in many phases of the project. Thanks also to the Municipality of Lucca and Opera delle Mura of Lucca for the support provided, especially during the installation phase. A special thanks to Barbara Leporini, Carmen Santoro and Antonello Calabrò of the Italian National Research Council, who developed the very first version of the application on a Symbian-based mobile terminal (Fanucci et al., 2011).

Thanks to Luigi Rosi, CEO of the company Veret srl, Capannori (LU), who designed and implemented the fiberglass mechanical structure of the smart cane.

References

Apice System. (n.d.). *Tiles for the visually impaired*. Retrieved from http://www.s-tiles.org/s-tiles/articoli.nsf/VSNW04E/B5937E10AFED7A80C1256F0E002DAC4C
Biader Ceipidor U., Medaglia C. M., Rizzo F., & Serbanati A. (2006). *RadioVirgilio/Sesamonet: an RFID-based Navigation system for visually impaired*.
BlindSquadre Website. (n.d.). Retrieved from http://www.blindsquare.com/about
Braille to Note GPS Website. (n.d.). Retrieved from https://store.humanware.com/hus/braillenote-gps-software-and-receiver-package.html
Brilhault A., Kammoun S., Gutierrez O., Truillet P., & Jouffrais C. (2011). Fusion of artificial vision and GPS to improve blind pedestrian positioning. *Proceedings of the 4th IFIP International Conference on New Technologies, Mobility and Security (NTMS), Paris*.
Corsair App Repository. (n.d.). Retrieved from https://snigle.github.io/corsaire
Dhruv J.. Path-guided indoor navigation for the visually impaired using minimal building retrofitting. *Proceedings of the 16th International ACM SIGACCESS Conference on Computers & Accessibility* (ASSETS'14), *New York*; 2014
Easy Walk. (n.d.). Retrieved from http://easywalk.ilvillage.it/en
Elmannai, W., & Elleithy, K. (2017). Sensor-based assistive devices for visually-impaired people: Current status, challenges, and future directions. *Sensors, 17*(3), pii: E565.
European Blind Union 2008 European Blind Union newsletter, No. 64, September–October 2008. Retrieved from http://euroblindstatic.eplica.is/fichiersGB/nl64.htm
Fanucci L., Roncella R., Iacopetti F., Donati M., Calabrò A., Leporini B., & Santoro C.. (2011). Improving mobility of pedestrian visually-impaired users. *Proceedings of the 11th European Conference for the Advancement of Assistive Technology (AAATE), Maastricht*.
Fanucci L., Roncella R., Iacopetti F., Donati M., & Giannelli N.. (2014). A mobility aid system for visually impaired people on the historical walls of Lucca city, Tuscany, Italy. *22nd Mediterranean Conference on Control and Automation, Palermo*.

Farcy, R., & Damaschini, R. (n.d.). *Guidance – Assist system for the blind*. CNRS Orsay Cedex: Laboratoire Aimé Cotton.

Fontanesi, S., Frigerio, A., Fanucci, L., & Li, W. (2015). Real-time pedestrian crossing recognition for assistive outdoor navigation. *Stud Health Technol Inform, 217*, 963–968.

GPS for the Visually Impaired. (n.d.). Retrieved from https://en.wikipedia.org/wiki/GPS_for_the_visually_impaired

Guide Dogs for Visually Impaired and Blind People. (n.d.). Retrieved from http://www.livingblind.com/guide-dogs-for-visually-impaired.html

Horus System Website. (n.d.). Retrieved from https://horus.tech/horus

Istituto Poligrafico e Zecca dello Stato. (2007). *Indagine multiscopo sulle famiglie. Condizioni di salute e ricorsi ai servizi sanitari (2004–2005)*. Rome: Istituto Poligrafico e Zecca dello Stato. (in Italian).

Kwiatkowski P., Jaeschke T., Starke D., Piotrowsky L., Deis H., & Pohl N. (2017). A concept study for a radar-based navigation device with sector scan antenna for visually impaired people. *First IEEE MTT-S International Microwave Bio Conference (IMBIOC), Gothenburg.*

LetiSmart LUCE System Website. (n.d.). Retrieved from http://www.letismart.com

Li-fi Based Blind Indoor Navigation System for Visually Impaired People. (n.d.). Retrieved from https://www.pantechsolutions.net/projects/li-fi-based-blind-indoor-navigation-system-for-visually-impaired-people#product_tabs_description_tabbed

Loges system Tiles for the visually impaired. (n.d.). Retrieved from http://www.s-tiles.org/s-tiles/articoli.nsf/VSNW04E/5F1E432D15468CB0C1256F0E002DAC3D

Malavasi M., Fanucci L., Evert-Jan H., Iacopetti F., Francesca Neccia, Matteo Rimondini et al. Giancarlo Varacalli (2009). A step forward towards increasing the mobility and participation of people with disabilities utilizing Satellite Navigation Technology Applications. *10th European Conference for the Advancement of Assistive Technology in Europe (AAATE); Florence.*

Pollicino Light System Website. (n.d.). Retrieved from https://bel108.it/index.php/apparecchiature-bel/14-scheda-tecnica-pollicino-ligth

Saaid M. F., Ismail I., Noor M. Z. H.. (2009). Radio frequency identification walking stick (RFIWS): A device for the blind. *Proceedings of the 5th International Colloquium on Signal Processing & Its Applications, Kuala Lumpur.*

Safewalk System Website. (n.d.). Retrieved from http://www.safewalk.it/it/index.html

StepInside System Website. (n.d.). Retrieved from https://senion.com/indoor-positioning-system

The Cittabile Project. (n.d.). Retrieved from http://www.sestosg.net/sportelli/sestoprogetta/agenda21/scheda/1144 (in Italian)

The MAPPED Project. (n.d.). Retrieved from http://services.txt.it/MAPPED/index.jsp

Tom Pouce II System Website. (n.d.). Retrieved from https://bel108.it/index.php/apparecchiature-bel/3-scheda-tecnica-pollicino

Trekker Breeze Plus Website. (n.d.). Retrieved from https://store.humanware.com/hau/trekker-breeze-plus-handheld-talking-gps.html

Ultracane System Website. (n.d.). Retrieved from https://www.bel108.it/index.php/apparecchiature-bel/31-ultracane

Vítek S., Klima M., Husnik L., & Spirk D. (2011). New possibilities for blind people navigation. *Proceedings of the 2011 International Conference on Applied Electronics (AE); Pilsen.*

Xiao J., Ramdath K., Losilevish M., Sigh D. and Tsakas A. (2013). A low cost outdoor assistive navigation system for blind people; *Proceedings of the 2013 8th IEEE Conference on Industrial Electronics and Applications (ICIEA) Melbourne.*

Index

© Springer Nature Switzerland AG 2020

S. Paiva (ed.), *Technological Trends in Improved Mobility of the Visually Impaired*,
EAI/Springer Innovations in Communication and Computing,
https://doi.org/10.1007/978-3-030-16450-8

.

Printed by Printforce, the Netherlands